P9-CJS-772

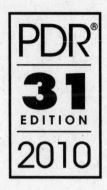

PDR®

for Nonprescription Drugs,
Dietary Supplements, and Herbs

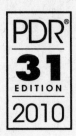

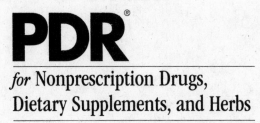

for Nonprescription Drugs,
Dietary Supplements, and Herbs

CEO: Edward Fotsch, MD
President: David Tanzer
Chief Medical Officer: Henry DePhillips, MD
General Manager, HCNN: Debra Del Guidice
Vice President, Publishing & Operations: Valerie Berger
Vice President, New Product Strategies: Cy Caine
Vice President, Finance: Dawn Carfora
**Vice President, Corporate Development
& General Counsel:** Andrew Gelman
Vice President, Engineering: Nick Krym
Vice President, Clinical Relations: Mukesh Mehta, RPh
Vice President, Marketing: Maria Robinson
Vice President, Product Management: Leslie Yuan
Senior Director, Copy Sales: Bill Gaffney

Director, Marketing: Kim Marich
Senior Promotion Manager: Linda Levine

Senior Director, Editorial & Publishing: Bette Kennedy
Senior Director, Client Services: Stephanie Struble

Director, Clinical Services: Sylvia Nashed, PharmD
Manager, Clinical Services: Nermin Shenouda, PharmD
Drug Information Specialists: Kristine Mecca, PharmD;
 Anila Patel, PharmD; Christine Sunwoo, PharmD
Manager, Editorial Services: Lori Murray
Associate Editor: Jennifer Reed
Manager, Art Department: Livio Udina
Electronic Publishing Designer: Carrie Spinelli Faeth
Project Managers: Deana DiVizio, Gary Lew

Director, PDR Production: Jeffrey D. Schaefer
Production Manager, PDR: Steven Maher
Manager, Production Purchasing: Thomas Westburgh
Senior Print Production Manager: Dawn Dubovich
Operations Database Manager: Noel Deloughery
Senior Index Editor: Allison O'Hare
Index Editor: Julie L. Cross
Senior Production Coordinator: Yasmin Hernández
Production Coordinators: Eric Udina, Christopher Whalen
Manager, Customer Service: Todd Taccetta

ISBN: 978-1-56363-750-6

FOREWORD TO THE 31ST EDITION

Announcing PDR Network

After more than 60 years of providing unparalleled drug information, *Physicians' Desk Reference®* has become part of the first national drug information and safety Alert service—**PDR Network**. This new service combines the expertise of *PDR* with the Health Care Notification Network (HCNN), the only network that delivers FDA-required drug Alerts and REMS programs to physicians and other prescribers online. PDR Network provides prescribers with a single, end-to-end drug information service, including:

- FDA-approved drug labeling
- FDA-required drug Alerts
- Product-safety Alerts and recalls
- Information on the new FDA-required Risk Evaluation and Mitigation Strategies (REMS) program

By improving communication of important drug information and FDA safety alerts, PDR Network's one-of-a-kind service can help enhance patient safety, reduce medical liability, and ensure FDA compliance. For more information, visit **www.PDRNetwork.net**.

About This Book

PDR® for Nonprescription Drugs, Dietary Supplements, and Herbs features four indices and a full-color Product Identification Guide followed by two distinct sections of product information. The first of these, entitled Nonprescription Drug Information, presents manufacturer-supplied labeling as published in the 2010 *PDR®* or 2010 *PDR® for Ophthalmic Medicines*, for products marketed in compliance with the Code of Federal Regulations labeling requirements for OTC drugs. The other product section, Dietary and Herbal Supplement Information, contains manufacturer-supplied labeling as published in the 2010 *PDR* or 2010 *PDR for Ophthalmic Medicines*. Please note that these products are marketed under the Dietary Supplement Health and Education Act of 1994 and therefore have not been evaluated by the Food and Drug Administration. Such products are not intended to diagnose, treat, cure, or prevent any disease.

PDR for Nonprescription Drugs, Dietary Supplements, and Herbs also includes clinical profiles on common dietary supplements and herbal medicines, including information on approved uses as well as warnings and drug interactions. The last section of the book features product comparison tables that cover various OTC therapeutic categories, allowing for easy comparison of active ingredients, drug strengths, and dosages.

PDR for Nonprescription Drugs, Dietary Supplements, and Herbs is published by PDR Network, LLC. The information on each product described in sections 5, 6, and 7 of the book has been supplied by the manufacturer for publication in the 2010 *PDR* or 2010 *PDR for Ophthalmic Medicines*. The function of the publisher is the compilation, organization, and distribution of this information. During compilation of this information, the publisher has emphasized the necessity of describing products comprehensively in order to provide all the facts necessary for sound and intelligent decision-making. Descriptions seen here include all information made available by the manufacturers.

In organizing and presenting the material in *PDR for Nonprescription Drugs, Dietary Supplements, and Herbs*, the publisher does not warrant or guarantee any of the products described, or perform any independent analysis in connection with any of the product information contained herein. *Physicians' Desk Reference* does not assume, and expressly disclaims, any obligation to obtain and include any information other than that provided by the manufacturer. It should be understood that by making this material available the publisher is not advocating the use of any product described herein, nor is the publisher responsible for misuse of a product due to typographical error. Additional information on any product may be obtained from the manufacturer.

This edition of *PDR for Nonprescription Drugs, Dietary Supplements, and Herbs* contains the latest information available when the book went to press. As new products are released, and new research data, clinical findings, and safety information emerge throughout the year, it is the responsibility of the manufacturer to provide that information to the medical community and revise that information in the *PDR* database accordingly. These revisions are published twice annually in the *PDR Supplements* and more regularly on PDR.net. To be certain that you have the most current data, healthcare providers should always consult PDR.net or the *PDR Supplements* before administering any product described in the following pages.

Register for Product Safety Alerts at HCNN

Physicians and other prescribers may register to receive electronic Alerts online at **HCNN.net**, through participating medical societies and other HCNN partners, or by returning the qualification form distributed with

physician copies of this year's *PDR*. Free to all licensed U.S. physicians and their staff, the HCNN is used exclusively for FDA-required product safety Alerts—not advertising or marketing—and fulfills FDA guidance for electronic delivery of Alerts.

Web-Based Clinical Resources

PDR.net, a web portal designed specifically for health-care professionals, provides a wealth of clinical information, including full FDA-approved labeling as well as concise drug information, disease monographs, specialty-specific resource centers, patient education, clinical news, and conference information. PDR.net gives prescribers online access to authoritative, evidence-based information they need to support or confirm diagnosis and treatment decisions.

PDR.net is also home to our **Clinical Resource Centers**, giving you the latest medical news and disease information all in one easy place. Online access is free for U.S.-based MDs, DOs, dentists, NPs, and PAs in full-time patient practice, as well as for medical students, residents, and other select prescribing allied health professionals. Register today at *www.PDR.net*.

Other Products from PDR

The *PDR® for Nutritional Supplements, Second Edition* offers scientific consensus on hundreds of popular products, including amino acids, fatty acids, probiotics, phytoestrogens, phytosterols, over-the-counter hormones, and much more. Focused on the clinical evidence for each supplement's claims, this unique reference offers you today's most detailed, informed, and objective overview of a burgeoning area in the field of self-treatment.

Likewise, the *PDR® for Herbal Medicines, Fourth Edition* provides evidence-based assessments of more than 700 botanicals. Indexed by scientific and common names (as well as Western, Asian, and homeopathic indications), this volume also includes a Side Effects Index, a Drug/Herb Interactions Guide, an Herb Identification Guide with nearly 400 color photos, and a Safety Guide that lists herbs to be avoided during pregnancy and those to be used only under professional supervision. Although botanical products are not officially regulated or monitored in the United States, *PDR for Herbal Medicines* provides you with authoritative information—the findings of the German Regulatory Authority's expert committee on herbal medicines, Commission E.

For more information on these or any other members of the growing family of *PDR* products, please call, toll-free, 800-232-7379 or fax 201-722-2680, or visit *PDRbookstore.com*.

HOW TO USE THIS BOOK

The 2010 edition of *PDR® for Nonprescription Drugs, Dietary Supplements, and Herbs* features a format designed to help you find the information you need as quickly and easily as possible. In addition to consulting the four indices, you can go directly to a specific product comparison table to find the relevant over-the-counter (OTC) products for a particular condition. Details of this organization are outlined below.

FOUR INDICES

- **Manufacturers' Index** lists all pharmaceutical manufacturers that provided OTC drug labeling for the 2010 *Physicians' Desk Reference®* or 2010 *PDR® for Ophthalmic Medicines*. Each entry contains addresses, phone numbers, and emergency contacts, as well as a listing of that manufacturer's products and the corresponding page numbers for labeling information.

- **Product Name Index** provides the page number of each product description in the Nonprescription Drug Information and Dietary and Herbal Supplement Information sections. Listings appear alphabetically by brand name.

- **Product Category Index** lists all fully described products according to therapeutic or pharmaceutical drug category (eg, acetaminophen combinations).

- **Active Ingredients Index** contains product cross references by generic ingredient.

PRODUCT IDENTIFICATION GUIDE
Organized alphabetically by manufacturer name. This section shows full-color, actual-sized photos of tablets and capsules, plus a variety of other dosage forms and packages.

NONPRESCRIPTION DRUG INFORMATION
Organized alphabetically by manufacturer name. The product labeling in this section includes brand-name OTC products marketed for home use. **Please keep in mind that the product information included herein is valid as of press time (September 2009).** Additional information, as well as updates to the product labeling, can be obtained from the manufacturer.

DIETARY AND HERBAL SUPPLEMENT INFORMATION
Organized alphabetically by manufacturer name. This section contains product labeling for dietary and herbal supplements marketed under the Dietary Supplement Health and Education Act of 1994. Be aware that these products are not federally regulated and are not intended to diagnose, treat, cure, or prevent any disease.

DIETARY SUPPLEMENT PROFILES
Organized alphabetically by common name. This section provides information on commonly used dietary supplements. The profiles are derived from monographs appearing in *PDR® for Nutritional Supplements* and have been updated based on recent scientific findings and reviewed by PDR's clinical staff. Each profile includes the supplement's pharmacological effects, common usage, contraindications, warnings/precautions, drug interactions, food interactions, adverse reactions, and administration and dosage (including pediatric, when available). Be aware that these products are not federally regulated and are not intended to diagnose, treat, cure, or prevent any disease.

HERBAL MEDICINE PROFILES
Organized alphabetically by common name. This section covers information on commonly used herbs. The profiles are derived from monographs appearing in *PDR® for Herbal Medicines* and have been updated based on recent scientific findings and reviewed by PDR's clinical staff. When available, the profiles also list the herb's accepted uses as determined by Commission E—Germany's regulatory agency that reviews clinical evidence on herbal medicines.

Also included are the herb's pharmacological effects, contraindications, warnings/precautions, drug interactions and food interactions, adverse reactions, and administration and dosage (including pediatric, when available). Be aware that these products are not federally regulated and are not intended to diagnose, treat, cure, or prevent any disease.

PRODUCT COMPARISON TABLES
Organized alphabetically by therapeutic category and brand name. These tables provide a quick and easy way to compare the active ingredients and dosages of common brand-name OTC drugs. Therapeutic categories covered include antacid and heartburn agents; laxatives; and cough, cold, and flu products.

CONTENTS

(Continued on next page)

Product Comparison Tables

SECTION 1

MANUFACTURERS' INDEX

This index lists manufacturers that have supplied information for the 2010 *PDR®* or 2010 *PDR® for Ophthalmic Medicines*. Each company's entry includes the address, phone, and fax number of its headquarters and regional offices, as well as company contacts for inquiries, orders, and emergency information.

Products with entries in the Nonprescription Drug Information section are listed with their page numbers under the heading "OTC Products Described." Products with entries in the Dietary Supplement Information section are listed with their page numbers under the heading "Dietary Supplements Described."

If an entry in the index lists multiple page numbers, the first one shown refers to the photograph of the product, the last one to its prescribing information.

- The ◆ symbol marks drugs shown in the Product Identification Guide.

- *Italic page numbers* signify partial information.

ALCON LABORATORIES, INC.   502

Alcon Laboratories, Inc.
And its affiliates
Corporate Headquarters
6210 South Freeway
Fort Worth, TX 76134
Address Inquiries to:
Pharmaceuticals/Consumer: (800) 451-3937
(Therapeutic Drugs/Lens Care)
Surgical: (800) 862-5266
(Instrumentation/Surgical Meds)
(817) 293-0450 (Main Switchboard)

OTC Products Described:
Systane Ultra Lubricant Eye Drops 502

ALTO PHARMACEUTICALS, INC.   402, 502

P.O. Box 271150
Tampa, FL 33688-1150
3172 Lake Ellen Drive
Tampa, FL 33618
Direct Inquiries to:
John J. Cullaro
Customer Service
altopharma@aol.com
Tel: (800) 330-2891
Fax: (813) 968-0527

OTC Products Described:
◆ Zinc-220 Capsules 402, 502

AMERICA PHARMA CO.   402, 502

750 Stimson Avenue
City of Industry, CA 91745
Direct Inquiries to:
Phone: (626) 336-8889
Fax: (626) 336-1299
E-mail: ac.usa.inc@gmail.com
http://www.acusainc.net

OTC Products Described:
◆ Happycode Spray 402, 502

Dietary Supplements Described:
◆ Heplive Softgel Capsules 402, 568
◆ Meili Clear Soft Capsules 402, 568
◆ Meili Soft Capsules 402, 568
◆ Springcode Spray 402, 568

BAUSCH & LOMB INCORPORATED   402, 503

One Bausch & Lomb Place
Rochester, NY 14604
7 Giralda Farms
Madison, NJ 07940
Direct Inquiries to:
Main Office
(585) 338-6000
Consumer Affairs
(800) 553-5340

OTC Products Described:
◆ Bausch & Lomb Alaway Eye Drops 402, 503
Muro 128 Ophthalmic Ointment 503
Muro 128 Ophthalmic Solution 2%
    and 5% 504
◆ Soothe Lubricant Eye Drops 402, 504
◆ Soothe XP Eye Drops 402, 505

(◆) **Shown in Product Identification Guide**

Italic Page Number **Indicates Brief Listing**

BAUSCH & LOMB INCORPORATED—cont.

BAYER HEALTHCARE LLC CONSUMER CARE

402, 505

36 Columbia Road
P.O. Box 1910
Morristown, NJ 07962-1910
Direct Inquiries to:
Consumer Relations
(800) 331-4536
www.BayerAspirin.com

BEACH PHARMACEUTICALS

403, 572

Division of Beach Products, Inc.
5220 S. Manhattan Avenue
Tampa, FL 33611
Direct Inquiries to:
Richard Stephen Jenkins
(813) 839-6565
FAX: (813) 837-2511
Manufacturing and Distribution:
1700 Perimeter Road
Greenville, SC 29605
(800) 845-8210

J. R. CARLSON LABORATORIES, INC.

403, 572

15 College Drive
Arlington Heights, IL 60004-1985
Direct Inquiries to:
Customer Service
(888) 234-5656
FAX: (847) 255-1605
www.carlsonlabs.com
For Medical Information Contact:
In Emergencies:
Customer Service
(888) 234-5656
FAX: (847) 255-1605

FLEET LABORATORIES

508

Division of C.B. Fleet Company, Incorporated
Lynchburg, VA 24502
Direct Inquiries to:
Sherrie McNamara, RN, MSN, MBA
Director of Medical Affairs and Product Safety
1-866-255-6960

GORDON LABORATORIES

403, 517

6801 Ludlow Street
Upper Darby, PA 19082
Direct Inquiries to:
Customer Service
(610) 734-2011
FAX: (610) 734-2049
www.gordonlabs.net
E-mail: gordonlabs@worldnet.att.net
For Medical Emergencies Contact:
David Dercher
(610) 734-2011
FAX: (610) 734-2049

GUARDIAN LABORATORIES

518

a division of United-Guardian, Inc.
P.O. Box 18050
Hauppauge, NY 11788
For Medical Information Contact:
Director of Product Development
(631) 273-0900
(800) 645-5566

HEEL INC.

518

10421 Research Road SE
Albuquerque, NM 87123
Direct Inquiries to:
Medical Department
(800) 621-7644
FAX: (800) 217-6934
www.heelusa.com
info@heelusa.com

HISAMITSU PHARMACEUTICAL CO., INC.

403, 518

408 Tashiro-Daikanmachi
Tosu Saga 841-0017
Japan
Direct Inquiries to:
Tel: +81-3-5293-1720
Fax: +81-3-5293-1724

UNICITY INTERNATIONAL   404, 564

The Make Life Better Company
1201 North 800 East
Orem, UT 84097
Direct Inquiries to:
(800) 226-2600
www.unicity.net
science@unicity.net
Products of Unicity International are distributed
through independent distributors.

OTC Products Described:

Dietary Supplements Described:

UPSHER-SMITH   565
LABORATORIES, INC.

6701 Evenstad Drive
Minneapolis, MN 55369
For Medical Information Contact:
Write: Professional Services Department
or call: (800) 654-2299
(during business hours-8 a.m. to 5 p.m. CST)

OTC Products Described:

Dietary Supplements Described:

U.S. PHARMACEUTICAL   565
CORPORATION

2401 Mellon Court, Suite C
Decatur, GA 30035
Direct Inquiries to:
Allison Krebs-Bensch
Vice President
(770) 987-4745
a.krebs@uspco.com

OTC Products Described:

USANA HEALTH SCIENCES, INC.   583

3838 West Parkway Boulevard
Salt Lake City, UT 84120-6336
Direct Inquiries to:
(801) 954-7860
FAX: (801) 954-7658

Dietary Supplements Described:

WESTLAKE   404, 565
LABORATORIES, INC.

24700 Center Ridge Road
Cleveland, OH 44145
www.westlake-labs.com
Direct Inquiries to:
Customer Service
(888) WSTLAKE (978-5253)
FAX: (440) 835-2177

OTC Products Described:

SECTION 2

PRODUCT NAME INDEX

This index includes all entries in the Product Information sections. Products are listed alphabetically by brand name.

If an entry in the index lists multiple page numbers, the first one shown refers to the photograph of the product, the last one to its prescribing information.

- **Bold page numbers** indicate that the entry contains full product information.
- *Italic page numbers* signify partial information.

Italic Page Number Indicates Brief Listing

Italic Page Number **Indicates Brief Listing**

SECTION 3

PRODUCT CATEGORY INDEX

This index cross-references each brand by pharmaceutical category. All fully described products in the Product Information sections are included.

If an entry in the index lists multiple page numbers, the first one shown refers to the photograph of the product, the last one to its prescribing information.

The classification of each product is determined by the publisher in cooperation with the product's manufacturer or, when necessary, by the publisher alone.

SECTION 4

ACTIVE INGREDIENTS INDEX

This index cross-references each brand by its generic ingredients. All entries in the Product Information sections are included.

If an entry in the index lists multiple page numbers, the first one shown refers to the photograph of the product, the last one to its prescribing information.

- **Bold page numbers** indicate full product information.
- *Italic page numbers* signify partial information.

Classification of products under these headings has been determined in cooperation with the products' manufacturers or, if necessary, by the publisher alone.

Italic Page Number Indicates Brief Listing

POISON CONTROL CENTERS

The American Association of Poison Control Centers (AAPCC) uses a single, nationwide emergency number to automatically link callers with their regional poison center. This toll-free number, **800-222-1222**, also works for **teletype lines (TTY)** for the hearing-impaired and **telecommunication devices (TTD)** for individuals who are deaf. However, a few local poison centers and the ASPCA/Animal Poison Control Center are not part of this nationwide system and continue to use separate numbers.

Most of the centers listed below are accredited by the AAPCC. **Certified centers are marked by an asterisk after the name**. Each has to meet certain criteria. It must, for example, serve a large geographic area; it must be open 24 hours a day and provide direct-dial or toll-free access; it must be supervised by a medical director; and it must have registered pharmacists or nurses available to answer questions from the public.

Within each state, centers are listed alphabetically by city. Some state poison centers also list their original emergency numbers (including TTY/TDD) that only work within that state. For these listings, callers may use either the state number or the nationwide 800 number.

ALABAMA

BIRMINGHAM

Regional Poison Control Center (*)
Children's Hospital of Alabama

1600 7th Ave. South
Birmingham, AL 35233
Business: 205-939-6334
Emergency: 800-222-1222
www.chsys.org

TUSCALOOSA

Alabama Poison Center (*)

2503 Phoenix Dr.
Tuscaloosa, AL 35405
Business: 800-462-0609
Emergency: 800-222-1222
               800-462-0800 (AL)
www.alapoisoncenter.org

ALASKA

JUNEAU

Alaska Poison Control System
Section of Injury Prevention and EMS

410 Willoughby Ave., Room 103
Box 110616
Juneau, AK 99811-0616
Business: 907-465-3027
Emergency: 800-222-1222
www.chems.alaska.gov

(PORTLAND, OR)

Oregon Poison Center (*)
Oregon Health and Science University

3181 SW Sam Jackson Park Rd.
CB550
Portland, OR 97239
Business: 503-494-8600
Emergency: 800-222-1222
www.oregonpoison.com

ARIZONA

PHOENIX

Banner Poison Control Center (*)
Banner Good Samaritan Medical Center

1111 E. McDowell
Phoenix, AZ 85006
Business: 602-495-4884
Emergency: 800-222-1222
www.bannerpoisoncontrol.com

TUCSON

Arizona Poison and Drug Information Center (*)
Arizona Health Sciences Center

1295 N. Martin Ave., Room B308
Tucson, AZ 85721
Business: 520-626-7899
Emergency: 800-222-1222
www.pharmacy.arizona.edu/outreach/poison

ARKANSAS

LITTLE ROCK

Arkansas Poison and Drug Information Center (*)
College of Pharmacy - UAMS

4301 West Markham St.
Mail Slot 522-2
Little Rock, AR 72205
Business: 501-686-6161
Emergency: 800-222-1222
               800-376-4766 (AR)
TDD/TTY: 800-641-3805

ASPCA/ANIMAL POISON CONTROL CENTER

1717 South Philo Rd.
Suite 36
Urbana, IL 61802
Business: 217-337-5030
Emergency: 888-426-4435
               800-548-2423
www.aspca.org/apcc

CALIFORNIA

FRESNO/MADERA

California Poison Control System-Fresno/Madera Div. (*)
Children's Hospital Central California

9300 Valley Children's Place, MB 15
Madera, CA 93638-8762
Business: 559-622-2300
Emergency: 800-222-1222
               800-876-4766 (CA)
TDD/TTY: 800-972-3323
www.calpoison.org

SACRAMENTO

California Poison Control System-Sacramento Div. (*)
UC Davis Medical Center

2315 Stockton Blvd.
Sacramento, CA 95817
Business: 916-227-1400
Emergency: 800-222-1222
               800-876-4766 (CA)
TDD/TTY: 800-972-3323
www.calpoison.org

SAN DIEGO

California Poison Control System-San Diego Div. (*)
UC San Diego Medical Center

200 West Arbor Dr.
San Diego, CA 92103-8925
Business: 858-715-6300
Emergency: 800-222-1222
               800-876-4766 (CA)
TDD/TTY: 800-972-3323
www.calpoison.org

SAN FRANCISCO

California Poison Control System-San Francisco Div. (*)
University of California San Francisco

Box 1369
San Francisco, CA 94143-1369
Business: 415-502-6000
Emergency: 800-222-1222
               800-876-4766 (CA)
TDD/TTY: 800-972-3323
www.calpoison.org

COLORADO

DENVER

Rocky Mountain Poison and Drug Center (*)

777 Bannock St., Mail Code 0180
Denver, CO 80204
Business: 303-739-1100
Emergency: 800-222-1222
TDD/TTY: 303-739-1127 (CO)
www.RMPDC.org

CONNECTICUT

FARMINGTON

Connecticut Poison Control Center (*)
University of Connecticut Health Center

263 Farmington Ave.
Farmington, CT 06030-5365
Business: 860-679-4540
Emergency: 800-222-1222
TDD/TTY: 866-218-5372
http://poisoncontrol.uchc.edu

DELAWARE

(PHILADELPHIA, PA)

The Poison Control Center (*)
Children's Hospital of Philadelphia

34th St. & Civic Center Blvd.
Philadelphia, PA 19104-4399
Business: 215-590-2003
Emergency: 800-222-1222
TDD/TTY: 215-590-8789
www.poisoncontrol.chop.edu

DISTRICT OF COLUMBIA

WASHINGTON, DC

National Capital Poison Center (*)

3201 New Mexico Ave., NW
Suite 310
Washington, DC 20016
Business: 202-362-3867
Emergency: 800-222-1222
www.poison.org

FLORIDA

JACKSONVILLE

Florida Poison Information Center-Jacksonville (*)

655 West 8th St.
Box C23
Jacksonville, FL 32209
Business: 904-244-4465
Emergency: 800-222-1222
http://fpicjax.org

MIAMI

Florida Poison Information Center (*)
University of Miami, Dept. of Pediatrics

P.O. Box 016960 (R-131)
Miami, FL 33101
Business: 305-585-5250
Emergency: 800-222-1222
www.med.miami.edu/poisoncontrol

TAMPA

Florida Poison Information Center (*)
Tampa General Hospital

P.O. Box 1289
Tampa, FL 33601-1289
Business: 813-844-7044
Emergency: 800-222-1222
www.poisoncentertampa.org

GEORGIA

ATLANTA

Georgia Poison Center (*)
Hughes Spalding Children's Hospital, Grady Health System

80 Jesse Hill Jr. Dr., SE
P.O. Box 26066
Atlanta, GA 30303-3050
Business: 404-616-9237
Emergency: 800-222-1222
                404-616-9000 (Atlanta)
TDD: 404-616-9287
www.georgiapoisoncenter.org

HAWAII

(DENVER, CO)

Rocky Mountain Poison and Drug Center (*)

777 Bannock St., Mail Code 0180
Denver, CO 80204
Business: 303-739-1100
Emergency: 800-222-1222
TDD/TTY: 303-739-1127 (CO)
www.RMPDC.org

IDAHO

(DENVER, CO)

Rocky Mountain Poison and Drug Center (*)

777 Bannock St., Mail Code 0180
Denver, CO 80204
Business: 303-739-1100
Emergency: 800-222-1222
TDD/TTY: 303-739-1127 (CO)
www.RMPDC.org

ILLINOIS

CHICAGO

Illinois Poison Center (*)

222 South Riverside Plaza
Suite 1900
Chicago, IL 60606
Business: 312-906-6136
Emergency: 800-222-1222
TDD/TTY: 312-906-6185
www.mchc.org/ipc

INDIANA

INDIANAPOLIS

Indiana Poison Control Center (*)
Methodist Hospital, Clarian Health Partners

I-65 at 21st St.
P.O. Box 1367
Indianapolis, IN 46206-1367
Business: 317-962-2335
Emergency: 800-222-1222
                800-382-9097
                317-962-2323
                (Indianapolis)
www.clarian.org/poisoncontrol

IOWA

SIOUX CITY

Iowa Statewide Poison Control Center (*)
Iowa Health System and the University of Iowa Hospitals and Clinics

401 Douglas St., Suite 402
Sioux City, IA 51101
Business: 712-279-3710
Emergency: 800-222-1222
                712-277-2222 (IA)
www.iowapoison.org

KANSAS

KANSAS CITY

University of Kansas
Poison Control Hospital Center

3901 Rainbow Blvd.
Delp - Room 4043
Kansas City, KS 66160-7231
Business: 913-588-6638
Emergency: 800-222-1222
                800-332-6633 (KS)
www.kumed.com/poison

KENTUCKY

LOUISVILLE

Kentucky Regional Poison Center (*)
Medical Towers South

234 E Gray St, Suite 847
Louisville, KY 40202
Business: 502-629-7264
Emergency: 800-222-1222
www.krpc.com

LOUISIANA

SHREVEPORT

Louisiana Poison Center (*)
LSUHSC - Shreveport
Dept. of Emergency Medicine
Section of Clinical Toxology

1455 Wilkinson St
Shreveport, LA 71130
Business: 318-813-3314
Emergency: 800-222-1222

MAINE

PORTLAND

Northern New England Poison Center (*)

22 Bramhall St.
Portland, ME 04102
Business: 207-662-7042
Emergency: 800-222-1222
           800-442-6035
           207-871-2879 (ME)
TDD/TTY: 207-662-2879 (ME)
www.nnepc.org

MARYLAND

BALTIMORE

Maryland Poison Center (*)
University of Maryland at Baltimore
School of Pharmacy

220 Arch St.
Office Level 01
Baltimore, MD 21201
Business: 410-706-7604
Emergency: 800-222-1222
TDD: 410-528-7530
www.mdpoison.com

(WASHINGTON, DC)

National Capital Poison Center (*)

3201 New Mexico Ave., NW
Suite 310
Washington, DC 20016
Business: 202-362-3867
Emergency: 800-222-1222
www.poison.org

MASSACHUSETTS

BOSTON

Regional Center for Poison Control and Prevention (*)
(Serving Massachusetts and Rhode Island)

300 Longwood Ave.
Boston, MA 02115
Business: 617-355-6609
Emergency: 800-222-1222
TDD/TTY: 888-244-5313
www.maripoisoncenter.com

MICHIGAN

DETROIT

Regional Poison Control Center (*)
Children's Hospital of Michigan

4160 John R. Harper Professional Office Bldg.
Suite 616
Detroit, MI 48201
Business: 313-745-5335
Emergency: 800-222-1222
www.mitoxic.org/pcc

MINNESOTA

MINNEAPOLIS

Hennepin Regional Poison Center (*)
Hennepin County Medical Center

701 Park Ave.
Mail Code RL
Minneapolis, MN 55415
Business: 612-873-3144
Emergency: 800-222-1222
www.mnpoison.org

MISSISSIPPI

JACKSON

Mississippi Regional Poison Control Center
University of Mississippi Medical Center

2500 North State St.
Jackson, MS 39216
Business: 601-984-1680
Emergency: 800-222-1222
http://poisoncontrol.umc.edu

MISSOURI

ST. LOUIS

Missouri Regional Poison Center (*)

7980 Clayton Rd. Suite 200
St. Louis, MO 63117
Business: 314-772-8300
Emergency: 800-222-1222
www.cardinalglennon.com

MONTANA

(DENVER, CO)

Rocky Mountain Poison and Drug Center (*)

777 Bannock St., Mail Code 0180
Denver, CO 80204
Business: 303-739-1100
Emergency: 800-222-1222
TDD/TTY: 303-739-1127 (CO)
www.RMPDC.org

NEBRASKA

OMAHA

Nebraska Regional Poison Center (*)

8401 W. Dodge Rd., Suite 115
Omaha, NE 68114
Business: 402-390-5555
Emergency: 800-222-1222
www.nebraskapoison.com

NEVADA

(DENVER, CO)

Rocky Mountain Poison and Drug Center (*)

777 Bannock St., Mail Code 0180
Denver, CO 80204
Business: 303-739-1100
Emergency: 800-222-1222
TDD/TTY: 303-739-1127 (CO)
www.RMPDC.org

NEW HAMPSHIRE

(PORTLAND, ME)

Northern New England Poison Center
Maine Medical Center

22 Bramhall St.
Portland, ME 04102
Business: 207-662-0111
Emergency: 800-222-1222
www.nnepc.org

NEW JERSEY

NEWARK

New Jersey Poison Information and Education System (*)
UMDNJ

140 Bergen St. PO Box 1709
Newark, NJ 07101
Business: 973-972-9280
Emergency: 800-222-1222
TDD/TTY: 973-926-8008
www.njpies.org

NEW MEXICO

ALBUQUERQUE

New Mexico Poison and Drug Information Center (*)

MSC09/5080
1 University of New Mexico
Albuquerque, NM 87131-0001
Business: 505-272-4261
Emergency: 800-222-1222
http://hsc.unm.edu/pharmacy/poison

NEW YORK

MINEOLA

Long Island Regional Poison and Drug Information Center (*)
Winthrop University Hospital

259 First St.
Mineola, NY 11501
Business: 516-663-4574
Emergency: 800-222-1222
www.lirpdic.org

NEW YORK CITY

New York City Poison Control Center (*)
NYC Bureau of Public Health

455 First Ave., Room 123, Box 81
New York, NY 10016
Business: 212-447-8152
Emergency: 800-222-1222
(English)   212-340-4494
               212-POISONS
               (212-764-7667)
Emergency: 212-venenos
(Spanish)   (212-836-3667)
TDD: 212-689-9014
www.nyc.gov/html/doh/html/poison/
poison.shtml

ROCHESTER

The Ruth A. Lawrence Regional Poison and Drug Information Center (*)
University of Rochester Medical Center

601 Elmwood Ave.
Box 321
Rochester, NY 14642
Business: 585-273-4155
Emergency: 800-222-1222
TTY: 585-273-3854
www.fingerlakespoison.org

SYRACUSE

Upstate New York Poison Center (*)
SUNY Upstate Medical University

750 East Adams St.
Syracuse, NY 13210
Business: 315-464-7078
Emergency: 800-222-1222
TTY: 315-464-5424
www.upstatepoison.org

NORTH CAROLINA

CHARLOTTE

Carolinas Poison Center (*)
Carolinas Medical Center

PO Box 32861
Charlotte, NC 28232-2861
Business: 704-512-3795
Emergency: 800-222-1222
www.ncpoisoncenter.org

NORTH DAKOTA

(MINNEAPOLIS, MN)

Hennepin Regional Poison Center (*)
Hennepin County Medical Center

701 Park Ave., Mail Code RL
Minneapolis, MN 55415
Business: 612-873-3144
Emergency: 800-222-1222
www.mnpoison.org

OHIO

CINCINNATI

Cincinnati Drug and Poison Information Center (*)

3333 Burnet Ave., MLC 9004
Cincinnati, OH 45229
Business: 513-636-5063
Emergency: 800-222-1222
www.cincinnatichildrens.org/dpic

CLEVELAND

Northern Ohio Poison Center
Rainbow Babies and Children's Hospital

11100 Euclid Ave.
B261 MP 6007
Cleveland, OH 44106-6010
Business: 216-844-1573
Emergency: 800-222-1222
www.uhhospitals.org/rainbowchildren/
tabid/195/Default.aspx

COLUMBUS

Central Ohio Poison Center (*)

700 Children's Dr.
Columbus, OH 43205
Business: 614-355-0435
Emergency: 800-222-1222
TTY: 866-688-0088
www.bepoisonsmart.com

OKLAHOMA

OKLAHOMA CITY

Oklahoma Poison Control Center (*)
OU Health Sciences Center

940 Northeast 13th St.
Room 3N3510
Oklahoma City, OK 73104
Business: 405-271-5062
Emergency: 800-222-1222
www.oklahomapoison.org

OREGON

PORTLAND

Oregon Poison Center (*)
Oregon Health and Science University

3181 S.W. Sam Jackson Park Rd.
CB550
Portland, OR 97239
Business: 503-494-8600
Emergency: 800-222-1222
www.ohsu.edu/poison

PENNSYLVANIA

PHILADELPHIA

The Poison Control Center (*)
Children's Hospital of Philadelphia

34th Street & Civic Center Blvd.
Philadelphia, PA 19104
Business: 215-590-2003
Emergency: 800-222-1222
             215-386-2100 (PA)
TDD/TTY: 215-590-8789
www.poisoncontrol.chop.edu

PITTSBURGH

Pittsburgh Poison Center (*)
University of Pittsburgh

200 Lothrop Street
Pittsburgh, PA 15213
Business: 412-390-3300
Emergency: 800-222-1222
             412-681-6669
www.upmc.com/services/poisoncenter

RHODE ISLAND

(BOSTON, MA)

Regional Center for Poison Control and Prevention (*)
(Serving Massachusetts and Rhode Island)

300 Longwood Ave.
Boston, MA 02115
Business: 617-355-6609
Emergency: 800-222-1222
TDD/TTY: 888-244-5313
www.maripoisoncenter.com

SOUTH CAROLINA

COLUMBIA

Palmetto Poison Center (*)
South Carolina College of Pharmacy
University of South Carolina

Columbia, SC 29208
Business: 803-777-7909
Emergency: 800-222-1222
http://poison.sc.edu

SOUTH DAKOTA

(MINNEAPOLIS, MN)

Hennepin Regional Poison Center (*)
Hennepin County Medical Center

701 Park Ave., Mail Code RL
Minneapolis, MN 55415
Business: 612-873-3144
Emergency: 800-222-1222
www.mnpoison.org

TENNESSEE

NASHVILLE

Tennessee Poison Center (*)

1161 21st Ave. South
501 Oxford House
Nashville, TN 37232-4632
Business: 615-936-0760
Emergency: 800-222-1222
www.tnpoisoncenter.org

TEXAS

AMARILLO

Texas Panhandle Poison Center (*)

1501 S. Coulter Dr.
Amarillo, TX 79106
Business: 806-354-1630
Emergency: 800-222-1222
www.poisoncontrol.org

DALLAS

North Texas Poison Center (*)
Texas Poison Center Network
Parkland Memorial Hospital

5201 Harry Hines Blvd.
Dallas, TX 75235
Business: 214-589-0911
Emergency: 800-222-1222
www.poisoncontrol.org

EL PASO

West Texas Regional Poison Center (*)
At University Medical Center of El Paso

4815 Alameda Ave.
El Paso, TX 79905
Business   915-534-3800
Emergency: 800-222-1222
www.poisoncontrol.org

GALVESTON

Southeast Texas Poison Center (*)
The University of Texas Medical Branch

3.112 Trauma Center
Galveston, TX 77555-1175
Business: 409-772-3332
Emergency: 800-222-1222
www.utmb.edu/setpc

SAN ANTONIO

South Texas Poison Center (*)
The University of Texas Health Science Center–San Antonio
Dept. of Surgery

7703 Floyd Curl Dr., MSC 7849
San Antonio, TX 78229-3900
Business: 210-567-5762
Emergency: 800-222-1222
www.texaspoison.com

TEMPLE

Central Texas Poison Center (*)
Scott & White Memorial Hospital

2401 South 31st St.
Temple, TX 76508
Business: 254-724-7405
Emergency: 800-222-1222
http://www.sw.org/web/
patientsAndVisitors/iwcontent/
public/poison/en_us/html/poison.jsp

UTAH

SALT LAKE CITY

Utah Poison Control Center (*)
University of Utah

585 Komas Dr. Suite #200
Salt Lake City, UT 84108-1234
Business: 801-587-0600
Emergency: 800-222-1222
http://uuhsc.utah.edu/poison

VERMONT

(PORTLAND, ME)

Northern New England Poison Center (*)
Maine Medical Center

22 Bramhall St.
Portland, ME 04102
Business: 207-662-0111
Emergency: 800-222-1222
www.nnepc.org

VIRGINIA

CHARLOTTESVILLE

Blue Ridge Poison Center (*)
Jefferson Park Place

1222 Jefferson Park Ave.
Charlottesville, VA 22908-0774
Business: 434-924-0347
Emergency: 800-222-1222
www.healthsystem.virginia.edu/brpc

RICHMOND

Virginia Poison Center (*)
Medical College of Virginia Hospitals
Virginia Commonwealth University Health System

P.O. Box 980522
Richmond, VA 23298-0522
Business: 804-828-4780
Emergency: 800-222-1222
www.poison.vcu.edu

WASHINGTON

SEATTLE

Washington Poison Center (*)

155 NE 100th St.
Seattle, WA 98125-8007
Business: 206-517-2350
Emergency: 800-222-1222
www.wapc.org

WEST VIRGINIA

CHARLESTON

West Virginia Poison Center (*)
WVU Charleston Division

3110 MacCorkle Ave. SE
Charleston, WV 25314
Business: 304-347-1212
Emergency: 800-222-1222
www.wvpoisoncenter.org

WISCONSIN

MILWAUKEE

Wisconsin Poison Center

Mail Station 660
P.O. Box 1997
Milwaukee, WI 53201-1997
Business: 414-266-6973
Emergency: 800-222-1222
www.wisconsinpoison.org

WYOMING

(OMAHA, NE)

Nebraska Regional Poison Center (*)

8401 W. Dodge St., Suite 115
Omaha, NE 68114
Business: 402-390-5555
Emergency: 800-222-1222
www.nebraskapoison.com

PRODUCT IDENTIFICATION GUIDE

For quick identification, this section provides full-color reproductions of product packaging, as well as some actual-sized photographs of tablets and capsules.

Products in this section are arranged alphabetically by manufacturer. In some instances, not all dosage forms and sizes are pictured. For more information on any of the products in this section, please turn to the page indicated above the product's photo or check directly with the product's manufacturer.

While every effort has been made to guarantee faithful reproduction of the photos in this section, changes in size, color, and design are always a possibility. Be sure to confirm a product's identity with the manufacturer or your pharmacist.

MANUFACTURER'S INDEX

ALTO

ALTO PHARMACEUTICALS, INC.   P. 502

220 mg

Zinc-220®
(zinc sulfate)

AMERICA PHARMA CO.

AMERICA PHARMA CO.   P. 502

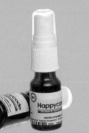

Sublingual Spray

Happycode

AMERICA PHARMA CO.   P. 568

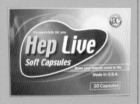

HepLive Soft Capsules

AMERICA PHARMA CO.   P. 568

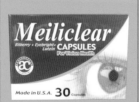

Meiliclear Capsules

AMERICA PHARMA CO.   P. 568

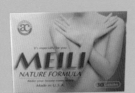

Meili Nature Formula

AMERICA PHARMA CO.   P. 568

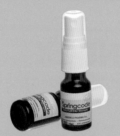

Sublingual Spray

Springcode

BAUSCH & LOMB

BAUSCH & LOMB INCORPORATED   P. 503

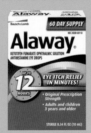

Antihistamine Eye Drops

Alaway®
(ketotifen fumarate
ophthalmic solution 0.025%)

BAUSCH & LOMB INCORPORATED   P. 570

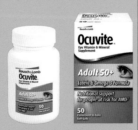

Adult 50+ Formula
Eye Vitamin and Mineral Supplement

Ocuvite® Adult 50+ Formula

BAUSCH & LOMB INCORPORATED   P. 571

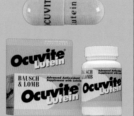

Eye Vitamin and Mineral Supplement

Ocuvite® Lutein

BAUSCH & LOMB INCORPORATED   P. 569

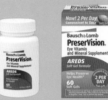

Eye Vitamin and Mineral Supplement

**PreserVision® AREDS
Soft Gels**

BAUSCH & LOMB INCORPORATED   P. 569

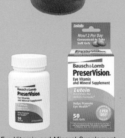

Eye Vitamin and Mineral Supplement
Available in 50 ct and 120 ct

**PreserVision® Lutein
Soft Gels**

BAUSCH & LOMB INCORPORATED   P. 504

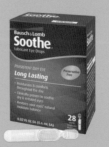

Single-Use Dispensers
Lubricant Eye Drops

Soothe®
(glycerin and propylene glycol 0.6%)

BAUSCH & LOMB INCORPORATED   P. 505

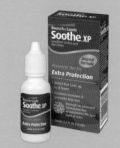

15 mL
Lubricant Eye Drops

Soothe® XP
(light mineral oil 1% and mineral oil 4.5%)

BAYER HEALTHCARE LLC, CONSUMER CARE

BAYER HEALTHCARE LLC,
CONSUMER CARE   P. 505

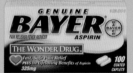

325 mg

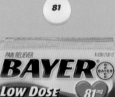

81 mg

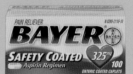

325 mg

BAYER® Aspirin

BAYER HEALTHCARE LLC,
CONSUMER CARE　　　P. 505

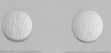

81 mg
Low dose, chewable aspirin
Cherry and Orange flavors

**Aspirin Regimen
BAYER® Chewable**

BEACH

BEACH PHARMACEUTICALS　　P. 572

600 mg/25 mg
Dietary Supplement

Beelith
(magnesium oxide/vitamin B6)

CARLSON LABORATORIES

CARLSON LABORATORIES　　P. 572

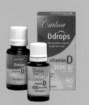

400 IU/1000 IU/2000 IU
Dietary Supplement

Ddrops®

GORDON LABORATORIES

GORDON LABORATORIES　　P. 517

25%
30 mL

Gordochom
(undecylenic acid)

HISAMITSU PHARMACEUTICAL

HISAMITSU　　P. 518, 519
PHARMACEUTICAL CO., INC.

Pain Relief Patch　　Arthritis Pain
Available in packs of 5 and 15 patches.

SALONPAS®

JOHNSON & JOHNSON HEALTHCARE PRODUCTS DIVISION OF MCNEIL-PPC, INC.

JOHNSON & JOHNSON　　P. 520
HEALTHCARE PRODUCTS
DIVISION OF MCNEIL-PPC, INC.

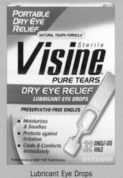

Lubricant Eye Drops

**VISINE® PURE TEARS®
Preservative Free Singles**

J&J-MERCK CONSUMER

J&J-MERCK CONSUMER　　P. 520

10 mg Tablets

**ORIGINAL STRENGTH
PEPCID® AC®**
(famotidine)

J&J-MERCK CONSUMER　　P. 520

20 mg Tablets

**MAXIMUM STRENGTH
PEPCID® AC®**
(famotidine)

J&J-MERCK CONSUMER　　P. 520

20 mg
Cool Mint and Berries 'n' Cream
Chewable Tablets

**MAXIMUM STRENGTH
PEPCID® AC® EZ CHEWS®**
(famotidine)

J&J-MERCK CONSUMER　　P. 521

10 mg/800 mg/165 mg
Berry, Cool Mint, and Tropical Fruit
Chewable Tablets

PEPCID® COMPLETE®
(famotidine/calcium carbonate/
magnesium hydroxide)

KYOWA WELLNESS CO.

KYOWA WELLNESS CO., LTD.　　P. 575

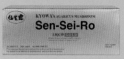

KYOWA's Agaricus Mushroom Extract
Dietary Supplement

Sen-Sei-Ro Liquid Gold™

KYOWA WELLNESS CO., LTD　　P. 575

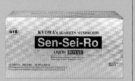

KYOWA's Agaricus Mushroom Extract
Dietary Supplement

Sen-Sei-Ro Liquid Royal™

KYOWA WELLNESS CO., LTD　　P. 575

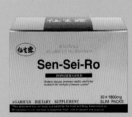

KYOWA's Agaricus Mushroom Powder
Dietary Supplement

Sen-Sei-Ro Powder Gold™

MERICON INDUSTRIES

MERICON INDUSTRIES　　P. 577

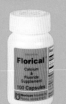

3.75 mg/145 mg

Florical®
(sodium fluoride/calcium carbonate)

PADDOCK LABORATORIES

PADDOCK LABORATORIES   P. 558

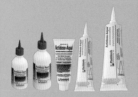

Available in 25 g/120 mL and 50 g/240 mL bottles; and 15 g/72 mL, 25 g/120 mL, and 50 g/240 mL tubes.

Actidose® -Aqua
(activated charcoal suspension)

PADDOCK LABORATORIES   P. 558

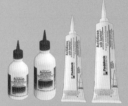

Available in 25 g/120 mL and 50 g/240 mL bottles; and 25 g/120 mL and 50 g/240 mL tubes.

Actidose® with Sorbitol
(activated charcoal suspension)

PADDOCK LABORATORIES   P. 558

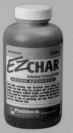

25 g

EZ-Char®
(activated charcoal pellets)

PADDOCK LABORATORIES   P. 559

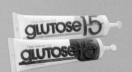

15 g
Available in lemon & grape flavors.

Glutose 15™
(oral glucose gel)

PADDOCK LABORATORIES   P. 559

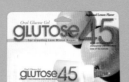

45 g
Available in lemon flavor.

Glutose 45™
(oral glucose gel)

STANDARD HOMEOPATHIC

STANDARD HOMEOPATHIC   P. 560

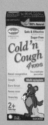

Hyland's Cold 'n Cough 4 Kids

STANDARD HOMEOPATHIC   P. 561

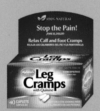

Caplets

Hyland's Leg Cramps with Quinine

TOPICAL BIOMEDICS, INC.

TOPICAL BIOMEDICS, INC.   P. 563

Homeopathic cream
Available in 2 oz. tube, 4 oz. jar, and 8 oz pump.
Topricin Jr. 1.5 oz. and Topricin Foot Therapy 8 oz.
Professional sizes of 16 and 32 oz. pump bottles.

Topricin®

UNICITY INTERNATIONAL

UNICITY INTERNATIONAL   P. 580

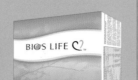

Dietary Supplement

Bios Life C™

UNICITY INTERNATIONAL   P. 564

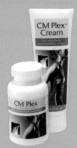

Dietary Supplement

CM Plex™

UNICITY INTERNATIONAL   P. 564

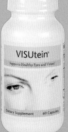

Dietary Supplement

VISUtein®

WESTLAKE LABORATORIES

WESTLAKE LABORATORIES, INC.   P. 565

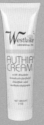

2 oz.

Authia® Cream

WESTLAKE LABORATORIES, INC.   P. 566

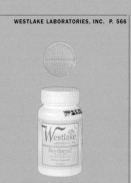

400 mcg-3 mg-1000 mcg

Bevitamel®
(folic acid/melatonin/vitamin B$_{12}$)

SECTION 6

NONPRESCRIPTION DRUG INFORMATION

This section presents information on nonprescription products marketed for home use by consumers. The information on each product described has been prepared, edited, and approved by the regulatory department, medical department, medical director, and/or counsel of its manufacturer for publication in the 2010 *PDR* or 2010 *PDR for Ophthalmic Medicines*.

Pharmaceutical product descriptions in this section must be in compliance with the Code of Federal Regulations' labeling requirements for over-the-counter drugs. The descriptions are designed to provide all information necessary for informed use, including, when applicable, active ingredients, inactive ingredients, indications, actions, warnings, cautions, drug interactions, symptoms

and treatment of oral overdosage, dosage and directions for use, professional labeling, and how supplied. In some cases, additional information has been supplied to complement the standard labeling.

In compiling this section, the publisher has emphasized the necessity of describing products comprehensively. The descriptions seen here include all information made available by the manufacturer. The publisher does not warrant or guarantee any product described here, and does not perform any independent analysis of the information provided. Inclusion of a product in this book does not represent an endorsement, and the publisher does not advocate the use of any product listed.

Alcon Laboratories, Inc.
AND ITS AFFILIATES
CORPORATE HEADQUARTERS
6201 SOUTH FREEWAY
FORT WORTH, TX 76134

Address Inquiries to:
6201 South Freeway
Fort Worth, TX 76134
(800) 757-9195
Outside the U.S. call (817) 568-6725
medinfo@alconlabs.com

SYSTANE® ULTRA LUBRICANT   OTC
EYE DROPS

Drug Facts
Active Ingredients   *Purpose*
Polyethylene Glycol 400 0.4% .... Lubricant
Propylene Glycol 0.3% .... Lubricant

USES
• For the temporary relief of burning and irritation due to dryness of the eye

WARNINGS
For external use only.
Do not use
• if this product changes color or becomes cloudy
• if you are sensitive to any ingredient in this product
When using this product
• do not touch tip of container to any surface to avoid contamination
• replace cap after each use
Stop use and ask a doctor if
• you feel eye pain
• changes in vision occur
• redness or irritation of the eye(s) gets worse, persists or lasts more than 72 hours
Keep out of reach of children.
If swallowed, get medical help or contact a Poison Control Center right away.

DIRECTIONS
• Shake well before using.
• Instill 1 or 2 drops in the affected eye(s) as needed.
Other Information
• Store at room temperature.
Inactive Ingredients:
Aminomethylpropanol, boric acid, hydroxypropyl guar, POLYQUAD® (polyquaternium-1) 0.001% preservative, potassium chloride, purified water, sodium chloride, sorbitol. May contain hydrochloric acid and/or sodium hydroxide to adjust pH.
Questions:
In the U.S. call **1-800-757-9195**
www.systane.com
TAMPER EVIDENT: For your protection, this bottle has an imprinted seal around the neck. Do not use if seal is damaged or missing at time of purchase.
Open your eyes to a breakthrough in comfort with SYSTANE® ULTRA Lubricant Eye Drops. SYSTANE® ULTRA elevates the science of dry eye therapy to a new level. From first blink, eyes feel lubricated and refreshed. Feel the difference in dry eye relief with SYSTANE® ULTRA.
U.S. Patent Nos. 6,403,609, 6,583,124 and 6,838,449.
©2008-2009 Alcon, Inc.

Alcon Laboratories, Inc.
Fort Worth, TX 76134 USA

Alto Pharmaceuticals, Inc.
P.O. BOX 271150
TAMPA, FL 33688-1150
3172 - LAKE ELLEN DRIVE
TAMPA, FL 33618

Direct Inquiries to:
John J. Cullaro
Customer Service
ALTOPHARM@AOL.COM
Tel (800) 330-2891
Fax (813) 968-0527

ZINC-220® CAPSULES   OTC
[zĭnk]
(zinc sulfate 220 mg.)

COMPOSITION
Each opaque blue and pink capsule contains zinc sulfate 220 mg. delivering 78.5 mg. of elemental zinc. Zinc-220 Capsules do not contain dextrose or glucose. Inactive Ingredients dicalcium phosphate, cellulose, magnesium stearate, magnesium trisilicate and gelatin (capsule shell).

ACTION AND USES
Zinc-220 Capsules are indicated as a dietary supplement. Normal growth and tissue repair are directly dependent upon an adequate supply of zinc in the diet. Zinc functions as an integral part of a number of enzymes important to protein and carbohydrate metabolism. Zinc-220 Capsules are recommended for deficiencies or the prevention of deficiencies of zinc.

WARNINGS
Zinc-220 if administered in stat dosages of 2 grams (9 capsules) will cause an emetic effect. This product should not be used by pregnant or lactating women.

PRECAUTION
It is recommended that Zinc-220 Capsules be taken with meals or milk to avoid gastric distress.

DOSAGE
One capsule daily with milk or meals. One capsule daily provides approximately 523% times the recommended adult requirement for zinc.

HOW SUPPLIED

Product	NDC	SIZE
Zinc-220® Capsules	0731-0401-06	Unit Dose Boxes ... 100 (5×10×2)

Each Zinc-220® capsule is identified by the "ALTO" logo on one side and the number "401" on the other side of the capsule.
ALTO® Pharmaceuticals, Inc.
Shown in Product Identification Guide, page 402

America Pharma Co.
750 STIMSON AVENUE
CITY OF INDUSTRY, CA 91745

Direct Inquiries to:
Phone: (626) 336-8889
Fax: (626) 336-1299
Email: ac.usa.inc@gmail.com
http://www.acusainc.net

HAPPYCODE SPRAY   OTC

The thymus gland, one of the most significant immune organs, degrades gradually as one ages, and it will gradually or completely loses its function of secreting thymus after the age of fifty.

The main ingredient of this product is obtained from healthy cows by employing microdialysis technique to extract thymus peptide. This product can thus effectively enhance a patient's immunity and cure immunity-related diseases. So it is considered the ideal and perfect preparation for bi-directional immune modulation and it's also the covet product in anti-aging medicine.

Employing the latest technology of Polymer Matrix Delivery (PMD), Happycode Spray can easily be absorbed directly via mouth, sublingual mucosa. It has the absolute advantages of portability, fast absorption, effectiveness and allergy-free and toxic-free properties over other thymus products.

Applicable to:
1. Repetitive respiratory tract infection
2. Allergic rhinitis, asthma, bronchitis and pneumonia.
3. Combination therapy and adjuvant therapy for the pre-symptomatic stage of various malignant tumors, chemo-therapy and radiation therapy
4. Chronicle hepatitis therapy
5. Autoimmune diseases, such as rheumatoid arthritis and systemic lupus erythematosus (SLE)
6. Herpes zoster, psoriasis, climacteric syndrome and melancholia.
7. Senior and weak persons with lower immunity

Application

Each bottle contains 10 ml. Use two to three times daily, apply two sprays each time to sublingual mucosa and swallow it after two minutes. For the amount taken for different physical constitution and illness, please follow the directions of doctors or professionals.

DOSAGE

10ml/bottle 1ml/40mg
Shown in Product Identification Guide, page 402

Bausch & Lomb Incorporated
ONE BAUSCH & LOMB PLACE
ROCHESTER NY 14604

7 GIRALDA FARMS
MADISON, NJ 07940

Direct Inquiries to:
Main Office
(585) 338-6000
Consumer Affairs
1-800-553-5340

BAUSCH & LOMB ALAWAY®   OTC
Ketotifen Fumarate Ophthalmic Solution
Antihistamine Eye Drops

DESCRIPTION

Alaway® (ketotifen fumarate ophthalmic solution 0.025%) Antihistamine Eye Drops are indicated for temporary relief for itchy eyes due to ragweed, pollen, grass, animal hair and dander. The original prescription strength, now available over-the-counter, stops the itch within minutes and provides up to 12 hours of symptom relief.

Drug Facts:
Active Ingredient: Ketotifen 0.025%
(equivalent to ketotifen fumarate 0.035%)
Purpose: Antihistamine
Inactive ingredients: Benzalkonium chloride, 0.01%, glycerin, sodium hydroxide and/or hydrochloric acid and water for injection.

USES

For the temporary relief of itchy eyes due to ragweed, pollen, grass, animal hair and dander.

WARNINGS

Do not use:
- if you are sensitive to any ingredient in this product
- if the solution changes color or becomes cloudy
- to treat contact lens related irritation

When using this product
- remove contact lenses before use
- wait at least 10 minutes before re-inserting contact lenses after use
- do not touch the tip of the container to any surface to avoid contamination
- replace cap after each use

Stop use and ask a doctor if you experience any of the following:
- eye pain
- changes in vision
- redness of the eyes
- itching that worsens or lasts for more than 72 hours

Keep out of reach of children. If swallowed, get medical help or contact a Poison Control Center right away.

DIRECTIONS

Adults and children 3 years and older: put 1 drop in the affected eye(s) twice daily, every 8-12 hours, no more than twice per day.

Children under 3 years of age: consult a doctor

Other information
STORE AT 4-25°C (39-77°F)

HOW SUPPLIED

NDC 24208-601-10 Sterile 0.34 FL OZ (10mL) plastic dispenser bottle

Questions or Comments?
Toll Free Product Information
Call: 1-800-553-5340
Distributed by: Bausch & Lomb Incorporated.
Rochester, NY 14609
Bausch & Lomb and Alaway are registered trademarks of Bausch & Lomb Incorporated
© Bausch & Lomb Incorporated
Rochester, NY 14609
Shown in Product Identification Guide, page 402

MURO® 128® 2%   OTC
[mŭ 'rō 128]
Sodium Chloride Hypertonicity
Ophthalmic Solution, 2%
STERILE OPHTHALMIC SOLUTION

MURO® 128® 5%   OTC
Sodium Chloride Hypertonicity
Ophthalmic Solution, 5%
STERILE OPHTHALMIC SOLUTION

DESCRIPTION

Muro® 128® 2% Solution is a sterile ophthalmic solution hypertonicity agent.

Each mL Contains: ACTIVE: Sodium Chloride 2%; INACTIVES: Boric Acid, Hypromellose, Propylene Glycol, Purified Water, Sodium Borate. Sodium Hydroxide and/ or Hydrochloric Acid may be added to adjust pH.
PRESERVATIVES: Methylparaben   0.028%, Propylparaben 0.012%

DESCRIPTION

Muro® 128® 5% Solution is a sterile ophthalmic solution hypertonicity agent.

Each mL Contains: ACTIVE: Sodium Chloride 5%; INACTIVES: Boric Acid, Hypromellose, Propylene Glycol, Purified Water, Sodium Borate. Sodium Hydroxide and/ or Hydrochloric Acid may be added to adjust pH.
PRESERVATIVES: Methylparaben   0.023%, Propylparaben 0.01%

USES

For the temporary relief of corneal edema.

WARNINGS

Do not use this product except under the advice and supervision of a doctor.

If you experience eye pain, changes in vision, continued redness or irritation of the eye, or if the condition worsens or persists for more than 72 hours, consult a doctor.

To avoid contamination of the product, do not touch the tip of the container to any surface.

Continued on next page

Muro 128 Solution—Cont.

Replace cap after use.
This product may cause temporary burning and irritation on being instilled into the eye.
If the solution changes color or becomes cloudy, do not use.
In case of accidental ingestion, seek professional assistance or contact a Poison Control Center immediately.

DIRECTIONS

Instill 1 or 2 drops in the affected eye(s) every 3 or 4 hours, or as directed by a doctor.
FOR OPHTHALMIC USE ONLY

HOW SUPPLIED

Muro® 128® 2% Solution is supplied in a plastic controlled drop tip bottle in the following size:
½ Fl. Oz. (15 mL) (NDC 24208-276-15)—Prod. No. AB15511

HOW SUPPLIED

Muro® 128® 5% Solution is supplied in ½ Fl. Oz. (15 mL) or 1 Fl. Oz. (30 mL) plastic controlled dropper tip bottles.
15 mL [NDC 24208-277-15]—Prod. No. AB15611
30 mL [NDC 24208-277-30]—Prod. No. AB15616

> **DO NOT USE IF IMPRINTED
> PROTECTIVE SEAL WITH YELLOW
> IS NOT INTACT**

Storage: Store between 15°–30°C [59°–86°F].
KEEP TIGHTLY CLOSED. **STORE UPRIGHT AND IMMEDIATELY REPLACE CAP AFTER USE.**
KEEP OUT OF REACH OF CHILDREN.
**Bausch & Lomb
Incorporated**
Tampa, FL 33637
MURO 128 is a registered trademark of Bausch & Lomb Incorporated

9082302
9081702
9082102

MURO® 128® 5% OINTMENT   OTC
[mŭ 'rō 128]
**Sodium Chloride Hypertonicity
Ophthalmic Ointment, 5%
FOR TEMPORARY RELIEF OF CORNEAL EDEMA
STERILE OPHTHALMIC OINTMENT**

DESCRIPTION

Muro™ 128® 5% Ointment is a sterile ophthalmic ointment hypertonicity agent.
Each Gram Contains: ACTIVE: Sodium Chloride 50mg (5%) INACTIVES: Lanolin, Mineral Oil, Purified Water, White Petrolatum.

USES

For the temporary relief of corneal edema.

WARNINGS

Do not use this product except under the advice and supervision of a doctor.
If you experience eye pain, changes in vision, continued redness or irritation of the eye, or if the condition worsens or persists for more than 72 hours, consult a doctor.
To avoid contamination of the product, do not touch the tip of the container to any surface.
Replace cap after using.
This product may cause temporary burning and irritation on being instilled into the eye.
In case of accidental ingestion, seek professional assistance or contact a Poison Control Center immediately.

DIRECTIONS

Pull down lower lid of the affected eye(s) and apply a small amount (approximately ¼ inch) of the ointment to the inside of the eyelid every 3 or 4 hours, or as directed by a doctor.
FOR OPHTHALMIC USE ONLY

HOW SUPPLIED

Muro™ 128® 5% Ointment is supplied in ⅛ oz (3.5 g) tube.
[NDC 24208-385-55]—Prod. No. AB15834
TWIN PACK: 2 x ⅛ oz (2 x 3.5 g)
[NDC 24208-385-56]—Prod. No. AB15899
NOTE: Tubes are filled by weight (⅛ oz/3.5g) not volume. See Crimp of tube or carton for Lot Number and Expiration Date.

> **DO NOT USE IF BOTTOM RIDGE OF
> TUBE CAP IS EXPOSED AND
> IMPRINTED SEAL ON BOX
> IS BROKEN OR MISSING.**

KEEP OUT OF REACH OF CHILDREN.
Storage: Store at 15°–30°C (59°–86°F). DO NOT FREEZE.
KEEP TIGHTLY CLOSED.
Bausch & Lomb Incorporated
Tampa, FL 33637
™/® denotes trademark of Bausch & Lomb Incorporated

9043603

SOOTHE®   OTC
Lubricant Eye Drops

PERSISTENT DRY EYE

DESCRIPTION

Preservative-Free, Long Lasting Relief. This revolutionary advance in dry eye therapy provides soothing comfort and long lasting lubrication, keeping eyes feeling fresh throughout the day. This unique new formula restores the natural moisture in your eyes, providing effective, long lasting dry eye relief. Preservative-Free so it's gentle enough to use as often as needed

DRUG FACTS

Active Ingredients	*Purpose*
Glycerin (0.6%)	Lubricant
Propylene Glycol (0.6%)	Lubricant

Purpose: Lubricant Eye Drops
Inactive Ingredients
Boric acid, hydroxyalkylphosphonate, purified water, sodium alginate, sodium borate

USES

- relieves dryness of the eye
- prevents further irritation

WARNINGS

Do not use
- if solution changes color or becomes cloudy
- if single-unit dispenser is not intact

When using this product
- do not touch the tip of container to any surface to avoid contamination
- once opened, discard
- do not reuse

Stop and ask a doctor if
- you experience eye pain, changes in vision, continued redness or irritation of the eye
- condition worsens or persists for more than 72 hours

Keep out of reach of children. If swallowed, get medical help or contact a Poison Control Center right away.

DIRECTIONS

Easy to use sterile dispenser
- To open, completely twist tab off
- Instill 1 to 2 drops in the affected eye(s) as needed
- Discard dispenser immediately after use.

Other Information
STORE AT 20°-25°C (68°-77°F)
DO NOT USE IF TAPE SEALS IMPRINTED WITH B&L TAPE SEAL ARE NOT INTACT

HOW SUPPLIED

NDC # 24208-475-28
4 ct. sample: 24208-495-95
28 sterile single-use dispensers 0.02 FL OZ EA (0.6mL EA)

Questions or Comments?
Toll Free product information or to report a serious side effect associated with use of this product call: 1-800-553-5340.
Bausch & Lomb and Soothe are registered trademarks of Bausch & Lomb Incorporated.
Patents pending.
Manufactured for:
Bausch & Lomb Incorporated
Rochester, NY 14609
Made in USA
www.bausch.com
Shown in Product Identification Guide, page 402

SOOTHE® XP   OTC
Emollient (Lubricant) Eye Drops

DESCRIPTION

Original Formula, Persistent Dry Eye, Extra Protection
• Relief that lasts up to 8 hours
• Restores moisture & prevents tear loss.
Restoryl®, an advanced formulation that re-establishes the lipid layer of tears.
Ordinary lubricant eye drops simply provide moisture which can evaporate quickly from the surface of the eye. While Soothe®XP also provides moisture, it contains Restoryl®, the advanced lipid restorative which provides a barrier to tear loss for relief that lasts up to 8 hours. Expect temporarily blurred vision upon application, as Soothe®XP eye drops seal in moisture.

Drug Facts:

Active Ingredients	*Purpose*
Light mineral oil (1.0%)	Emollient
Mineral oil (4.5%)	Emollient

Purpose: Emollient (Lubricant) Eye Drops for persistent dry eye

Inactive Ingredients
edetate disodium, octoxynol-40, poly-hexamethylene biguanide (preservative), polysorbate-80, purified water, sodium chloride, sodium hydroxide and/or hydrochloric acid (to adjust pH), sodium phosphate dibasic, sodium phosphate monobasic.

USES

■ temporary relief of burning and irritation due to dryness of the eye
■ temporary relief of discomfort due to minor irritations of the eye or to exposure to wind or sun
■ as a protectant to prevent further irritation or to relieve dryness of the eye

WARNINGS

For external use only.
Do not use
■ if solution changes color
When using this product
■ do not touch the tip of container to any surface
■ replace cap after using
Stop use and ask a doctor if
■ you experience eye pain, changes in vision, continued redness or irritation of the eye, or if condition worsens or persists for more than 72 hours
Keep out of reach of children. If swallowed, get medical help or contact a Poison Control Center right away.

DIRECTIONS

■ remove contact lenses before use
■ shake well before using
■ instill 1 or 2 drop(s) in the affected eye(s) as needed or as directed by your doctor
Other Information
■ temporarily blurred vision is typical upon application
■ drops appear as a milky white solution
■ store at 15°-30°C (59°-86°F)

> **TAMPER EVIDENT: DO NOT USE IF IMPRINTED "Protective Seal" WITH YELLOW (MORTAR & PESTAL IMAGE) IS NOT INTACT.**

HOW SUPPLIED

NDC # 24208-490-15
Sterile 0.5 FL OZ (15mL)
2.5 mL sample 24208-490-95
2.5 mL travel size 24208-490-04

Questions or Comments?
Toll Free Product Information or to report a serious side effect associated with use of this product call: 1-800-553-5340.
Bausch & Lomb and Soothe and Restoryl are registered trademarks of Bausch & Lomb Incorporated.
US Patent #5,578,586
© Bausch & Lomb Incorporated
Rochester, NY 14609
Manufactured by:
Bausch & Lomb Incorporated
Tampa, FL 33637
Made in USA
www.bausch.com
Shown in Product Identification Guide, page 402

Bayer HealthCare LLC
Consumer Care
36 COLUMBIA ROAD
P.O. BOX 1910
MORRISTOWN, NJ 07962-1910

Direct Inquiries to:
Consumer Relations
(800) 331-4536
www.BayerAspirin.com

BAYER® ASPIRIN   OTC
Comprehensive Prescribing Information

DESCRIPTION

Aspirin for Oral Administration
Regular Strength 325 mg and Low Strength 81 mg Tablets
Antiplatelet, Antiarthritic

Aspirin

$C_9H_8O_4$
Mol. Wt.: 180.16
C 60.00 %; H 4.48 %; O 35.52%

Aspirin is an odorless white, needle-like crystalline or powdery substance. When exposed to moisture, aspirin hydrolyzes into salicylic and acetic acids, and gives off a vinegary-odor. It is highly lipid soluble and slightly soluble in water.

CLINICAL PHARMACOLOGY

Mechanism of Action
Aspirin is a more potent inhibitor of both prostaglandin synthesis and platelet aggregation than other salicylic acid derivatives. The differences in activity between aspirin and salicylic acid are thought to be due to the acetyl group on the aspirin molecule. This acetyl group is responsible for the inactivation of cyclo-oxygenase via acetylation.

Pharmacokinetics
Absorption: In general, immediate release aspirin is well and completely absorbed from the gastrointestinal (GI) tract. Following absorption, aspirin is hydrolyzed to salicylic acid with peak plasma levels of salicylic acid occurring within 1-2 hours of dosing (see **Pharmacokinetics**—Metabolism). The rate of absorption from the GI tract is dependent

Continued on next page

Bayer Aspirin—Cont.

upon the dosage form, the presence or absence of food, gastric pH (the presence or absence of GI antacids or buffering agents), and other physiologic factors. Enteric coated aspirin products are erratically absorbed from the GI tract.

Distribution: Salicylic acid is widely distributed to all tissues and fluids in the body including the central nervous system (CNS), breast milk, and fetal tissues. The highest concentrations are found in the plasma, liver, renal cortex, heart, and lungs. The protein binding of salicylate is concentration-dependent, i.e., non-linear. At low concentrations (< 100 micrograms/milliliter (mcg/mL)), approximately 90 percent of plasma salicylate is bound to albumin while at higher concentrations (>400 mcg/mL), only about 75 percent is bound. The early signs of salicylic overdose (salicylism), including tinnitus (ringing in the ears), occur at plasma concentrations approximating 200 mcg/mL. Severe toxic effects are associated with levels >400 mcg/mL. (See **ADVERSE REACTIONS** and **OVERDOSAGE**.)

Metabolism: Aspirin is rapidly hydrolyzed in the plasma to salicylic acid such that plasma levels of aspirin are essentially undetectable 1–2 hours after dosing. Salicylic acid is primarily conjugated in the liver to form salicyluric acid, a phenolic glucuronide, an acyl glucuronide, and a number of minor metabolites. Salicylic acid has a plasma half-life of approximately 6 hours. Salicylate metabolism is saturable and total body clearance decreases at higher serum concentrations due to the limited ability of the liver to form both salicyluric acid and phenolic glucuronide. Following toxic doses (10–20 grams (g)), the plasma half-life may be increased to over 20 hours.

Elimination: The elimination of salicylic acid follows zero order pharmacokinetics; (i.e., the rate of drug elimination is constant in relation to plasma concentration). Renal excretion of unchanged drug depends upon urine pH. As urinary pH rises above 6.5, the renal clearance of free salicylate increases from < 5 percent to >80 percent. Alkalinization of the urine is a key concept in the management of salicylate overdose. (See **OVERDOSAGE**.) Following therapeutic doses, approximately 10 percent is found excreted in the urine as salicylic acid, 75 percent as salicyluric acid, 10 percent phenolic and 5 percent acyl glucuronides of salicylic acid.

Pharmacodynamics

Aspirin affects platelet aggregation by irreversibly inhibiting prostaglandin cyclo-oxygenase. This effect lasts for the life of the platelet and prevents the formation of the platelet aggregating factor thromboxane A2. Non-acetylated salicylates do not inhibit this enzyme and have no effect on platelet aggregation. At somewhat higher doses, aspirin reversibly inhibits the formation of prostaglandin I2 (prostacyclin), which is an arterial vasodilator and inhibits platelet aggregation. At higher doses aspirin is an effective anti-inflammatory agent, partially due to inhibition of inflammatory mediators via cyclo-oxygenase inhibition in peripheral tissues. In vitro studies suggest that other mediators of inflammation may also be suppressed by aspirin administration, although the precise mechanism of action has not been elucidated. It is this nonspecific suppression of cyclo-oxygenase activity in peripheral tissues following large doses that leads to its primary side effect of gastric irritation. (See **ADVERSE REACTIONS**.)

CLINICAL STUDIES

Ischemic Stroke and Transient Ischemic Attack (TIA): In clinical trials of subjects with TIA's due to fibrin platelet emboli or ischemic stroke, aspirin has been shown to significantly reduce the risk of the combined endpoint of stroke or death and the combined endpoint of TIA, stroke, or death by about 13–18 percent.

Suspected Acute Myocardial Infarction (MI): In a large, multi-center study of aspirin, streptokinase, and the combination of aspirin and streptokinase in 17,187 patients with suspected acute MI, aspirin treatment produced a 23-percent reduction in the risk of vascular mortality. Aspirin was also shown to have an additional benefit in patients given a thrombolytic agent.

Prevention of Recurrent MI and Unstable Angina Pectoris: These indications are supported by the results of six large, randomized, multi-center, placebo-controlled trials of pre-dominantly male post-MI subjects and one randomized placebo-controlled study of men with unstable angina pectoris. Aspirin therapy in MI subjects was associated with a significant reduction (about 20 percent) in the risk of the combined endpoint of subsequent death and/or nonfatal reinfarction in these patients. In aspirin-treated unstable angina patients the event rate was reduced to 5 percent from the 10 percent rate in the placebo group.

Chronic Stable Angina Pectoris: In a randomized, multi-center, double-blind trial designed to assess the role of aspirin for prevention of MI in patients with chronic stable angina pectoris, aspirin significantly reduced the primary combined endpoint of nonfatal MI, fatal MI, and sudden death by 34 percent. The secondary endpoint for vascular events (first occurrence of MI, stroke, or vascular death) was also significantly reduced (32 percent).

Revascularization Procedures: Most patients who undergo coronary artery revascularization procedures have already had symptomatic coronary artery disease for which aspirin is indicated. Similarly, patients with lesions of the carotid bifurcation sufficient to require carotid endarterectomy are likely to have had a precedent event. Aspirin is recommended for patients who undergo revascularization procedures if there is a preexisting condition for which aspirin is already indicated.

Rheumatologic Diseases: In clinical studies in patients with rheumatoid arthritis, juvenile rheumatoid arthritis, ankylosing spondylitis and osteoarthritis, aspirin has been shown to be effective in controlling various indices of clinical disease activity.

ANIMAL TOXICOLOGY

The acute oral 50 percent lethal dose in rats is about 1.5 g/kilogram (kg) and in mice 1.1 g/kg. Renal papillary necrosis and decreased urinary concentrating ability occur in rodents chronically administered high doses. Dose-dependent gastric mucosal injury occurs in rats and humans. Mammals may develop aspirin toxicosis associated with GI symptoms, circulatory effects, and central nervous system depression. (See **OVERDOSAGE**.)

INDICATIONS AND USAGE

Vascular Indications (Ischemic Stoke, TIA, Acute MI, Prevention of Recurrent MI, Unstable Angina Pectoris, Chronic Stable Angina Pectoris): Aspirin is indicated to: (1) Reduce the combined risk of death and nonfatal stroke in patients who have had ischemic stroke or transient ischemia of the brain due to fibrin platelet emboli, (2) reduce the risk of vascular mortality in patients with a suspected acute MI, (3) reduce the combined risk of death and nonfatal MI in patients with a previous MI or unstable angina pectoris, (4) reduce the combined risk of MI and sudden death in patients with chronic stable angina pectoris.

Revascularization Procedures (Coronary Artery Bypass Graft (CABG), Percutaneous Transluminal Coronary Angioplasty (PTCA), and Carotid Endarterectomy): Aspirin is indicated in patients who have undergone revascularization procedures (i.e., CABG, PTCA, or carotid endarterectomy) when there is a preexisting condition for which aspirin is already indicated.

Rheumatologic Disease Indications (Rheumatoid Arthritis, Juvenile Rheumatoid Arthritis, Spondyloarthropathies, Osteoarthritis, and the Arthritis and Pleurisy of Systemic Lupus Erythematosus (SLE)): Aspirin is indicated for the relief of the signs and symptoms of rheumatoid arthritis, juvenile rheumatoid arthritis, osteoarthritis, spondyloarthropathies, and arthritis and pleurisy associated with SLE.

CONTRAINDICATIONS

Allergy: Aspirin is contraindicated in patients with known allergy to nonsteroidal anti-inflammatory drug products and in patients with the syndrome of asthma, rhinitis, and nasal polyps. Aspirin may cause severe urticaria, angioedema, or bronchospasm (asthma).

Reye's Syndrome: Aspirin should not be used in children or teenagers for viral infections, with or without fever, because of the risk of Reye's syndrome with concomitant use of aspirin in certain viral illnesses.

WARNINGS

Alcohol Warning: Patients who consume three or more alcoholic drinks every day should be counseled about the

bleeding risks involved with chronic, heavy alcohol use while taking aspirin.

Coagulation Abnormalities: Even low doses of aspirin can inhibit platelet function leading to an increase in bleeding time. This can adversely affect patients with inherited (hemophilia) or acquired (liver disease or vitamin K deficiency) bleeding disorders.

GI Side Effects: GI side effects include stomach pain, heartburn, nausea, vomiting, and gross GI bleeding. Although minor upper GI symptoms, such as dyspepsia, are common and can occur anytime during therapy, physicians should remain alert for signs of ulceration and bleeding, even in the absence of previous GI symptoms. Physicians should inform patients about the signs and symptoms of GI side effects and what steps to take if they occur.

Peptic Ulcer Disease: Patients with a history of active peptic ulcer disease should avoid using aspirin, which can cause gastric mucosal irritation and bleeding.

PRECAUTIONS
General
Renal Failure: Avoid aspirin in patients with severe renal failure (glomerular filtration rate less than 10 mL/minute).
Hepatic Insufficiency: Avoid aspirin in patients with severe hepatic insufficiency.
Sodium Restricted Diets: Patients with sodium-retaining states, such as congestive heart failure or renal failure, should avoid sodium-containing buffered aspirin preparations because of their high sodium content.

Laboratory Tests
Aspirin has been associated with elevated hepatic enzymes, blood urea nitrogen and serum creatinine, hyperkalemia, proteinuria, and prolonged bleeding time.

Drug Interactions
Angiotensin Converting Enzyme (ACE) Inhibitors: The hyponatremic and hypotensive effects of ACE inhibitors may be diminished by the concomitant administration of aspirin due to its indirect effect on the renin-angiotensin conversion pathway.

Acetazolamide: Concurrent use of aspirin and acetazolamide can lead to high serum concentrations of acetazolamide (and toxicity) due to competition at the renal tubule for secretion.

Anticoagulant Therapy (Heparin and Warfarin): Patients on anticoagulation therapy are at increased risk for bleeding because of drug-drug interactions and the effect on platelets. Aspirin can displace warfarin from protein binding sites, leading to prolongation of both the prothrombin time and the bleeding time. Aspirin can increase the anticoagulant activity of heparin, increasing bleeding risk.

Anticonvulsants: Salicylate can displace protein-bound phenytoin and valproic acid, leading to a decrease in the total concentration of phenytoin and an increase in serum valproic acid levels.

Beta Blockers: The hypotensive effects of beta blockers may be diminished by the concomitant administration of aspirin due to inhibition of renal prostaglandins, leading to decreased renal blood flow, and salt and fluid retention.

Diuretics: The effectiveness of diuretics in patients with underlying renal or cardiovascular disease may be diminished by the concomitant administration of aspirin due to inhibition of renal prostaglandins, leading to decreased renal blood flow, and salt and fluid retention.

Methotrexate: Salicylate can inhibit renal clearance of methotrexate, leading to bone marrow toxicity, especially in the elderly or renal impaired.

Nonsteroidal Anti-inflammatory Drugs (NSAID's): The concurrent use of aspirin with other NSAID's should be avoided because this may increase bleeding or lead to decreased renal function.

Oral Hypoglycemics: Moderate doses of aspirin may increase the effectiveness of oral hypoglycemic drugs, leading to hypoglycemia.

Uricosuric   Agents   (Probenecid   and Sulfinpyrazone): Salicylates antagonize the uricosuric action of uricosuric agents.

Carcinogenesis, Mutagenesis, Impairment of Fertility
Administration of aspirin for 68 weeks at 0.5 percent in the feed of rats was not carcinogenic. In the Ames Salmonella assay, aspirin was not mutagenic; however, aspirin did induce chromosome aberrations in cultured human fibroblasts. Aspirin inhibits ovulation in rats. (See **Pregnancy**).

Pregnancy
Pregnant women should only take aspirin if clearly needed. Because of the known effects of NSAIDs on the fetal cardiovascular system (closure of the ductus arteriosus), use during the third trimester of pregnancy should be avoided. Salicylate products have also been associated with alterations in maternal and neonatal hemostasis mechanisms, decreased birth weight, and with perinatal mortality.

Labor and Delivery
Aspirin should be avoided 1 week prior to and during labor and delivery because it can result in excessive blood loss at delivery. Prolonged gestation and prolonged labor due to prostaglandin inhibition have been reported.

Nursing Mothers
Nursing mothers should avoid using aspirin because salicylate is excreted in breast milk. Use of high doses may lead to rashes, platelet abnormalities, and bleeding in nursing infants.

Pediatric Use
Pediatric dosing recommendations for juvenile rheumatoid arthritis are based on well-controlled clinical studies. An initial dose of 90–130 mg/kg/day in divided doses, with an increase as needed for anti-inflammatory efficacy (target plasma salicylate levels of 150–300 mcg/mL) are effective. At high doses (i.e., plasma levels of greater than 200 mcg/mL), the incidence of toxicity increases.

ADVERSE REACTIONS
Many adverse reactions due to aspirin ingestion are dose-related. The following is a list of adverse reactions that have been reported in the literature. (See **WARNINGS**.)

Body as a Whole: Fever, hypothermia, thirst.
Cardiovascular: Dysrhythmias, hypotension, tachycardia.
Central Nervous System: Agitation, cerebral edema, coma, confusion, dizziness, headache, subdural or intracranial hemorrhage, lethargy, seizures.
Fluid and Electrolyte: Dehydration, hyperkalemia, metabolic acidosis, respiratory alkalosis.
Gastrointestinal: Dyspepsia, GI bleeding, ulceration and perforation, nausea, vomiting, transient elevations of hepatic enzymes, hepatitis, Reye's syndrome, pancreatitis.
Hematologic: Prolongation of the prothrombin time, disseminated intravascular coagulation, coagulopathy, thrombocytopenia.
Hypersensitivity: Acute   anaphylaxis,   angioedema, asthma, bronchospasm, laryngeal edema, urticaria.
Musculoskeletal: Rhabdomyolysis.
Metabolism: Hypoglycemia (in children), hyperglycemia.
Reproductive: Prolonged pregnancy and labor, stillbirths, lower birth weight infants, antepartum and postpartum bleeding.
Respiratory: Hyperpnea, pulmonary edema, tachypnea.
Special Senses: Hearing loss, tinnitus. Patients with high frequency hearing loss may have difficulty perceiving tinnitus. In these patients, tinnitus cannot be used as a clinical indicator of salicylism.
Urogenital: Interstitial nephritis, papillary necrosis, proteinuria, renal insufficiency and failure.

DRUG ABUSE AND DEPENDENCE
Aspirin is nonnarcotic. There is no known potential for addiction associated with the use of aspirin.

OVERDOSAGE
Salicylate toxicity may result from acute ingestion (overdose) or chronic intoxication. The early signs of salicylic overdose (salicylism), including tinnitus (ringing in the ears), occur at plasma concentrations approaching 200 mcg/mL. Plasma concentrations of aspirin above 300 mcg/mL are clearly toxic. Severe toxic effects are associated with levels above 400 mcg/mL. (See **CLINICAL PHARMACOLOGY**). A single lethal dose of aspirin in adults is not known with certainty but death may be expected at 30 g. For real or suspected overdose, a Poison Control Center should be contacted immediately. Careful medical management is essential.

Signs and Symptoms: In acute overdose, severe acid-base and electrolyte disturbances may occur and are complicated by hyperthermia and dehydration. Respiratory alkalosis occurs early while hyperventilation is present, but is quickly followed by metabolic acidosis.

Continued on next page

Bayer Aspirin—Cont.

Treatment: Treatment consists primarily of supporting vital functions, increasing salicylate elimination, and correcting the acid-base disturbance. Gastric emptying and/or lavage is recommended as soon as possible after ingestion, even if the patient has vomited spontaneously. After lavage and/or emesis, administration of activated charcoal, as a slurry, is beneficial, if less than 3 hours have passed since ingestion. Charcoal adsorption should not be employed prior to emesis and lavage.

Severity of aspirin intoxication is determined by measuring the blood salicylate level. Acid-base status should be closely followed with serial blood gas and serum pH measurements. Fluid and electrolyte balance should also be maintained.

In severe cases, hyperthermia and hypovolemia are the major immediate threats to life. Children should be sponged with tepid water. Replacement fluid should be administered intravenously and augmented with correction of acidosis. Plasma electrolytes and pH should be monitored to promote alkaline diuresis of salicylate if renal function is normal. Infusion of glucose may be required to control hypoglycemia. Hemodialysis and peritoneal dialysis can be performed to reduce the body drug content. In patients with renal insufficiency or in cases of life-threatening intoxication, dialysis is usually required. Exchange transfusion may be indicated in infants and young children.

DOSAGE AND ADMINISTRATION

Each dose of aspirin should be taken with a full glass of water unless patient is fluid restricted. Anti-inflammatory and analgesic dosages should be individualized. When aspirin is used in high doses, the development of tinnitus may be used as a clinical sign of elevated plasma salicylate levels except in patients with high frequency hearing loss.

Ischemic Stroke and TIA:
50–325 mg once a day. Continue therapy indefinitely.

Suspected Acute MI:
The initial dose of 160–162.5 mg is administered as soon as an MI is suspected. The maintenance dose of 160–162.5 mg a day is continued for 30 days post-infarction. After 30 days, consider further therapy based on dosage and administration for prevention of recurrent MI.

Prevention of Recurrent MI:
75–325 mg once a day. Continue therapy indefinitely.

Unstable Angina Pectoris:
75–325 mg once a day. Continue therapy indefinitely.

Chronic Stable Angina Pectoris:
75–325 mg once a day. Continue therapy indefinitely.

CABG:
325 mg daily starting 6 hours post-procedure. Continue therapy for one year post-procedure.

PTCA:
The initial dose of 325 mg should be given 2 hours presurgery. Maintenance dose is 160–325 mg daily. Continue therapy indefinitely.

Carotid Endarterectomy:
Doses of 80 mg once daily to 650 mg twice daily, started pre-surgery, are recommended. Continue therapy indefinitely.

Rheumatoid Arthritis:
The initial dose is 3 g a day in divided doses. Increase as needed for anti-inflammatory efficacy with target plasma salicylate levels of 150–300 mcg/mL. At high doses (i.e., plasma levels of greater than 200 mcg/mL), the incidence of toxicity increases.

Juvenile Rheumatoid Arthritis:
Initial dose is 90–130 mg/kg/day in divided doses. Increase as needed for anti-inflammatory efficacy with target plasma salicylate levels of 150–300 mcg/mL. At high doses (i.e., plasma levels of greater than 200 mcg/mL), the incidence of toxicity increases.

Spondyloarthropathies:
Up to 4 g per day in divided doses.

Osteoarthritis:
Up to 3 g per day in divided doses.

Arthritis and Pleurisy of SLE:
The initial dose is 3 g a day in divided doses. Increase as needed for anti-inflammatory efficacy with target plasma

salicylate levels of 150–300 mcg/mL. At high doses (i.e., plasma levels of greater than 200 mcg/mL), the incidence of toxicity increases.

Storage Conditions
Store at room temperature.
Bayer HealthCare LLC
Consumer Care
36 Columbia Road
PO Box 1910
Morristown, NJ 07962-1910
Shown in Product Identification Guide, page 402 & 403

Fleet Laboratories
Division of C. B. Fleet Company, Incorporated
LYNCHBURG, VA 24502

Direct Inquiries to:
Sherrie McNamara, RN, MSN, MBA
Director of Medical Affairs and Product Safety
1-866-255-6960

FLEET® GLYCERIN LAXATIVES: OTC
FLEET® SUPPOSITORIES, FLEET® BABYLAX® AND FLEET® PEDIA-LAX® SUPPOSITORIES AND FLEET® LIQUID GLYCERIN SUPPOSITORIES
A HYPEROSMOTIC LAXATIVE

COMPOSITION

FLEET® Pedia-Lax® and Babylax® Liquid Glycerin Suppositories—Each rectal applicator delivers 2.8 g of glycerin.
FLEET® Liquid Glycerin Suppositories for Adults and Children 6 years of age and over—Each rectal applicator delivers 5.4 g of glycerin.
FLEET® Maximum-Strength Glycerin Suppositories for Adults—Each suppository contains 3 g of glycerin.
FLEET® Glycerin Suppositories for Adults—Each suppository contains 2 g of glycerin.
FLEET® Pedia-Lax® Glycerin Suppositories for Children 2 years to under 6—Each suppository contains 1 g of glycerin.

ACTIONS AND USES

Glycerin is a hyperosmotic laxative, given rectally, which usually produces a bowel movement within 15 minutes to 1 hour. Hyperosmotic laxatives encourage bowel movements by drawing water into the bowel from surrounding tissues. This produces a softer stool mass and increased bowel action. These products are used for fast, predictable relief of occasional constipation. However, rectal irritation may occur with its use.

INFORMATION FOR PATIENT

WARNINGS

This product may cause rectal discomfort or a burning sensation.

GENERAL LAXATIVE WARNINGS

Do not use a laxative product when nausea, vomiting or abdominal pain is present unless directed by a physician. If you notice a sudden change in bowel habits that persists over a period of 2 weeks, consult a physician before using a laxative. Rectal bleeding or failure to have a bowel movement after 1 hour of using this laxative product may indicate a serious condition. Discontinue use and consult a physician. Laxative products should not be used longer than 1 week unless directed by a physician.

Keep this and all drugs out of the reach of children. In case of accidental overdose or ingestion, seek professional assistance or contact a Poison Control Center right away.

DOSAGE AND ADMINISTRATION

FLEET® Pedia-Lax® and Babylax® Liquid Glycerin Suppositories—Children 2 to under 6 years: 1 suppository or as directed by a physician. Children under 2 years: Consult a physician.

Preferred position: Place child on left side with knees bent and arms resting comfortably, or have child kneel, then lower head and chest forward until left side of face is resting on surface with left arm folded comfortably.

CAUTION: REMOVE ORANGE PROTECTIVE SHIELD FROM TIP BEFORE INSERTING. Hold the unit upright, grasping the bulb with fingers. Grasp the orange protective shield with the other hand; pull gently to remove. With steady pressure, gently insert the tip into the rectum with a slight side-to-side movement, with the tip pointing towards navel. **DISCONTINUE USE IF RESISTANCE IS ENCOUNTERED. FORCING THE TIP CAN RESULT IN INJURY.** Insertion may be easier if child receiving the liquid suppository bears down as if having a bowel movement. This helps relax the muscles around the anus. Squeeze the bulb until nearly all liquid has been expelled. While continuing to squeeze the bulb, remove the tip from the rectum and discard the unit. It is not necessary to empty the unit completely. The unit contains more than the amount of liquid needed for effective use. A small amount of liquid will remain in the unit after squeezing.

FLEET® Liquid Glycerin Suppositories for Adults and Children 6 years of age and older: One suppository or as directed by a physician. Children 2 years to under 6 use Fleet® Pedia-Lax® or Fleet® Babylax® Liquid Glycerin Suppositories. Children under 2 years, consult a physician.

Preferred position: Lie on left side with right knee bent and arms resting comfortably, or kneel, then lower head and chest forward until left side of face is resting on surface with left arm folded comfortably.

CAUTION: REMOVE ORANGE PROTECTIVE SHIELD BEFORE INSERTING. Hold the unit upright, grasping the bulb with fingers. Grasp the orange protective shield with the other hand; pull gently to remove. With steady pressure, insert the tip into the rectum with a slight side-to-side movement, with the tip pointing toward the navel. **DISCONTINUE USE IF RESISTANCE IS ENCOUNTERED. FORCING THE TIP CAN RESULT IN INJURY.** Insertion may be easier if person receiving the liquid suppository bears down as if having a bowel movement. This helps relax the muscles around the anus. Squeeze the bulb until nearly all liquid has been expelled. While continuing to squeeze the bulb, remove the tip from the rectum and discard the unit. It is not necessary to empty the unit completely. The unit contains more than the amount of liquid needed for use. A small amount of liquid will remain in the unit after squeezing.

FLEET® Maximum-Strength Glycerin Suppositories—Adults and Children 6 years of age and older: One suppository.

Remove the foil wrapper and insert one suppository fully into the rectum. The suppository need not melt completely to produce laxative action. Keep away from excessive heat.

FLEET® Glycerin Suppositories—Adults and Children 6 years of age and older: One suppository or as directed by a doctor.

If foil-wrapped, remove the foil wrapper. Insert one suppository fully into the rectum. The suppository need not melt completely to produce laxative action. Store the container tightly closed and keep away from excessive heat.

FLEET® Pedia-Lax® Glycerin Suppositories—Children 2 to under 6 years: One suppository or as directed by a doctor. Children under 2 years: Consult a physician.

Insert suppository fully into the rectum. The suppository need not melt completely to produce laxative action. Store the container tightly closed and keep away from excessive heat.

HOW SUPPLIED

FLEET® Pedia-Lax® and Babylax® Liquid Glycerin Suppositories for children 2 to under 6 years—Each box contains 6 child rectal applicators (4 mL each).

FLEET® Liquid Glycerin Suppositories for Adults and Children 6 years of age and over—Each box contains 4 adult rectal applicators (7.5 mL each).

FLEET® Maximum-Strength Glycerin Suppositories—Each box contains 18 individually foil-wrapped adult suppositories.

FLEET® Glycerin Suppositories—Available in jars of 12, 24, 50 and 100 adult suppositories as well as a box containing 12 individually foil-wrapped adult suppositories.

FLEET® Pedia-Lax® Glycerin Suppositories—Available in jars of 12.

IS THIS PRODUCT OTC? Yes.

QUESTIONS? Call 1-866-255-6960 or visit www.fleetlabs.com

FLEET® BISACODYL LAXATIVES: OTC ENEMA, SUPPOSITORIES, AND TABLETS
A STIMULANT LAXATIVE

COMPOSITION

Latex-free FLEET® Bisacodyl Enema - 10 mg bisacodyl enema solution in a 37-mL ready-to-use squeeze bottle with a 2 inch, pre-lubricated Comfortip®. It is disposable after a single use.

FLEET® Stimulant Laxative Tablets - Enteric-coated 5 mg bisacodyl each tablet.

FLEET® Laxative Suppositories - 10 mg bisacodyl each suppository.

ACTION AND USES

Bisacodyl is a stimulant laxative given either orally or rectally, acting directly on the colonic mucosa where it stimulates sensory nerve endings to produce parasympathetic reflexes resulting in increased peristaltic contractions of the colon. The contact action of the drug is restricted to the colon, and motility in the small intestine is not appreciably influenced. FLEET® Stimulant Laxative Tablets usually work within 6–12 hours. FLEET® Bisacodyl Suppositories produce a bowel movement within 15 minutes to 1 hour, and the **latex-free** FLEET® Bisacodyl Enema produces a bowel movement within 5–20 minutes. Bisacodyl is useful as a laxative for relief of occasional constipation and in bowel cleansing in preparation for x-ray or endoscopic examination. Bisacodyl may be used as a laxative in postoperative, antepartum, or postpartum care or in preparation for delivery under guidance of a healthcare professional.

Store at temperatures not above 86°F (30°C)

WARNING Do not administer Fleet® Bisacodyl Enema to children under 12 years of age.

GENERAL LAXATIVE WARNINGS
INFORMATION FOR PATIENT

Do not use a laxative product when nausea, vomiting or abdominal pain is present unless directed by a physician. If you notice a sudden change in bowel habits that persists over a period of 2 weeks, consult a physician before using a laxative. Rectal bleeding or failure to have a bowel movement after use of a laxative may indicate a serious condition. Discontinue use and consult a physician. Laxative products should not be used longer than 1 week unless directed by a physician. As with any drug, if you are pregnant or nursing a baby, seek the advice of a healthcare professional before using this product. All bisacodyl products may cause abdominal discomfort, faintness and mild cramps. Rectal products may also cause rectal burning.

Keep this and all drugs out of the reach of children. In case of accidental overdose or ingestion, seek professional assistance or contact a Poison Control Center right away.

DOSAGE AND ADMINISTRATION
Enema
SHAKE BEFORE USING.
Dosage:
Adults and children 12 years of age and over: Use one 1.25 fl. oz. bottle (30-mL delivered dose) as a single daily dose.

Children under 12 years of age: DO NOT USE.

Preferred position: Lie on left side with right knee bent and arms resting comfortably, or kneel, then lower head and chest forward until left side of face is resting on surface with left arm folded comfortably. Fleet® Bisacodyl Enema should be used at room temperature.

REMOVE ORANGE PROTECTIVE SHIELD FROM TIP BEFORE ADMINISTERING. With steady pressure, gently insert the tip into the rectum with a slight side-to-side movement,

Continued on next page

Fleet Bisacodyl—Cont.

with the tip pointing towards naval. **DISCONTINUE USE IF RESISTANCE IS ENCOUNTERED, FORCING THE TIP CAN RESULT IN INJURY.** Insertion may be easier if person receiving the enema bears down as if having a bowel movement. This helps relax the muscles around the anus. The diaphragm at the base of the tube prevents reflux and assures controlled flow of the enema solution. It is not necessary to empty the unit completely. The unit contains more than the amount of liquid needed for effective use. A small amount of liquid will remain in the unit after squeezing.
IMPORTANT: FLEET® Bisacodyl Enema IS NOT INTENDED FOR ORAL CONSUMPTION in any dosage size.

Tablets
Adults and children 12 years of age and over: Take 1 to 3 tablets (usually 2) in a single dose once daily.
Children 6 to under 12 years of age: Take 1 tablet once daily.
Expect results in 6–12 hours if taken at bedtime or within 6 hours if taken before breakfast. Swallow tablets whole. Do not chew or crush tablets. Do not administer tablets within 1 hour after taking an antacid, milk, or milk products.
Children under 6 years of age: Consult a physician.

Suppositories
Adults and children 12 years of age and over: Use 1 suppository once daily. Remove foil wrapper. Lie on your side and, with pointed end first, insert the suppository towards the navel and well up into the rectum. Make sure the suppository touches the bowel wall.
Children 6 to under 12 years of age: One-half of one 10 mg. suppository once daily.
Children under 6 years of age: Consult a physician.

PROFESSIONAL ADMINISTRATION
FLEET® Bisacodyl Enema should not be used in children under 12 years of age. Careful consideration of the use of enemas in children in general is recommended. Proper and safe use of FLEET® enemas also requires that the products be administered according to the directions. Healthcare professionals should remember when administering the product to gently insert the enema into the rectum with the tip pointing toward the navel. Insertion may be made easier by having the patient bear down as if having a bowel movement. Care during insertion is necessary due to lack of sensory innervation of the rectum and due to the possibility of bowel perforation. Once inserted, squeeze the bottle until nearly all the liquid is expelled. If resistance is encountered on insertion of the nozzle or in administering the solution, the procedure should be discontinued. **Forcing the enema can result in perforation and/or abrasion of the rectum.**

HOW SUPPLIED
Enema
FLEET® Bisacodyl Enema is supplied in a 1.25 fl. oz. (37-mL) ready-to-use squeeze bottle.
Tablets
FLEET® Stimulant Laxative Tablets are supplied in cartons of 25 tablets (5 mg bisacodyl in each tablet) wrapped in a foil seal.
Suppositories
FLEET® Bisacodyl Suppositories are supplied in cartons of 4 individually foil-wrapped suppositories (10 mg bisacodyl in each suppository).
IS THIS PRODUCT OTC? Yes.
QUESTIONS? Call 1-866-255-6960 or visit www.fleetlabs.com

FLEET® ENEMA, A SALINE LAXATIVE   OTC
FLEET® ENEMA EXTRA®, A SALINE LAXATIVE
FLEET® PEDIA-LAX® ENEMA, A SALINE LAXATIVE, FLEET® ENEMA FOR CHILDREN, A SALINE LAXATIVE

FLEET® enemas are designed for quick, convenient administration by nurse, patient or parent according to instructions. Each is disposable after a single use.

COMPOSITION
FLEET® ENEMA: Each **latex-free** FLEET® Enema unit, with a 2 inch, pre-lubricated Comfortip®, contains 4.5 fl. oz. (133 mL) of enema solution in a ready-to-use squeeze bottle.

Each enema unit delivers a dose of 118 mL, which contains 19 g monobasic sodium phosphate monohydrate and 7 g dibasic sodium phosphate heptahydrate. Each Fleet® Enema 118 mL delivered dose contains 4.4 grams sodium.
FLEET® ENEMA EXTRA®: Each **latex-free** FLEET® Enema EXTRA® unit, with a 2 inch, pre-lubricated Comfortip®, contains 7.8 fl. oz. (230 mL) of enema solution in a ready-to-use squeeze bottle. Each enema unit delivers a dose of 197 mL, which contains 19 g monobasic sodium phosphate monohydrate and 7 g dibasic sodium phosphate heptahydrate. Each Fleet® Enema EXTRA® 197 mL delivered dose contains 4.4 grams sodium.
Fleet® Pedia-Lax® Enema and FLEET® ENEMA FOR CHILDREN: Each **latex-free** Fleet® Pedia-Lax® Enema and FLEET® Enema for Children unit, with a 2 inch, pre-lubricated Comfortip®, contains 2.25 fl. oz. (66 mL) of enema solution in a ready-to-use squeeze bottle. Each enema unit delivers a dose of 59 mL, which contains 9.5 g monobasic sodium phosphate monohydrate and 3.5 g dibasic sodium phosphate heptahydrate. Each Fleet® Enema for Children and Fleet® Pedia-Lax® Enema 59 mL delivered dose contains 2.2 grams sodium.

ELEMENTAL AND ELECTROLYTIC CONTENT (Fleet® Enema, Fleet® Pedia-Lax® Enema and Fleet® Enema for Children)

mEq Phosphate (PO$_4$) per mL	4.15
mEq Sodium (Na) per mL	1.61
mg Sodium (Na) per mL	37
mmole Phosphorus (P) per mL	1.38

ELEMENTAL AND ELECTROLYTIC CONTENT (Fleet® Enema EXTRA®)

mEq Phosphate (PO$_4$) per mL	2.484
mEq Sodium (Na) per mL	0.961
mg Sodium (Na) per mL	22.1
mmole Phosphorus (P) per mL	0.828

ACTION AND USES
FLEET® Enema, FLEET® Enema EXTRA® Fleet® Pedia-Lax® Enema and FLEET® Enema for Children are useful as laxatives in the relief of occasional constipation and as part of a bowel cleansing regimen in preparing the colon for surgery, x-ray or endoscopic examination.
When used as directed, FLEET® Enema, FLEET® Enema EXTRA®, Fleet® Pedia-Lax® Enema and FLEET® Enema for Children provide thorough yet safe cleansing action and induce complete emptying of the left colon, usually within 1 to 5 minutes, without pain or spasm.

INFORMATION FOR PATIENT
WARNINGS
Using more than one enema in 24 hours can be harmful.
AFTER THE ENEMA SOLUTION IS ADMINISTERED, THE RETENTION TIME SHOULD NOT EXCEED 10 MINUTES. IF THE RETENTION TIME EXCEEDS 10 MINUTES OR THERE IS NO RETURN OF ENEMA SOLUTION, CONTACT A PHYSICIAN IMMEDIATELY, AS ELECTROLYTE DISTURBANCES AND CONSEQUENT SERIOUS SIDE EFFECTS COULD OCCUR.
DO NOT USE ANY FLEET® ENEMA IN CHILDREN UNDER 2 YEARS OF AGE.
DO NOT ADMINISTER THE 4.5 FL. OZ. ADULT SIZE OR THE 7.8 FL.OZ. EXTRA® SIZE TO CHILDREN UNDER 12 YEARS OF AGE.
DO NOT ADMINISTER A FULL 2.25 FL. OZ. CHILDREN'S SIZE TO CHILDREN UNDER 5 YEARS OF AGE. FOR CHILDREN 2 TO UNDER 5 YEARS, USE ONE-HALF BOTTLE OF 2.25 FL. OZ. CHILDREN'S SIZE. (SEE **DOSAGE AND ADMINISTRATION**).
IMPORTANT: FLEET® Enema (Adult size), FLEET® Enema EXTRA®, Fleet® Pedia-Lax® Enema and Fleet® Enema for Children ARE NOT INTENDED FOR ORAL CONSUMPTION in any dosage size.
When using any of these Fleet® enemas, patient may experience anal discomfort.

GENERAL LAXATIVE WARNINGS
Do not use laxative products when nausea, vomiting or abdominal pain is present unless directed by a physician. If you notice a sudden change in bowel habits that persists over a period of 2 weeks, consult a physician. Fleet® enemas should be administered according to the instructions for use and handling. Stop use if resistance is encountered as forced administration of the enema may cause injury. Stop using this product and consult a doctor if you have rectal bleeding

following the use of this product as this may indicate a serious condition. Failure to have bowel movement within 30 minutes of using this product may also indicate a serious condition. Discontinue use and consult a physician. Laxative products should not be used longer than 1 week unless directed by a physician. As with any drug, if you are pregnant or nursing a baby, seek the advice of a healthcare professional before using this product. As sodium phosphate may pass into the breast milk, it is advised that breast milk is expressed and discarded for at least 24 hours after receiving the Fleet® enema.

Keep this and all drugs out of the reach of children. In case of accidental overdose or ingestion, seek professional assistance or contact a Poison Control Center right away.

PROFESSIONAL USE INFORMATION
CONTRAINDICATIONS

Do not use in patients with
- Congestive heart failure
- Clinically significant impairment of renal function
- Known or suspected gastrointestinal obstruction
- Megacolon (congenital or acquired)
- Paralytic ileus
- Perforation
- Active inflammatory bowel disease
- Imperforate anus
- Dehydration
- Generally in all cases where absorption capacity is increased or elimination capacity is decreased
- Children under 2 years of age
- Hypersensitivity to active ingredients or to any of the excipients of the product

PRECAUTIONS

Use with caution in patients
- With impaired renal function
- With pre-existing electrolyte disturbances or who are taking diuretics or other medications which may affect electrolyte levels
- Who are taking medications known to prolong the QT interval
- Ascites
- With a colostomy
- In children 2-11 years of age
- 65 or older and under a doctor's care for any medical condition
- Who are pregnant or nursing a baby

Patients with conditions that may predispose to dehydration or those taking medications which may decrease glomerular filtration rate, such as diuretics, angiotensin converting enzyme inhibitors (ACE-Is), angiotensin receptor blockers (ARBs), or non-steroidal anti-inflammatory drugs (NSAIDs), should be assessed for hydration status prior to use and managed appropriately.

Fleet® Pedia-Lax® Enema and Fleet® Enema for Children should be used with caution in children of any age. Careful consideration of the use of enemas in children in general is recommended.

Careful consideration of the use of sodium phosphates enemas in the elderly with co-morbidities is also recommended. See PROFESSIONAL USE WARNINGS. In those cases where complications have been reported, elderly patients with co-morbidities are often involved.

Since FLEET® enemas contain sodium phosphates, in all patients there is a risk of elevated serum levels of sodium and phosphate and decreased levels of calcium and potassium, and consequently hypernatremia, hyperphosphatemia, hypocalcemia and hypokalemia may occur which could result in metabolic acidosis, tetany, renal failure, QT prolongation and/or, in more severe cases, multi-organ failure, cardiac arrhythmia/arrest and death. This is of particular concern in children with megacolon or any other condition where there is retention of enema solution, and in patients with co-morbidities, particularly gastrointestinal, renal and neurological disorders. If any patient develops vomiting and/or signs of dehydration, measure post-administration labs (phosphate, calcium, potassium, sodium, creatinine, GFR and BUN.)

SINCE FLEET® BRAND ENEMAS ARE AVAILABLE IN ADULT, ADULT EXTRA, AND CHILDREN'S SIZES, PRESCRIBE CAREFULLY.

DRUG INTERACTIONS

NO OTHER SODIUM PHOSPHATES PREPARATIONS INCLUDING SODIUM PHOSPHATES ORAL SOLUTION OR TABLETS SHOULD BE GIVEN CONCOMITANTLY. Electrolyte disturbances and hypovolemia from purgation may be exacerbated by inadequate oral fluid intake, nausea, vomiting, loss of appetite, or use of diuretics, angiotensin converting enzyme inhibitors (ACE-Is), angiotensin receptor blockers (ARBs), non-steroidal anti-inflammatory drugs (NSAIDs), and lithium or other medications that may affect electrolyte levels, and may result in metabolic acidosis, tetany, renal failure, QT prolongation and, in more severe cases, multi-organ failure, cardiac arrhythmia/arrest and death.

As hypernatremia is associated with lower lithium levels, concomitant use of Fleet® enemas and lithium therapy could lead to a fall in serum lithium levels with a lessening of effectiveness.

POSSIBLE SIDE EFFECTS

Hypersensitivity
Pruritis
Dehydration
Hyperphosphatemia
Hypocalcemia
Hypokalemia
Hypernatremia
Metabolic Acidosis
Nausea
Vomiting
Abdominal Pain
Abdominal Distension
Diarrhea
Gastrointestinal Pain
Chills
Blistering
Stinging
Anal Discomfort
Protalgia

HYDRATION

Additional liquids by mouth are recommended.
Encourage patients to drink large amounts of clear liquids to prevent dehydration. Inadequate fluid intake when using any effective purgative may lead to excessive fluid loss, possibly producing dehydration and hypovolemia.

OVERDOSAGE OR RETENTION

Overdosage (more than one enema in a 24 hour period), no return of enema solution, retention time greater than 10 minutes or failure to have a bowel movement within 30 minutes of enema use may lead to severe electrolyte disturbances, including hypernatremia, hyperphosphatemia, hypocalcemia, and hypokalemia, as well as dehydration and hypovolemia, with attendant signs and symptoms of these disturbances (such as metabolic acidosis, renal failure, and tetany), QT prolongation and/or, in more severe cases, multi-organ failure, cardiac arrhythmia/arrest and death. The patient who has taken an overdose or who has retained the product for more than 10 minutes should be monitored carefully. If any patient develops vomiting and/or signs of dehydration, measure post-procedure labs (phosphate, calcium, potassium, sodium, creatinine, GFR and BUN.) **Treatment of electrolyte imbalance may require immediate medical intervention with appropriate electrolyte and fluid replacement therapy.**

DOSAGE AND ADMINISTRATION

Dosage: FLEET® Enema (Adult size) and FLEET® Enema EXTRA®:
Do not use more unless directed by a doctor. See Warnings. Do not use if taking another sodium phosphates product.

adults and children 12 years and older	one bottle
children 2 to 11 years	use Fleet® Pedia-Lax® Enema or FLEET® Enema for Children (See below)
children under 2 years	**DO NOT USE**

Continued on next page

Fleet Enema—Cont.

REMOVE ORANGE PROTECTIVE SHIELD FROM TIP BEFORE INSERTING.
Preferred position: Lie on left side with knee slightly bent and the right leg drawn up, or in knee-chest position.
The diaphragm at base of tube prevents reflux and assures controlled flow of the enema solution. FLEET® Enema should be used at room temperature.

Dosage: Fleet® Pedia-Lax® Enema and FLEET® Enema for Children:
Do not use more unless directed by a doctor. See Warnings. Do not use if child is taking another sodium phosphates product.

children 5 to 11 years	one bottle or as directed by a doctor
children 2 to under 5 years	one-half bottle (see below) or as directed by a doctor
children under 2 years	**DO NOT USE**

One-half bottle preparation: Unscrew cap and remove 2 Tablespoons of liquid with a measuring spoon. Replace cap and follow DIRECTIONS on back of carton.
REMOVE ORANGE PROTECTIVE SHIELD FROM TIP BEFORE INSERTING.
Preferred position: Lie on left side with knee slightly bent and the right leg drawn up, or in knee-chest position.
The diaphragm at base of tube prevents reflux and assures controlled flow of the enema solution. Fleet® Pedia-Lax® Enema and FLEET® Enema for Children should be used at room temperature.

PROFESSIONAL DOSAGE AND ADMINISTRATION

Administration of more than one enema in 24 hours can be harmful. In those cases where complications have been reported, overdoses are often involved.
NO OTHER SODIUM PHOSPHATES PREPARATIONS INCLUDING SODIUM PHOSPHATES ORAL SOLUTION OR TABLETS SHOULD BE GIVEN CONCOMITANTLY.
FLEET® Enema (Adult size) and FLEET® Enema EXTRA® should not be used in children under 12 years of age. In those cases where complications have been reported, infants and young children are often involved. Fleet® Pedia-Lax® Enema and FLEET® Enema for Children should be used with caution in children of any age. Careful consideration of the use of enemas in children in general is recommended.
Careful consideration of the use of sodium phosphates enemas in the elderly with co-morbidities is also recommended. See PROFESSIONAL USE WARNINGS. In those cases where complications have been reported, elderly patients with co-morbidities are often involved.
See **DOSAGE AND ADMINISTRATION** for dosing detail. Proper and safe use of FLEET® Enemas also requires that the products be administered according to the Directions. Healthcare professionals should remember when administering the product to <u>gently</u> insert the enema into the rectum with the tip pointing toward the navel. Insertion may be made easier by having the patient bear down as if having a bowel movement. Care during insertion is necessary due to lack of sensory innervation of the rectum and due to possibility of bowel perforation. Once inserted, squeeze the bottle until nearly all the liquid is expelled. If resistance is encountered on insertion of the nozzle or in administering the solution, the procedure should be discontinued. **Forcing the enema can result in perforation and/or abrasion of the rectum.**
If an enema containing phosphate or sodium is not advised, consider using FLEET® Bisacodyl Enema.

HOW SUPPLIED

FLEET® Enema is supplied in a 4.5 fl. oz. (133-mL) ready-to-use squeeze bottle. Fleet® Enema EXTRA® is supplied in a 7.8 fl. oz. (230-mL) ready-to-use squeeze bottle. Fleet®

Pedia-Lax® Enema and Fleet® Enema for Children are supplied in a 2.25 fl. oz. (66 mL) ready-to-use squeeze bottle.
QUESTIONS?   Call   1-866-255-6960   or   visit www.fleetlabs.com

---

FLEET® MINERAL OIL ENEMA   OTC
A LUBRICANT LAXATIVE

COMPOSITION

Latex-free FLEET® Mineral Oil Enema unit, with a 2-inch, pre-lubricated Comfortip®, delivers 118 mL of mineral oil, 100%, in a ready-to-use squeeze bottle. FLEET® Mineral Oil Enema is sodium-free. The unit is disposable after a single use.

ACTION AND USES

FLEET® Mineral Oil Enema serves to soften and lubricate hard stools, easing their passage without irritating the mucosa. Results approximate a normal bowel movement in that only the rectum, sigmoid, and part or all of the descending colon are evacuated. FLEET® Mineral Oil Enema is indicated for relief of fecal impaction; is valuable in relief of occasional constipation when straining must be avoided (in hypertension, coronary occlusion, proctologic procedures, or postoperative care); is indicated for removal of barium sulfate residues from the colon after barium administration and is indicated for obtaining the laxative benefits of mineral oil while avoiding possible untoward effects of oral administration such as (1) interference with intestinal absorption of fat-soluble vitamins A, D, E and K and other nutrients, (2) danger of systemic absorption, or (3) possible risk of lipid pneumonia due to aspiration. It is generally effective in 2 to 15 minutes.

WARNINGS

DO NOT ADMINISTER TO CHILDREN UNDER 2 YEARS OF AGE.

GENERAL LAXATIVE WARNINGS
INFORMATION FOR PATIENT
Do not use laxative products when nausea, vomiting or abdominal pain is present unless directed by a physician. If you notice a sudden change in bowel habits that persists over a period of 2 weeks, consult a physician before using a laxative. Rectal bleeding or failure to have a bowel movement after use of a laxative may indicate a serious condition. Discontinue use and consult a physician. Laxative products should not be used longer than 1 week unless directed by a physician. As with any drug, if you are pregnant or nursing a baby, seek the advice of a healthcare professional before using this product.
Keep this and all drugs out of the reach of children. In case of accidental overdose or ingestion, seek professional assistance or contact a Poison Control Center right away.

DOSAGE AND ADMINISTRATION

Dosage: Adults and children 12 years of age and over—one 133-mL (4.5 fl. oz.) bottle (118-mL delivered dose) in a single daily dose. Children 2 to under 12 years of age—one-half bottle (59-mL delivered dose) in a single daily dose.
REMOVE ORANGE PROTECTIVE SHIELD FROM TIP BEFORE INSERTING.
Preferred position: Lie on left side with knee slightly bent and the right leg drawn up, or in knee-chest position.
The diaphragm at base of tube prevents reflux and assures controlled flow of the enema solution. The enema should be used at room temperature. For more thorough cleansing, follow with FLEET® Enema—**according to dosage instructions contained in PDR.**

PROFESSIONAL DOSAGE AND ADMINISTRATION

FLEET® Mineral Oil Enema should not be used in children under 2 years of age and should be used with caution in children of any age. In general, careful consideration of the use of enemas in children is recommended.
Proper and safe use of FLEET® Mineral Oil Enema also requires that the product be administered according to the Directions. Healthcare professionals should remember when administering the product to <u>gently</u> insert the enema into

the rectum with the tip pointing toward the navel. Insertion may be made easier by having the patient bear down as if having a bowel movement. Care during insertion is necessary due to lack of sensory innervation of the rectum and due to the possibility of bowel perforation. Once inserted, squeeze the bottle until nearly all the liquid is expelled. If resistance is encountered on insertion of the nozzle or in administering the solution, the procedure should be discontinued. **Forcing the enema can result in perforation and/or abrasion of the rectum.**

HOW SUPPLIED

FLEET® Mineral Oil Enema is supplied in 4.5 fl. oz. (133-mL) ready-to-use squeeze bottle.
IS THIS PRODUCT OTC? Yes.
QUESTIONS? Call 1-866-255-6960 or visit www.fleetlabs.com

FLEET® PEDIA-LAX® DOCUSATE SODIUM LIQUID STOOL SOFTENER　　OTC
Stool softener laxative

DRUG FACTS

Active ingredient (in each tablespoon – 15 mL)	Purpose
Docusate sodium 50 mg	Stool softener

USES
• to help prevent dry, hard stools
• to relieve occasional constipation

DESCRIPTION

Docusate sodium is a stool softener laxative, given orally, which usually produces a bowel movement within 12 to 72 hours. Stool softener laxatives penetrate and soften the stool, thereby promoting bowel movement.

INFORMATION FOR PATIENT
DRUG INTERACTION PRECAUTION: Do not give this product to child if child is presently taking mineral oil, unless directed by a doctor.

WARNINGS
Ask a doctor before using any laxative if your child has
• abdominal pain, nausea or vomiting
• a sudden change in bowel habits lasting more than 2 weeks
• already used a laxative for more than 1 week
Stop using this product and consult a doctor if your child has
• rectal bleeding
• no bowel movement within 72 hours of using this product
These symptoms may be signs of a serious condition.
Keep this and all drugs out of the reach of children. In case of overdose, get medical help or contact a Poison Control Center right away.

DIRECTIONS
Doses may be taken as a single daily dose or in divided doses.
Doses must be given in a 6-8 ounce glass of milk or juice, to prevent throat irritation.
Each tablespoon (15 mL) contains 13 mg sodium.

Dosing Chart

Age	Starting Dose	Maximum Dose per Day
Children 2 to 11 years	1–3 tablespoons	3 tablespoons
Children under 2	Ask a doctor	Ask a doctor

Inactive ingredients: citric acid, edetate disodium, FD&C Red #3, flavor, methylparaben, polyethylene glycol, povidone, propylene glycol, propylparaben, sodium citrate, sorbitol, sucralose, water, zanthan gum, xylitol.

HOW SUPPLIED
4 fl.oz. (118 mL) bottles with child-resistant cap, and sealed for your protection. Fruit punch flavor.
Is this product OTC?
Yes.
QUESTIONS? Call 1-866-255-6960 or visit www.Pedia-Lax.com

FLEET® PEDIA-LAX® MAGNESIUM HYDROXIDE CHEWABLE TABLETS　　OTC
Saline laxative

DRUG FACTS

Active ingredient (in each tablet):	Purpose
Magnesium hydroxide 400 mg	Saline laxative

USE
• to relieve occasional constipation

DESCRIPTION

Magnesium hydroxide is a saline laxative, given orally, which usually produces a bowel movement within 30 minutes to 6 hours. Saline laxatives increase water in the intestine thereby promoting bowel movement.

INFORMATION FOR PATIENT
WARNINGS
Ask a physician before using this product if child has a magnesium-restricted diet or kidney disease.
Ask a doctor before using any laxative if your child has
• abdominal pain, nausea or vomiting
• a sudden change in bowel habits lasting more than 2 weeks
• already used a laxative for more than 1 week
Stop using this product and consult a doctor if your child has
• rectal bleeding
• no bowel movement within 6 hours of taking this product
These symptoms may be signs of a serious condition.
Keep this and all drugs out of the reach of children. In case of overdose, get medical help or contact a Poison Control Center right away.

DIRECTIONS
Doses may be taken as a single daily dose or in divided doses. **Have child drink a full glass (8 fluid ounces) of liquid with each dose.**
Each tablet contains 170 mg magnesium.

Dosing Chart

Age	Starting Dose	Maximum Dose per Day
Children 6 to 11 years	3–6 tablets	6 tablets
Children 2 to 5 years	1–3 tablets	3 tablets
Children under 2	Ask a doctor	Ask a doctor

Inactive ingredients: colloidal silicon dioxide, FD&C Red #40 aluminum lake, flavor, magnesium stearate, maltodextrin, mannitol, sorbitol, stearic acid, sucralose

HOW SUPPLIED
30 Pedia-Lax Chewable Tablets per bottle with child-resistant cap, sealed for your protection. Watermelon flavor.
Is this product OTC?
Yes.

QUESTIONS?
Call 1-866-255-6960 or visit www.Pedia-Lax.com

Continued on next page

FLEET® PEDIA-LAX® SENNA QUICK DISSOLVE STRIPS
OTC

Stimulant laxative

DRUG FACTS

Active ingredient (in each strip)	Purpose
Standardized Sennosides 8.6 mg	Stimulant laxative

USE
• to relieve occasional constipation

DESCRIPTION
Senna is a stimulant laxative, given orally, which usually produces a bowel movement within 6 to 12 hours. Stimulant laxatives promote bowel movement by one or more direct actions on the intestine.

INFORMATION FOR PATIENT
WARNINGS
Ask a physician before using this product if child is taking non-steroidal anti-inflammatory drugs (NSAIDs).
Ask a doctor before using any laxative if your child has
• abdominal pain, nausea, or vomiting
• a sudden change in bowel habits lasting more than 2 weeks
• already used a laxative for more than 1 week
Stop using this product and consult a doctor if your child has
• rectal bleeding
• no bowel movement within 12 hours of taking this product
These symptoms may be signs of a serious condition.
Keep this and all drugs out of the reach of children. In case of overdose, get medical help or contact a Poison Control Center right away.

DIRECTIONS
Dosing Chart

Age	Starting Dose	Maximum Dose per Day
Children 6 to 11 years	2 strips	Do not exceed 4 strips in 24 hours
Children 2 to 5 years	1 strip	Do not exceed 2 strips in 24 hours
Children under 2	Ask a doctor	Ask a doctor

Place quick dissolve strip on child's tongue or have child place on the tongue. Allow strip to dissolve. Encourage child to drink plenty of liquids.
Inactive ingredients: butylated hydroxytoluene, FD&C Red #40, flavor, hydroxypropyl methylcellulose, malic acid, methylparaben, polydextrose, polyethylene oxide, simethicone, sodium bicarbonate, sucralose, white ink.

HOW SUPPLIED
12 individually-wrapped Pedia-Lax Quick Dissolve Strips per carton. Grape flavor.
Other Information: Color of strips may vary. Store at controlled room temperature 59°–86°F (15°–30°C).
Is this product OTC?
Yes.
QUESTIONS?
Call 1-866-255-6960 or
visit www.Pedia-Lax.com

FLEET® PREP KIT 3
OTC

Bowel Evacuant

COMPOSITION
FLEET® Prep Kit 3 contains:
1. FLEET® Phospho-soda® Oral Saline Laxative—1.5 fl. oz. (45 mL). Active Ingredients: Each Tablespoon (15 mL) contains monobasic sodium phosphate monohydrate 7.2 g and dibasic sodium phosphate heptahydrate 2.7 g. Natural ginger-lemon flavoring.
2. FLEET® Bisacodyl Tablets—4 laxative tablets. Active Ingredient: Each enteric-coated tablet contains 5 mg bisacodyl.
3. FLEET® Bisacodyl Enema 1.25 fl. oz. (37 mL)—1 laxative enema. Active Ingredient: Each 30-mL delivered dose contains 10 mg bisacodyl USP.
4. 1 Patient Instruction Sheet.
5. 1 Patient Information Sheet.
FLEET® Prep Kit 3 should not be used in children under 18 years of age.

PHARMACOKINETICS
Caswell M, Thompson WO, Kanapka JA, Galt DJB. The time course and effect on serum electrolytes of oral sodium phosphates solution in healthy male and female volunteers. Can J Clin Pharmacol 14(3):e260-e274, 2007
http://www.cjcp.ca/pdf/CJCP07005e260_e274.pdf
Each recommended dose (1.5 fl. oz.) (45 mL) of FLEET® Phospho-soda® oral saline laxative contains 5004 mg sodium.

ACTIONS AND USES
Bowel Cleansing System

INDICATIONS
For use as part of a bowel cleansing regimen in preparing the colon for surgery, x-ray or endoscopic examination.

PROFESSIONAL USE INFORMATION
WARNINGS
RENAL DISEASE AND ACUTE PHOSPHATE NEPHROPATHY: There have been rare, but serious reports of acute phosphate nephropathy (also known as nephrocalcinosis) in patients who received oral sodium phosphates products (solution and tablets) for bowel cleansing prior to colonoscopy or other medical procedures. Some cases resulted in permanent impairment of renal function, with some patients requiring long term dialysis and/or kidney transplant. The time to onset is typically within days; however, in some cases, the diagnosis of these events has been delayed up to several months after the ingestion of these products. While some cases occurred in patients without identifiable risk factors, patients at increased risk of acute phosphate nephropathy may include those with increased age, hypovolemia, increased bowel transit time (such as bowel obstruction), active colitis, or baseline kidney disease, and those using medicines that affect renal perfusion or function (such as diuretics, angiotensin converting enzyme [ACE] inhibitors, angiotensin receptor blockers [ARBs], and possibly nonsteroidal anti-inflammatory drugs [NSAIDs]). Patients at increased risk should be assessed for hydration status prior to use of purgative preparations and managed appropriately. See PRECAUTIONS. It is important to use the dose and dosing regimen as recommended.
ELECTROLYTE DISORDERS: Administration of sodium phosphate products prior to colonoscopy for colon cleansing or other medical procedures has resulted in fatalities due to significant fluid shifts, severe electrolyte abnormalities, and cardiac arrhythmias. These fatalities have been observed in elderly patients, in patients with renal insufficiency, in patients with bowel perforation, and in patients who misused or overdosed sodium phosphate products. The benefit/risk ratio of Fleet® Prep Kit 3 needs to be carefully considered before initiating treatment in this at-risk population. Special attention should be taken when prescribing Fleet® Prep Kit 3 to any patient with regard to known contraindications and risks, the importance of adequate hydration and, in at-risk populations (see below), the importance of also obtaining baseline and post-treatment serum electrolyte levels, and blood urea nitrogen and creatinine levels.
In all patients there is a risk of elevated serum levels of sodium and phosphate and decreased serum levels of calcium and potassium; consequently, hypernatremia, hyperphosphatemia, hypocalcemia, hypokalemia, and acidosis may occur.
CARDIAC ARRHYTHMIAS: There have been rare, but serious, reports of arrhythmias associated with the use of sodium phosphate products. Fleet® Prep Kit 3 should be used with caution in patients with prolonged QT, patients with a history of uncontrolled arrhythmias, and patients with a recent history of a myocardial infarction. Pre-dose and post-colonoscopy ECGs should be considered in patients with high risk of serious cardiac arrhythmias.
OTHER IMPORTANT SAFETY INFORMATION:
Renal Impact: Sodium phosphate is known to be substantially excreted by the kidney, and the risk of adverse reac-

tions with sodium phosphates may be greater in patients with impaired renal function. Since elderly patients are more likely to have impaired renal function, consider performing baseline and post-procedure labs (phosphate, calcium, potassium, sodium, creatinine, GFR and BUN) in these patients (see WARNINGS).

Hypersensitivity Reactions: There have been reports of hypersensitivity reactions (e.g., rash, urticaria, pruritus, tongue edema, throat tightness, and paresthesia of the lips) associated with the use of marketed sodium phosphates products.

Aphthoid Lesions: Single or multiple aphthoid-like punctiform lesions located in the rectosigmoid region have been observed by endoscopy. These were either lymphoid follicles or discrete inflammatory infiltrates or epithelial congestions/changes revealed by the colonic preparation. These abnormalities are not clinically significant and disappear spontaneously without any treatment.

Absorption of Medications: During the intake of Fleet® Prep Kit 3 the absorption of drugs from the gastrointestinal tract may be delayed or even completely prevented. The efficacy of regularly taken oral drugs (e.g. oral contraceptives, antiepileptic drugs, diabetic medications, antibiotics) may be reduced or completely absent.

Concomitant Medications: NO OTHER SODIUM PHOSPHATES PREPARATIONS INCLUDING SODIUM PHOSPHATES-BASED ENEMAS OR TABLETS SHOULD BE GIVEN CONCOMITANTLY.

CONTRAINDICATIONS

Do not use in patients with
- Biopsy proven acute phosphate nephropathy
- Congestive heart failure
- Clinically significant impairment of renal function
- Ascites
- Known or suspected gastrointestinal obstruction
- Megacolon (congenital or acquired)
- Perforation
- Hyperparathyroidism
- Ileus
- Active inflammatory bowel disease; Crohn's disease; ulcerative colitis.

Do not use
- In children under the age of 18 years
- When abdominal pain, nausea, or vomiting are present
- If there is a hypersensitivity to the active ingredients or any of the excipients

PRECAUTIONS

Use with caution in patients who are
- Elderly
- Debilitated
- Taking medications known to affect renal perfusion or function, or hydration status
- Taking medications known to prolong the QT interval
- Taking parathyroid hormone medications
- On a low-salt diet
- Pregnant or nursing a baby

And in patients with
- Heart disease
- Arrhythmia
- Cardiomyopathy
- Recent myocardial infarction
- Unstable angina
- Prolonged QT interval
- An increased risk for underlying renal impairment
- An increased risk for, or pre-existing, electrolyte disturbances, including patients with
  - Dehydration
  - Inability to take adequate oral fluid
  - Hypertension or other conditions in which the patients are taking products that affect electrolytes or may result in dehydration (see Hydration information below)
  - Gastric retention, hypomotility disorders, history of gastric bypass/stapling surgery; or
  - Colitis
- A colostomy or ileostomy

In at-risk patients, including elderly patients, the benefit/risk ratio of Fleet® Prep Kit 3 needs to be carefully considered before initiating treatment. Consider obtaining baseline and post-procedure serum sodium, potassium, calcium, chloride, bicarbonate, phosphate, blood urea nitrogen and creatinine values. If any patient develops vomiting and/or signs of dehydration, measure post-procedure labs (phosphate, calcium, potassium, sodium, creatinine, GFR and BUN.)

Patients with electrolyte abnormalities such as hypernatremia, hyperphosphatemia, hypokalemia, or hypocalcemia should have their electrolytes corrected before use of Fleet® Prep Kit 3.

Bisacodyl products may cause abdominal discomfort, faintness, and cramps. FLEET® Bisacodyl Tablets should be swallowed whole. Do not prescribe to patients who cannot swallow without chewing unless directed by a physician. Store at temperatures not above 86°F (30°C)

HYDRATION

Additional liquids by mouth are recommended with all bowel cleansing dosages. Encourage patients to drink large amounts of clear liquids before and during the bowel preparation process, and after the procedure, in order to prevent dehydration. Before the procedure, the patient should begin drinking plenty of clear liquids, such as 36 to 48 fl. oz. of a carbohydrate-electrolyte solution; during the preparation the patient should drink a minimum of 72 fl. oz. of clear liquids; during the procedure it is recommended that intravenous fluids (500–1,000 mL) be administered; and after the procedure the patient should drink as much liquid as possible to help prevent dehydration. Inadequate fluid intake when using any effective purgative may lead to excessive fluid loss, possibly producing dehydration and hypovolemia. Dehydration and hypovolemia from purgation may be exacerbated by inadequate oral liquid intake, nausea, vomiting, loss of appetite, or use of diuretics, ACE-Is, ARBs, NSAIDs, and lithium or other medications that may affect electrolyte levels, and may be associated with acute renal failure. There have been reports of acute renal failure associated with bowel purgatives. Drinking large amounts of clear liquids (at least 72 fl. oz. during the bowel preparation process) also helps ensure that your patient's bowel will be clean for the procedure. Instruct the patient to contact a physician if there is no bowel movement after six hours as electrolyte imbalance can occur. (See OVERDOSAGE OR NO BOWEL MOVEMENT below).

OVERDOSAGE OR NO BOWEL MOVEMENT

Overdosage (including shorter time intervals between doses than recommended) or no bowel movement may lead to severe electrolyte disturbances, including hypernatremia, hyperphosphatemia, hypocalcemia, and hypokalemia, as well as dehydration and hypovolemia, with attendant signs and symptoms of these disturbances (such as metabolic acidosis, renal failure, and tetany). Certain severe electrolyte disturbances may lead to cardiac arrhythmia and death. The patient who has taken an overdose or who fails to have a bowel movement after six hours should be monitored carefully. Patients experiencing overdose or no bowel movement have presented the following symptoms; dehydration, hypotension, tachycardia, bradycardia, tachypnoea, cardiac arrest, shock, respiratory failure, dyspnoea, convulsions, ileus paralytic, anxiety, and pain. Overdoses or no bowel movement can also lead to elevated serum levels of sodium and phosphate and decreased levels of calcium and potassium. In those cases, hypernatremia, hyperphosphatemia, hypocalcemia and hypokalemia may occur with resulting metabolic acidosis, renal failure, tetany and in severe cases, multi-organ failure, cardiac arrhythmia and death. **Treatment of electrolyte imbalance may require immediate medical intervention with appropriate electrolyte and fluid replacement therapy.**

INFORMATION FOR PATIENT

The patient should be instructed to open and read directions and patient information sheet at least two (2) days in advance of the examination.

Instruct the patient to use this product for bowel cleansing only as directed by a doctor, to discuss with the doctor the patient's health and warnings about use of this product for bowel cleansing, to follow the special directions from the doctor exactly and to take only the dose the doctor has recommended. The patient should be instructed to drink plenty of clear liquids before beginning the bowel preparation process; consider recommending the patient consume 36–48 fl.

Continued on next page

Fleet Prep Kit 3—Cont.

oz. of a carbohydrate-electrolyte solution in the six hours before the first dose is taken. During the bowel preparation process, the patient should be instructed to drink as much extra clear liquids as they can to replace the fluids lost during bowel movements: minimum 72 fl. oz. The patient should be instructed to drink as much liquid as possible after the procedure to help prevent dehydration.

WARNINGS FOR PATIENTS

DO NOT EXCEED RECOMMENDED DOSE UNLESS DIRECTED BY A PHYSICIAN. SERIOUS SIDE EFFECTS MAY OCCUR FROM EXCESS DOSAGE. IF THERE IS NO BOWEL MOVEMENT AFTER SIX HOURS, CONTACT A PHYSICIAN, AS ELECTROLYTE IMBALANCE AND CONSEQUENT SERIOUS SIDE EFFECTS COULD OCCUR.

During bowel preparation you will lose significant amounts of fluid. THIS IS NORMAL. It is very important that you replace this fluid to prevent dehydration. Early symptoms of dehydration include feeling thirsty, dizziness, urinating less often than normal, or vomiting. These symptoms may be signs of serious problems. Drink as much extra liquids as you can to help replace the fluids you are losing during bowel movements. Drinking large amounts of clear liquids also helps ensure that your bowel will be clean for the examination or procedure.

DO NOT TAKE MORE THAN 45 ML (1.5 FL. OZ.) OF FLEET® PHOSPHO-SODA® PER DOSE. NEVER TAKE MORE THAN 1 BOTTLE AT ONE TIME.

Swallow Fleet® Bisacodyl Tablets whole; do not chew tablets unless directed by a physician. Do not take tablets within one hour after taking antacids, milk, or milk products.

DO NOT USE if you have congestive heart failure, if you have serious kidney problems, or in children under 18 years of age. Ask a doctor before use if you are under a doctor's care for any medical condition, are on a low-salt diet or are pregnant or nursing a baby. Ask a doctor or pharmacist before use if you are taking any other prescription or nonprescription drugs. Ask a doctor before using any laxative if you have abdominal (belly) pain, nausea, or vomiting, have a change in your daily bowel movements that lasts more than 2 weeks, or have already used another laxative daily for constipation for more than 1 week. Stop using this product and consult a doctor if you have any rectal bleeding, do not have a bowel movement within 6 hours of taking this product or have any symptoms that your body is losing more fluids than you are drinking. This is called dehydration. Early symptoms of dehydration include feeling thirsty, dizziness, urinating less often than normal, or vomiting. These symptoms may be signs of serious problems.

Keep this and all drugs out of the reach of children. In case of accidental overdose or ingestion, seek professional assistance or contact a Poison Control Center right away.

PATIENT SAFETY INFORMATION GUIDE
FLEET® Prep Kit 3
This Patient Safety Information Guide should be shared with your patient before your patient uses FLEET® Prep Kit 3. The Patient Safety Information Guide should not take the place of any discussion between doctor and patient about the patient's medical condition or treatment. Encourage your patient to ask you questions about FLEET® Prep Kit 3.

What is the most important information I should know about FLEET® Prep Kit 3?
FLEET® Prep Kit 3 can cause serious side effects, including:
Serious kidney problems. Rare, but serious kidney problems can happen in people who take medicines made with sodium phosphate, including FLEET® Prep Kit 3, to clean your colon before a colonoscopy or other medical procedures. These kidney problems can sometimes lead to kidney failure, the need for dialysis for a long time or kidney transplant. These problems often happen within a few days, but sometimes may happen several months after taking FLEET® Prep Kit 3.
Conditions that can make you more at risk for having serious kidney problems with FLEET® Prep Kit 3 include if you:

- lose too much body fluid (dehydration)
- have slow moving bowel
- have bowel blocked with stool (constipation)
- have severe stomach pain or bloating
- have any disease that causes bowel irritation (colitis)
- have kidney disease
- have heart failure
- take water pills or non-steroidal anti-inflammatory drugs (NSAIDS).

Your age may also affect your risk for having kidney problems with FLEET® Prep Kit 3.
Before you start taking FLEET® Prep Kit 3, tell your doctor if you:
- have kidney problems
- take any medicines for blood pressure, heart disease, or kidney disease.

Severe fluid loss (dehydration). People who take medicines that contain sodium phosphate can have severe loss of body fluid, with severe changes in body salts in the blood, and abnormal heart rhythms. These problems can lead to death.
Tell your doctor if you have any of these symptoms of loss of too much body fluid (dehydration) while taking FLEET® Prep Kit 3:
- vomiting
- dizziness
- urinating less often than normal
- headache

See "What are the possible side effects of FLEET® Prep Kit 3?" for more information about side effects.

What is FLEET® Prep Kit 3?
FLEET® Prep Kit 3 is a medicine used in adults 18 years or older, to clean your colon before a colonoscopy or other medical procedure. FLEET® Prep Kit 3 cleans your colon by causing you to have diarrhea. Cleaning your colon helps your doctor see the inside of your colon more clearly during the colonoscopy or other medical procedure.
It is not known if FLEET® Prep Kit 3 is safe and works in children under age 18.

Who should not take FLEET® Prep Kit 3?
Do not take FLEET® Prep Kit 3 if:
- you have had a kidney biopsy that shows you have kidney problems because of too much phosphate
- you are allergic to sodium phosphate salts, bisacodyl or any of the ingredients in FLEET® Prep Kit 3

What should I tell my doctor before taking FLEET® Prep Kit 3?
Before taking FLEET® Prep Kit 3, tell your doctor about all your medical conditions, including if you have:
- any of the medical conditions listed in the section "What is the most important information I should know about FLEET® Prep Kit 3?"
- irritation of the bowel (colitis). FLEET® Prep Kit 3 can cause symptoms of irritable bowel disease to flare-up.
- damage to your bowel
- problems with abnormal heart beat
- had a recent heart attack or have other heart problems
- symptoms of too much body fluid loss (dehydration) including vomiting, dizziness, urinating less often than normal, or headache
- had stomach surgery
- a history of seizures
- if you drink alcohol
- are on a low salt diet
- are pregnant. It is not known if FLEET® Prep Kit 3 will harm your unborn baby.

Tell your doctor about all the medicines you take, including prescription and non-prescription medicines, vitamins, and herbal supplements. Any medicine that you take close to the time that you take FLEET® Prep Kit 3 may not work as well. Especially tell your doctor if you take:
- water pills (diuretics)
- medicines for blood pressure or heart problems
- medicines for kidney damage
- medicines for pain, such as aspirin or a non-steroidal anti-inflammatory drug (NSAID)

- a medicine for seizures
- a laxative for constipation in the last 7 days. You should not take another medicine that contains sodium phosphate while you take FLEET® Prep Kit 3.

Ask your doctor if you are not sure if your medicine is listed above.

Know the medicines you take. Keep a list of your medicines to show your doctor or pharmacist when you get a new prescription.

How should I take FLEET® Prep Kit 3?

- take FLEET® Prep Kit 3 exactly as prescribed by your doctor.
- **It is important for you to drink clear liquids before, during, and after taking FLEET® Prep Kit 3. This may help prevent kidney damage. Examples of clear liquids** are water, flavored water, lemonade (no pulp), ginger ale, or apple juice. Do not drink any liquids colored purple or red.
- Follow the detailed instructions enclosed.

Tell your doctor if you have any of these symptoms while taking FLEET® Prep Kit 3:

- vomiting, dizziness, or if you urinate less often than normal. These may be signs that you have lost too much fluid while taking FLEET® Prep Kit 3.
- trouble drinking clear fluids
- severe stomach cramping, bloating, nausea, or headache

If you take too much FLEET® Prep Kit 3, call your doctor or get medical help right away.

What should I avoid while taking FLEET® Prep Kit 3?

- You should not take other laxatives or enemas made with sodium phosphate while taking FLEET® Prep Kit 3.
- You should not use FLEET® Prep Kit 3 if you have already used it or any other sodium phosphate product for colon cleansing in the last 7 days.

What are the possible side effects of FLEET® Prep Kit 3?

FLEET® Prep Kit 3 can cause serious side effects, including:

- See "What is the most important information I should know about FLEET® Prep Kit 3?"
- Seizures or fainting (black-outs). People who take a medicine that contains sodium phosphate, such as FLEET® Prep Kit 3, can have seizures or faint (become unconscious) even if they have not had seizures before. Tell your doctor right away if you have a seizure or faint while taking FLEET® Prep Kit 3.
- abnormal heart beat (arrhythmias)
- changes in your blood levels of calcium, phosphate, potassium, sodium

The most common side effects of FLEET® Prep Kit 3 are:

- bloating
- stomach area (abdominal) pain
- nausea
- vomiting
- cramping
- fainting

These are not all the possible side effects of FLEET® Prep Kit 3. For more information, ask your doctor or pharmacist.

Call your doctor for medical advice about side effects. You may report side effects to FDA at 1- 800-FDA-1088.

How do I store FLEET® Prep Kit 3?

- Store FLEET® Prep Kit 3 at room temperature, between 59° F to 86° F (15° C to 30° C).
- Keep FLEET® Prep Kit 3 and all medicines out of the reach of children.

DOSAGE AND ADMINISTRATION

SEE PATIENT INSTRUCTION SHEET FOR 18-, AND 24-HOUR PREPARATION SCHEDULE IN EACH KIT. The patient should open and read the enclosed directions, patient information sheet and carton labels at least 48 hours in advance of examination.

Fleet® Prep Kit 3 or any of the sodium phosphates-based bowel preparations should not be used for colon cleansing within seven (7) days of previous administration.

FLEET® PREP KIT 3 SHOULD NOT BE USED IN CHILDREN UNDER 18 YEARS OF AGE.

Additional patient instruction and information sheets are available by calling 1-866-255-6960

HOW SUPPLIED

See "Description" for contents of each kit.

Shipping Unit: 48 FLEET® Prep Kits per case.

For additional information, see individual listings under FLEET® Bisacodyl Laxatives.

IS THIS PRODUCT OTC? Yes.

QUESTIONS? Call 1-866-255-6960

Gordon Laboratories
6801 LUDLOW STREET
UPPER DARBY, PA 19082

Direct inquiries to:
Customer Service
(610) 734-2011
Fax (610) 734-2049
Website: http://www.gordonlabs.net
E-mail: gordonlabs@worldnet.att.net
For medical emergencies contact:
David Dercher   (610) 734-2011
                                                          Fax (610) 734-2049

GORDOCHOM™ Solution   OTC
[gŏrdō'kŏm]

DESCRIPTION

Gordochom is an antifungal solution for topical use containing 25% Undecylenic Acid and 3% Chloroxylenol as its active ingredients in a penetrating oil base. Undecylenic Acid is chemically 10 hendecenoic acid having the empirical formula $C_{11}H_{20}O_2$ and the chemical bond structure $CH_2=CH$ $(CH_2)8$ CO_2H.

Undecylenic Acid is a colorless to pale yellow liquid. It is insoluble in water and soluble in alcohol, chloroform and ether.

Chloroxylenol is chemically 2-chloro-5-hydroxy-1,3-dimethylbenzene having the empirical formula C_8H_9ClO.

CLINICAL PHARMACOLOGY

Undecylenic Acid is a fungistatic agent employed in the treatment of tinea pedis, ringworm and dermatophytosis.

Chloroxylenol is a topical antiseptic, germicide and antifungal agent effective against a wide variety of causative fungi and yeast organisms. Among those affected by chloroxylenol are candida albicans, aspergillus niger, aspergillus flavus, trichophyton rubrum, trichophyton mentagrophytes, penicillum luteum and epidermophyton floccosum.

The penetrating oil base vehicle serves as a delivery system, enhancing the impregnation of Undecylenic Acid and Chloroxylenol as antimicrobial agents.

INDICATIONS

Cures athlete's foot (tinea pedis), and ringworm (tinea corporis).

CONTRAINDICATIONS

Gordochom is contraindicated in patients who are sensitive to Undecylenic Acid or Chloroxylenol.

Continued on next page

Gordochom—Cont.

WARNINGS

FOR EXTERNAL USE ONLY. Not for opthalmic or optic use. Avoid inhaling and contact with eyes or other mucous membranes. Not to be applied over blistered, raw or oozing areas of skin or over deep puncture wounds.

PRECAUTIONS

If a reaction suggesting sensitivity or chemical irritation should occur with the use of Gordochom, treatment should be discontinued. Use of Gordochom in pregnancy has not been established.

ADVERSE REACTIONS

No significant adverse reactions have been reported. However, attention should be paid to localized hypersensitivity.

DOSAGE AND ADMINISTRATION

Cleanse and dry affected areas. Apply a thin application twice a day (morning and night) to the affected area, or as recommended by your physician. Supervise children in the use of this product. For athlete's foot, pay special attention to the spaces between the toes; wear well-fitting, ventilated shoes, and change shoes and socks at least once daily. For athlete's foot and ringworm, use daily for 4 weeks. If condition persists longer, consult a physician. This product has not been proven effective on the scalp or nails.

HOW SUPPLIED

Gordochom is available in 1 oz. bottles with special brush applicator. (NDC 10481-8010-2)
Store at controlled room temperatures (59°–86°F).
For external use only.
Keep out of reach of children.
Shown in Product Identification Guide, page 403

Guardian Laboratories
a division of United-Guardian, Inc.
P.O. Box 18050
HAUPPAUGE, NY 11788

For Medical Information Contact:
Director of Product Development
(631) 273-0900
(800) 645-5566

CLORPACTIN® WCS-90　　　　　　　　OTC
[*klor-pak 'tin*]
(brand of sodium oxychlorosene)

COMPOSITION

Stabilized organic derivative of hypochlorous acid. A white, water soluble powder with a characteristic smell of hypochlorous acid. Active chlorine derived from calcium hypochlorite: 3–4%.

ACTION AND USES

For use as a topical antiseptic for treating localized infections, particularly when resistant organisms are present.

ADMINISTRATION AND DOSAGE

Generally applied as the 0.4% solution in water, or isotonic saline, but as the 0.1% to 0.2% in Urology and Ophthalmology.

CONTRAINDICATIONS

The use of this product is contraindicated where the site of the infection is not exposed to the direct contact with the solution. Not for systemic use.

HOW SUPPLIED

In boxes containing 5 x 2 gram bottles. NDC: 0327-0001-10
Store under refrigeration.

Heel Inc.
10421 RESEARCH RD. SE
ALBUQUERQUE, NM 87123

Direct Inquiries to:
Medical Department
800-621-7644
Fax: (800) 217-6934
www.heelusa.com
info@heelusa.com

TRAUMEEL® Gel	OTC
Anti-inflammatory	
TRAUMEEL® Tablets	OTC
Anti-inflammatory	
TRAUMEEL® Ointment	OTC
Anti-inflammatory	
TRAUMEEL® Oral Drops	OTC
Anti-inflammatory	
TRAUMEEL® Oral Liquid in Vials	OTC
Anti-inflammatory	
TRAUMEEL® Ear Drops	OTC
Anti-inflammatory	
TRAUMEEL® Injection Solution	℞
Anti-inflammatory	

Hisamitsu Pharmaceutical Co., Inc.
408 TASHIRO-DAIKANMACHI
TOSU SAGA 841-0017
JAPAN

Direct Inquiries to:
Tel: +81-3-5293-1720
Fax: +81-3-5293-1724

SALONPAS® ARTHRITIS PAIN　　　　OTC
Pain Relieving Patch

DRUG FACTS

Active ingredients: (in each patch) — **Purpose:**
Menthol 3% — Topical analgesic
Methyl Salicylate 10% (NSAID*) — Topical analgesic
*nonsteroidal anti-inflammatory drug

USES

Temporarily relieves mild to moderate aches & pains of muscles & joints associated with:
• arthritis • sprains • strains • bruises • simple backache

WARNINGS

For external use only
Stomach bleeding warning
This product contains an NSAID, which may cause stomach bleeding. The chance is small but higher if you:
• are age 60 or older
• have had stomach ulcers or bleeding problems
• take a blood thinning (anticoagulant) or steroid drug
• take other drugs containing an NSAID [aspirin, ibuprofen, naproxen, or others]
• have 3 or more alcoholic drinks every day while using this product
• take more or for a longer time than directed
Do not use
• on the face or rashes
• on wounds or damaged skin

- if allergic to aspirin or other NSAIDs
- with a heating pad
- when sweating (such as from exercise or heat)
- any patch from a pouch that has been open for 14 or more days
- right before or after heart surgery

Ask a doctor before use if
- you are allergic to topical products
- the stomach bleeding warning applies to you
- you have high blood pressure, heart disease, or kidney disease
- you are taking a diuretic

When using this product
- wash hands after applying or removing patch. Avoid contact with eyes. If eye contact occurs, rinse thoroughly with water.
- the risk of heart attack or stroke may increase if you use more than directed or for longer than directed

Stop use and ask a doctor if
- you feel faint, vomit blood, or have bloody or black stools. These are signs of stomach bleeding.
- rash, itching or skin irritation develops
- condition worsens
- symptoms last for more than 3 days
- symptoms clear up and occur again within a few days
- stomach pain or upset gets worse or lasts

If pregnant or breast-feeding, ask a doctor before use while breast-feeding and during the first 6 months of pregnancy. Do not use during the last 3 months of pregnancy because it may cause problems in the unborn child or complications during delivery.

Keep out of reach of children.
If put in mouth, get medical help or contact a Poison Control Center right away.
Package not child resistant.

DIRECTIONS

Adults 18 years and older:
- clean and dry affected area
- remove patch from backing film and apply to skin
- apply one patch to the affected area and leave in place for up to 8 to 12 hours
- if pain lasts after using the first patch, a second patch may be applied for up to another 8 to 12 hours
- only use one patch at a time
- do not use more than 2 patches per day
- do not use for more than 3 days in a row

Children under 18 years of age:
- do not use

Other Information:
- some individuals may not experience pain relief until several hours after applying the patch
- avoid storing product in direct sunlight
- protect product from excessive moisture
- store at 20-25°C (68-77°F)

Inactive ingredients: alicyclic saturated hydrocarbon resin, backing cloth, film, mineral oil, polyisobutylene, polyisobutylene 1,200,000, styrene-isoprene-styrene block copolymer, synthetic aluminum silicate
Questions or comments?
Toll free 1-87-SALONPAS
MON-FRI 9AM to 5PM (PST)

HOW SUPPLIED

Available in 5 patches & 15 patches 2 3/4 × 3 15/16 inch (7cm ×10cm)
Shown in Product Identification Guide, page 403

SALONPAS® PAIN RELIEF PATCH   OTC
Pain Relieving Patch

DRUG FACTS

Active ingredients: (in each patch):	Purpose:
Menthol 3%	Topical analgesic
Methyl salicylate 10% (NSAID*)	Topical analgesic

*nonsteroidal anti-inflammatory drug

USES

Temporarily relieves mild to moderate aches & pains of muscles & joints associated with:
- strains • sprains • simple backache • arthritis • bruises

WARNINGS
For external use only
Stomach bleeding warning:
This product contains an NSAID, which may cause stomach bleeding. The chance is small but higher if you:
- are age 60 or older
- have had stomach ulcers or bleeding problems
- take a blood thinning (anticoagulant) or steroid drug
- take other drugs containing an NSAID [aspirin, ibuprofen, naproxen, or others]
- have 3 or more alcoholic drinks every day while using this product
- take more or for a longer time than directed

Do not use
- on the face or rashes
- on wounds or damaged skin
- if allergic to aspirin or other NSAIDs
- with a heating pad
- when sweating (such as from exercise or heat)
- any patch from a pouch that has been open for 14 or more days
- right before or after heart surgery

Ask a doctor before use if
- you are allergic to topical products
- the stomach bleeding warning applies to you
- you have high blood pressure, heart disease, or kidney disease
- you are taking a diuretic

When using this product
- wash hands after applying or removing patch. Avoid contact with eyes. If eye contact occurs, rinse thoroughly with water.
- the risk of heart attack or stroke may increase if you use more than directed or for longer than directed

Stop use and ask a doctor if
- you feel faint, vomit blood, or have bloody or black stools. These are signs of stomach bleeding.
- rash, itching or skin irritation develops
- condition worsens
- symptoms last for more than 3 days
- symptoms clear up and occur again within a few days
- stomach pain or upset gets worse or lasts

If pregnant or breast-feeding, ask a doctor before use while breast-feeding and during the first 6 months of pregnancy. Do not use during the last 3 months of pregnancy because it may cause problems in the unborn child or complications during delivery.

Keep out of reach of children
If put in mouth, get medical help or contact a Poison Control Center right away.
Package not child resistant.

DIRECTIONS

Adults 18 years and older:
- clean and dry affected area
- remove patch from backing film and apply to skin
- apply one patch to the affected area and leave in place for up to 8 to 12 hours
- if pain lasts after using the first patch, a second patch may be applied for up to another 8 to 12 hours
- only use one patch at a time
- do not use more than 2 patches per day
- do not use for more than 3 days in a row

Children under 18 years of age:
- do not use

Other information:
- some individuals may not experience pain relief until several hours after applying the patch
- avoid storing product in direct sunlight
- protect product from excessive moisture
- store at 20-25°C (68-77°F)

Inactive ingredients: alicyclic saturated hydrocarbon resin, backing cloth, film, mineral oil, polyisobutylene, polyisobutylene 1,200,000, styrene-isoprene-styrene block copolymer, synthetic aluminum silicate
Questions or comments?
Toll free 1-87-SALONPAS
MON-FRI 9AM to 5PM (PST)

Continued on next page

Salonpas Pain Relief Patch—Cont.

HOW SUPPLIED

Available in 5 patches & 15 patches 2 3/4 × 3 15/16 inch (7cm ×10cm)

Shown in Product Identification Guide, page 403

Johnson & Johnson Healthcare Products Division of McNEIL-PPC, Inc.

**199 Grandview Road
Skillman, NJ 08558
©McNEIL-PPC, Inc. 2009**

Direct Inquiries to:
Consumer Affairs
1-888-734-7648

VISINE® PURE TEARS   OTC
**Dry Eye Relief
Lubricant Eye Drops
Preservative Free Singles**

DESCRIPTION

VISINE® Pure Tears Singles Preservative Free Lubricant Eye Drops cools and comforts your dry, scratchy irritated eyes, and helps them feel their best. It relieves the dryness caused by computer use, reading, wind, heat and air conditioning, while it protects your eyes from further irritation. Specially formulated for people whose eyes are sensitive to preservatives, VISINE® Pure Tears Singles is sealed in convenient single-use vials and is safe to use as often as needed. This "natural tears formula" contains 10 important ingredients found in your own natural tears.

Active Ingredients:	Purpose:
Glycerin 0.2%	Lubricant
Hypromellose 0.2%	Lubricant
Polyethylene glycol 400 1%	Lubricant

USES
• for the temporary relief of burning and irritation due to dryness of the eye
• for protection against further irritation

WARNINGS
When using this product
• remove contact lenses before using
• do not use if this solution changes color or becomes cloudy
• do not touch tip of container to any surface to avoid contamination
• do not reuse; once opened, discard
Stop use and ask a doctor if
• you feel eye pain
• changes in vision occur
• redness or irritation of the eye lasts
• condition worsens or lasts more than 72 hours
If pregnant or breast-feeding, ask a health professional before use.
Keep out of reach of children. If swallowed, get medical help or contact a Poison Control Center right away.

DIRECTIONS
• put 1 or 2 drops in the affected eye(s) as needed
• children under 6 years of age: ask a doctor
Other Information:
• store at 15° to 25°C (59° to 77°F)

INACTIVE INGREDIENTS

ascorbic acid, dextrose, disodium phosphate, glycine, magnesium chloride, potassium chloride, purified water, sodium chloride, sodium citrate, sodium lactate, and sodium phosphate
Questions? call **1-888-734-7648,** weekdays

Caution: Use only if single-use container is intact.

HOW SUPPLIED

1 box contains 32 single-use containers, 0.01 FL OZ (0.4 mL) each

Shown in Product Identification Guide, page 403

Johnson & Johnson • MERCK
**Consumer Pharmaceuticals Co.
CAMP HILL ROAD
FORT WASHINGTON, PA 19034**

Direct Inquiries to:
Consumer Relationship Center
Fort Washington, PA 19034
1-800-755-4008

PEPCID AC®   OTC
**ORIGINAL STRENGTH PEPCID® AC Tablets and Gelcaps
MAXIMUM STRENGTH PEPCID® AC Tablets
Acid reducer**

DESCRIPTION

Each Original Strength Pepcid AC Tablet and Gelcap contains famotidine 10 mg as an active ingredient.
Each Maximum Strength Pepcid AC Tablet contains famotidine 20 mg as an active ingredient.
INACTIVE INGREDIENTS (Orig. Strength Pepcid AC)
TABLETS: hydroxypropyl cellulose, hypromellose, magnesium stearate, microcrystalline cellulose, red iron oxide, starch, talc, titanium dioxide
GELCAPS: benzyl alcohol, black iron oxide, butylparaben, castor oil, edetate calcium disodium, FD&C red #40, gelatin, hypromellose, magnesium stearate, methylparaben, microcrystalline cellulose, pregelatinized corn starch, propylene glycol, propylparaben, sodium lauryl sulfate, sodium propionate, talc, titanium dioxide
INACTIVE INGREDIENTS (Max. Strength Pepcid AC.)
carnauba wax, hydroxypropyl cellulose, hypromellose, magnesium stearate, microcrystalline cellulose, pregelatinized starch, talc, titanium dioxide
Product Benefits:
• **1 Tablet or Gelcap** relieves heartburn associated with acid indigestion and sour stomach.
• ORIGINAL STRENGTH and MAXIMUM STRENGTH PEPCID AC prevent heartburn associated with acid indigestion and sour stomach brought on by eating or drinking certain food and beverages.
• They contain famotidine, a prescription-proven medicine. The ingredient in ORIGINAL STRENGTH PEPCID AC and MAXIMUM STRENGTH PEPCID AC, famotidine, has been prescribed by doctors for years to treat millions of patients safely and effectively. The active ingredient in ORIGINAL STRENGTH PEPCID AC and MAXIMUM STRENGTH PEPCID AC has been taken safely with many frequently prescribed medications.

ACTION

It is normal for the stomach to produce acid, especially after consuming food and beverages. However, acid in the wrong place (the esophagus), or too much acid, can cause burning pain and discomfort that interfere with everyday activities.
•**Heartburn—Caused by acid in the esophagus**

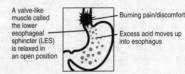

A valve-like muscle called the lower esophageal sphincter (LES) is relaxed in an open position

Burning pain/discomfort

Excess acid moves up into esophagus

USES
• **Relieves heartburn associated with acid indigestion and sour stomach;**

- **Prevents heartburn associated with acid indigestion and sour stomach brought on by eating or drinking certain food and beverages.**

Tips for Managing Heartburn:
- Do not lie flat or bend over soon after eating.
- Do not eat late at night, or just before bedtime.
- Certain foods or drinks are more likely to cause heartburn, such as rich, spicy, fatty, and fried foods, chocolate, caffeine, alcohol, and even some fruits and vegetables.
- Eat slowly and do not eat big meals.
- If you are overweight, lose weight.
- If you smoke, quit smoking.
- Raise the head of your bed.
- Wear loose fitting clothing around your stomach.

WARNINGS

Allergy alert: Do not use if you are allergic to famotidine or other acid reducers

Do not use:
- if you have trouble or pain swallowing food, vomiting with blood, or bloody or black stools. These may be signs of a serious condition. See your doctor.
- with other acid reducers
- if you have kidney disease, except under the advice and supervision of a doctor (Maximum Strength Pepcid AC).

Ask a doctor before use if you have
- had heartburn over 3 months. This may be a sign of a more serious condition.
- heartburn with **lightheadedness, sweating, or dizziness**
- chest pain or shoulder pain with shortness of breath; sweating; pain spreading to arms, neck or shoulder; or lightheadedness
- frequent **chest pain**
- frequent wheezing, particularly with heartburn
- unexplained weight loss
- nausea or vomiting
- stomach pain

Stop use and ask a doctor if
- your heartburn continues or worsens
- you need to take this product for more than 14 days

If pregnant or breast-feeding, ask a health professional before use.

Keep out of reach of children. In case of overdose, get medical help or contact a Poison Control Center right away. (1-800-222-1222)

DIRECTIONS

Original Strength Pepcid AC:
- adults and children 12 years and over:
- Tablet & Gelcap: To **relieve** symptoms, swallow 1 tablet or gelcap with a glass of water. Do not chew.
- Tablet & Gelcap: To **prevent** symptoms, swallow 1 tablet or gelcap with a glass of water at any time from **15 to 60 minutes before** eating food or drinking beverages that cause heartburn
- do not use more than 2 tablets or gelcaps in 24 hours
- children under 12 years: ask a doctor

Maximum Strength Pepcid AC:
- adults and children 12 years and over:
- to **relieve** symptoms, swallow 1 tablet with a glass of water. Do not chew.
- to **prevent** symptoms, swallow 1 tablet with a glass of water at any time from **10 to 60 minutes before** eating food or drinking beverages that cause heartburn
- do not use more than 2 tablets in 24 hours
- children under 12 years: ask a doctor

OTHER INFORMATION
- read the directions and warnings before use
- keep the carton. It contains important information.
- store at 20°–30°C (68°–86°F)
- protect from moisture

HOW SUPPLIED

Original Strength Pepcid AC Tablet is available as a rose-colored tablet identified as 'PEPCID AC'.

Original Strength Pepcid AC Gelcap is available as a rose and white gelatin coated, capsule shaped tablet identified as 'PEPCID AC'.

Maximum Strength Pepcid AC Tablet is a white, "D" shaped, film coated tablet identified as "PAC 20."

Shown in Product Identification Guide, page 403

PEPCID® COMPLETE   OTC
Acid Reducer + Antacid Chewable Tablets
DUAL ACTION:
Reduces and Neutralizes Acid

DESCRIPTION

Active Ingredients (in each chewable tablet):	Purpose:
Famotidine 10 mg	Acid Reducer
Calcium carbonate 800 mg	Antacid
Magnesium hydroxide 165 mg	Antacid

Inactive Ingredients:

Mint flavor: cellulose acetate, corn starch, flavors, hydroxypropyl cellulose, hypromellose, lactose, magnesium stearate, crospovidone, D&C yellow #10 aluminum lake, dextrose, FD&C blue #1 aluminum lake, gum arabic, maltodextrin, mineral oil, sucralose

Berry flavor: cellulose acetate, corn starch, flavors, hydroxypropyl cellulose, hypromellose, lactose, magnesium stearate, crospovidone, D&C red #7 calcium lake, dextrose, FD&C blue #1 aluminum lake, FD&C red #40 aluminum lake, gum arabic, maltodextrin, mineral oil, sucralose

Tropical Fruit flavor: cellulose acetate, corn starch, corn syrup solids, crospovidone, dextrose, FD&C yellow #5 aluminum lake (tartrazine), FD&C yellow #6 aluminum lake, flavors, gum arabic, hydroxypropyl cellulose, hypromellose, lactose, magnesium stearate, maltodextrin, mineral oil, sucralose, triacetin

Product Benefits: Pepcid Complete combines an acid reducer (famotidine) with antacids (calcium carbonate and magnesium hydroxide) to relieve heartburn in two different ways: Acid reducers decrease the production of new stomach acid; antacids neutralize acid that is already in the stomach. The active ingredients in PEPCID COMPLETE have been used for years to treat acid-related problems in millions of people safely and effectively.

USES: Relieves heartburn associated with acid indigestion and sour stomach.

ACTION

It is normal for the stomach to produce acid, especially after consuming food and beverages. However, acid in the stomach may move up into the wrong place (the esophagus), causing burning pain and discomfort that interfere with everyday activities.

Heartburn—Caused by acid in the esophagus

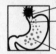

Burning pain/discomfort in esophagus

A valve-like muscle called the lower esophageal sphincter (LES) is relaxed in an open position

Acid moves up from stomach

Tips For Managing Heartburn
- Do not lie flat or bend over soon after eating.
- Do not eat late at night, or just before bedtime.
- Certain foods or drinks are more likely to cause heartburn, such as rich, spicy, fatty, and fried foods, chocolate, caffeine, alcohol, and even some fruits and vegetables.
- Eat slowly and do not eat big meals.
- If you are overweight, lose weight.
- If you smoke, quit smoking.
- Raise the head of your bed.
- Wear loose fitting clothing around your stomach.

WARNINGS
- **Allergy alert:** Do not use if you are allergic to famotidine or other acid reducers

Do not use
- if you have trouble or pain swallowing food, vomiting with blood, or bloody or black stools. These may be signs of a serious condition. See your doctor.
- with other acid reducers

Ask a doctor before use if you have
- had heartburn over 3 months. This may be a sign of a more serious condition.
- heartburn with **lightheadedness, sweating, or dizziness**
- chest pain or shoulder pain with shortness of breath; sweating; pain spreading to arms, neck or shoulders; or lightheadedness

Continued on next page

Pepcid Complete—Cont.

* frequent **chest pain**
* frequent wheezing, particularly with heartburn
* unexplained weight loss
* nausea or vomiting
* stomach pain

Ask a doctor or pharmacist before use if you are presently taking a prescription drug. Antacids may interact with certain prescription drugs.

Stop use and ask a doctor if
* your heartburn continues or worsens
* you need to take this product for more than 14 days
* **If pregnant or breast-feeding,** ask a health professional before use.
* **Keep out of reach of children.** In case of overdose, get medical help or contact a Poison Control Center right away. (1-800-222-1222)

DIRECTIONS

* adults and children 12 years and over:
  * **do not swallow tablet whole; chew completely**
  * to relieve symptoms, **chew** 1 tablet before swallowing
  * do not use more than 2 chewable tablets in 24 hours
* children under 12 years: ask a doctor

OTHER INFORMATION:

* each tablet contains: **calcium 320 mg; magnesium 70 mg.**
* read the directions and warnings before use
* keep the carton and package insert. They contain important information.
* read the bottle label. It contains important information.
* store at 20°–30°C (68°–86°F).
* protect from moisture

HOW SUPPLIED

Pepcid Complete is available as a rose-colored chewable tablet identified by 'P'.

Shown in Product Identification Guide, page 403

Eli Lilly and Company
**LILLY CORPORATE CENTER
INDIANAPOLIS, IN 46285**

Direct Inquiries to:
Lilly Corporate Center
Indianapolis, IN 46285
(317) 276-2000
www.lilly.com
For Medical Information Contact:
Lilly Research Laboratories
Lilly Corporate Center
Indianapolis, IN 46285
(800) 545-5979

HUMULIN® 50/50   OTC
[hŭ 'mŭ-lĭn]
**50% HUMAN INSULIN ISOPHANE SUSPENSION
AND
50% HUMAN INSULIN INJECTION (rDNA ORIGIN)
100 UNITS PER ML (U-100)**

INFORMATION FOR THE PATIENT
10 mL Vial (1000 Units per vial)

WARNINGS

THIS LILLY HUMAN INSULIN PRODUCT DIFFERS FROM ANIMAL-SOURCE INSULINS BECAUSE IT IS STRUCTURALLY IDENTICAL TO THE INSULIN PRODUCED BY YOUR BODY'S PANCREAS AND BECAUSE OF ITS UNIQUE MANUFACTURING PROCESS.
ANY CHANGE OF INSULIN SHOULD BE MADE CAUTIOUSLY AND ONLY UNDER MEDICAL SUPERVISION. CHANGES IN STRENGTH, MANUFACTURER, TYPE (E.G., REGULAR, NPH, ANALOG), SPECIES, OR METHOD OF MANUFACTURE MAY RESULT IN THE NEED FOR A CHANGE IN DOSAGE.

SOME PATIENTS TAKING HUMULIN® (HUMAN INSULIN, rDNA ORIGIN) MAY REQUIRE A CHANGE IN DOSAGE FROM THAT USED WITH OTHER INSULINS. IF AN ADJUSTMENT IS NEEDED, IT MAY OCCUR WITH THE FIRST DOSE OR DURING THE FIRST SEVERAL WEEKS OR MONTHS.

DIABETES

Insulin is a hormone produced by the pancreas, a large gland that lies near the stomach. This hormone is necessary for the body's correct use of food, especially sugar. Diabetes occurs when the pancreas does not make enough insulin to meet your body's needs.

To control your diabetes, your doctor has prescribed injections of insulin products to keep your blood glucose at a near–normal level. You have been instructed to test your blood and/or your urine regularly for glucose. Studies have shown that some chronic complications of diabetes such as eye disease, kidney disease, and nerve disease can be significantly reduced if the blood sugar is maintained as close to normal as possible. The American Diabetes Association recommends that if your pre–meal glucose levels are consistently above 130 mg/dL or your hemoglobin A_{1c} (HbA_{1c}) is more than 7%, you should talk to your doctor. A change in your diabetes therapy may be needed. If your blood tests consistently show below–normal glucose levels, you should also let your doctor know. Proper control of your diabetes requires close and constant cooperation with your doctor. Despite diabetes, you can lead an active and healthy life if you eat a balanced diet, exercise regularly, and take your insulin injections as prescribed by your doctor.

Always keep an extra supply of insulin as well as a spare syringe and needle on hand. Always wear diabetic identification so that appropriate treatment can be given if complications occur away from home.

50/50 HUMAN INSULIN
Description
Humulin is synthesized in a special non-disease-producing laboratory strain of *Escherichia coli* bacteria that has been genetically altered to produce human insulin. Humulin 50/50 is a mixture of 50% Human Insulin Isophane Suspension and 50% Human Insulin Injection (rDNA origin). It is an intermediate-acting insulin combined with the more rapid onset of action of Regular human insulin. The duration of activity may last up to 24 hours following injection. The time course of action of any insulin may vary considerably in different individuals or at different times in the same individual. As with all insulin preparations, the duration of action of Humulin 50/50 is dependent on dose, site of injection, blood supply, temperature, and physical activity. Humulin 50/50 is a sterile suspension and is for subcutaneous injection only. It should not be used intravenously or intramuscularly. The concentration of Humulin 50/50 is 100 units/mL (U-100).

Identification
Human insulin from Eli Lilly and Company has the trademark Humulin. Your doctor has prescribed the type of insulin that he/she believes is best for you.
DO NOT USE ANY OTHER INSULIN EXCEPT ON YOUR DOCTOR'S ADVICE AND DIRECTION.
Always check the carton and the bottle label for the name and letter designation of the insulin you receive from your pharmacy to make sure it is the same as prescribed by your doctor.

Always check the appearance of your bottle of Humulin 50/50 before withdrawing each dose. Before each injection the Humulin 50/50 bottle must be carefully shaken or rotated several times to completely mix the insulin. Humulin 50/50 suspension should look uniformly cloudy or milky after mixing. If not, repeat the above steps until contents are mixed.
Do not use Humulin 50/50:
* if the insulin substance (the white material) remains at the bottom of the bottle after mixing or
* if there are clumps in the insulin after mixing, or
* if solid white particles stick to the bottom or wall of the bottle, giving a frosted appearance.

If you see anything unusual in the appearance of Humulin 50/50 suspension in your bottle or notice your insulin requirements changing, talk to your doctor.

Storage
Not in-use (unopened): Humulin 50/50 bottles not in-use should be stored in a refrigerator, but not in the freezer.

In-use (opened): The Humulin 50/50 bottle you are currently using can be kept unrefrigerated as long as it is kept as cool as possible [below 86°F (30°C)] away from heat and light.

Do not use Humulin 50/50 after the expiration date stamped on the label or if it has been frozen.
INSTRUCTIONS FOR INSULIN VIAL USE
NEVER SHARE NEEDLES AND SYRINGES.
Correct Syringe Type
Doses of insulin are measured in **units**. U–100 insulin contains 100 units/mL (1 mL = 1 cc). With Humulin 50/50, it is important to use a syringe that is marked for U–100 insulin preparations. Failure to use the proper syringe can lead to a mistake in dosage, causing serious problems for you, such as a blood glucose level that is too low or too high.
Syringe Use
To help avoid contamination and possible infection, follow these instructions exactly.
Disposable syringes and needles should be used only once and then discarded by placing the used needle in a puncture-resistant disposable container. Properly dispose of the puncture-resistant container as directed by your Health Care Professional.
Preparing the Dose
1. Wash your hands.
2. Carefully shake or rotate the bottle of insulin several times to completely mix the insulin.
3. Inspect the insulin. Humulin 50/50 suspension should look uniformly cloudy or milky. Do not use Humulin 50/50 if you notice anything unusual in its appearance.
4. If using a new Humulin 50/50 bottle, flip off the plastic protective cap, but **do not** remove the stopper. Wipe the top of the bottle with an alcohol swab.
5. Draw an amount of air into the syringe that is equal to the Humulin 50/50 dose. Put the needle through rubber top of the Humulin 50/50 bottle and inject the air into the bottle.
6. Turn the Humulin 50/50 bottle and syringe upside down. Hold the bottle and syringe firmly in one hand and shake gently.
7. Making sure the tip of the needle is in the Humulin 50/50 suspension, withdraw the correct dose of Humulin 50/50 into the syringe.
8. Before removing the needle from the Humulin 50/50 bottle, check the syringe for air bubbles. If bubbles are present, hold the syringe straight up and tap its side until the bubbles float to the top. Push the bubbles out with the plunger and then withdraw the correct dose.
9. Remove the needle from the bottle and lay the syringe down so that the needle does not touch anything.
Injection Instructions
1. To avoid tissue damage, choose a site for each injection that is at least 1/2 inch from the previous injection site. The usual sites of injection are abdomen, thighs, and arms.
2. Cleanse the skin with alcohol where the injection is to be made.
3. With one hand, stabilize the skin by spreading it or pinching up a large area.
4. Insert the needle as instructed by your doctor.
5. Push the plunger in as far as it will go.
6. Pull the needle out and apply gentle pressure over the injection site for several seconds. **Do not rub the area.**
7. Place the used needle in a puncture-resistant disposable container and properly dispose of the puncture-resistant container as directed by your Health Care Professional.

DOSAGE

Your doctor has told you which insulin to use, how much, and when and how often to inject it. Because each patient's diabetes is different, this schedule has been individualized for you. Your usual dose of Humulin 50/50 may be affected by changes in your diet, activity, or work schedule. Carefully follow your doctor's instructions to allow for these changes. Other things that may affect your Humulin 50/50 dose are:
Illness
Illness, especially with nausea and vomiting, may cause your insulin requirements to change. Even if you are not eating, you will still require insulin. You and your doctor should establish a sick day plan for you to use in case of

illness. When you are sick, test your blood glucose frequently. If instructed by your doctor, test your ketones and report the results to your doctor.
Pregnancy
Good control of diabetes is especially important for you and your unborn baby. Pregnancy may make managing your diabetes more difficult. If you are planning to have a baby, are pregnant, or are nursing a baby, talk to your doctor.
Medication
Insulin requirements may be increased if you are taking other drugs with blood-glucose-raising activity, such as oral contraceptives, corticosteroids, or thyroid replacement therapy. Insulin requirements may be reduced in the presence of drugs that lower blood glucose or affect how your body responds to insulin, such as oral antidiabetic agents, salicylates (for example, aspirin), sulfa antibiotics, alcohol, certain antidepressants and some kidney and blood pressure medicines. Your Health Care Professional may be aware of other medications that may affect your diabetes control. Therefore, always discuss any medications you are taking with your doctor.
Exercise
Exercise may lower your body's need for insulin during and for some time after the physical activity. Exercise may also speed up the effect of an insulin dose, especially if the exercise involves the area of injection site (for example, the leg should not be used for injection just prior to running). Discuss with your doctor how you should adjust your insulin regimen to accommodate exercise.
Travel
When traveling across more than 2 time zones, you should talk to your doctor concerning adjustments in your insulin schedule.
COMMON PROBLEMS OF DIABETES
Hypoglycemia (Low Blood Sugar)
Hypoglycemia (too little glucose in the blood) is one of the most frequent adverse events experienced by insulin users. It can be brought about by:
1. **Missing or delaying meals.**
2. Taking too much insulin.
3. Exercising or working more than usual.
4. An infection or illness associated with diarrhea or vomiting.
5. A change in the body's need for insulin.
6. Diseases of the adrenal, pituitary, or thyroid gland, or progression of kidney or liver disease.
7. Interactions with certain drugs, such as oral antidiabetic agents, salicylates (for example, aspirin), sulfa antibiotics, certain antidepressants and some kidney and blood pressure medicines.
8. Consumption of alcoholic beverages.
Symptoms of mild to moderate hypoglycemia may occur suddenly and can include:

• sweating	• drowsiness
• dizziness	• sleep disturbances
• palpitation	• anxiety
• tremor	• blurred vision
• hunger	• slurred speech
• restlessness	• depressed mood
• tingling in the hands, feet, lips, or tongue	• irritability
• lightheadedness	• abnormal behavior
• inability to concentrate	• unsteady movement
• headache	• personality changes

Signs of severe hypoglycemia can include:

• disorientation	• seizures
• unconsciousness	• death

Therefore, it is important that assistance be obtained immediately.
Early warning symptoms of hypoglycemia may be different or less pronounced under certain conditions, such as long duration of diabetes, diabetic nerve disease, use of medica-

Continued on next page

Humulin 50/50—Cont.

tions such as beta–blockers, changing insulin preparations, or intensified control (3 or more insulin injections per day) of diabetes.

A few patients who have experienced hypoglycemic reactions after transfer from animal–source insulin to human insulin have reported that the early warning symptoms of hypoglycemia were less pronounced or different from those experienced with their previous insulin.

Without recognition of early warning symptoms, you may not be able to take steps to avoid more serious hypoglycemia. Be alert for all of the various types of symptoms that may indicate hypoglycemia. Patients who experience hypoglycemia without early warning symptoms should monitor their blood glucose frequently, especially prior to activities such as driving. If the blood glucose is below your normal fasting glucose, you should consider eating or drinking sugar–containing foods to treat your hypoglycemia.

Mild to moderate hypoglycemia may be treated by eating foods or drinks that contain sugar. Patients should always carry a quick source of sugar, such as hard candy or glucose tablets. More severe hypoglycemia may require the assistance of another person. Patients who are unable to take sugar orally or who are unconscious require an injection of glucagon or should be treated with intravenous administration of glucose at a medical facility.

You should learn to recognize your own symptoms of hypoglycemia. If you are uncertain about these symptoms, you should monitor your blood glucose frequently to help you learn to recognize the symptoms that you experience with hypoglycemia.

If you have frequent episodes of hypoglycemia or experience difficulty in recognizing the symptoms, you should talk to your doctor to discuss possible changes in therapy, meal plans, and/or exercise programs to help you avoid hypoglycemia.

Hyperglycemia (High Blood Sugar) and Diabetic Ketoacidosis (DKA)

Hyperglycemia (too much glucose in the blood) may develop if your body has too little insulin.

Hyperglycemia can be brought about by any of the following:

1. Omitting your insulin or taking less than your doctor has prescribed.
2. Eating significantly more than your meal plan suggests.
3. Developing a fever, infection, or other significant stressful situation.

In patients with type 1 or insulin-dependent diabetes, prolonged hyperglycemia can result in DKA (a life-threatening emergency). The first symptoms of DKA usually come on gradually, over a period of hours or days, and include a drowsy feeling, flushed face, thirst, loss of appetite, and fruity odor on the breath. With DKA, blood and urine tests show large amounts of glucose and ketones. Heavy breathing and a rapid pulse are more severe symptoms. If uncorrected, prolonged hyperglycemia or DKA can lead to nausea, vomiting, stomach pain, dehydration, loss of consciousness, or death. Therefore, it is important that you obtain medical assistance immediately.

Lipodystrophy

Rarely, administration of insulin subcutaneously can result in lipoatrophy (seen as an apparent depression of the skin) or lipohypertrophy (seen as a raised area of the skin). If you notice either of these conditions, talk to your doctor. A change in your injection technique may help alleviate the problem.

Allergy

Local Allergy—Patients occasionally experience redness, swelling, and itching at the site of injection. This condition, called local allergy, usually clears up in a few days to a few weeks. In some instances, this condition may be related to factors other than insulin, such as irritants in the skin cleansing agent or poor injection technique. If you have local reactions, talk to your doctor.

Systemic Allergy—Less common, but potentially more serious, is generalized allergy to insulin, which may cause rash over the whole body, shortness of breath, wheezing, reduction in blood pressure, fast pulse, or sweating. Severe cases of generalized allergy may be life threatening. If you think

you are having a generalized allergic reaction to insulin, call your doctor immediately.

ADDITIONAL INFORMATION

Information about diabetes may be obtained from your diabetes educator.

Additional information about diabetes and Humulin can be obtained by calling The Lilly Answers Center at 1-800-LillyRx (1-800-545-5979) or by visiting www.LillyDiabetes.com.

Patient Information revised August 22, 2007

Vials manufactured by

Eli Lilly and Company, Indianapolis, IN 46285, USA or Lilly France, F-67640 Fegersheim, France

for Eli Lilly and Company, Indianapolis, IN 46285, USA

PV 5703 AMP

HUMULIN® 70/30   OTC

[hū'mŭ-lĭn]

70% HUMAN INSULIN ISOPHANE SUSPENSION
AND
30% HUMAN INSULIN INJECTION (rDNA ORIGIN)
100 UNITS PER ML (U-100)

INFORMATION FOR THE PATIENT
10 mL Vial (1000 Units per vial)

WARNINGS

THIS LILLY HUMAN INSULIN PRODUCT DIFFERS FROM ANIMAL-SOURCE INSULINS BECAUSE IT IS STRUCTURALLY IDENTICAL TO THE INSULIN PRODUCED BY YOUR BODY'S PANCREAS AND BECAUSE OF ITS UNIQUE MANUFACTURING PROCESS.

ANY CHANGE OF INSULIN SHOULD BE MADE CAUTIOUSLY AND ONLY UNDER MEDICAL SUPERVISION. CHANGES IN STRENGTH, MANUFACTURER, TYPE (E.G., REGULAR, NPH, ANALOG), SPECIES, OR METHOD OF MANUFACTURE MAY RESULT IN THE NEED FOR A CHANGE IN DOSAGE.

SOME PATIENTS TAKING HUMULIN® (HUMAN INSULIN, rDNA ORIGIN) MAY REQUIRE A CHANGE IN DOSAGE FROM THAT USED WITH OTHER INSULINS. IF AN ADJUSTMENT IS NEEDED, IT MAY OCCUR WITH THE FIRST DOSE OR DURING THE FIRST SEVERAL WEEKS OR MONTHS.

DIABETES

Insulin is a hormone produced by the pancreas, a large gland that lies near the stomach. This hormone is necessary for the body's correct use of food, especially sugar. Diabetes occurs when the pancreas does not make enough insulin to meet your body's needs.

To control your diabetes, your doctor has prescribed injections of insulin products to keep your blood glucose at a near–normal level. You have been instructed to test your blood and/or your urine regularly for glucose. Studies have shown that some chronic complications of diabetes such as eye disease, kidney disease, and nerve disease can be significantly reduced if the blood sugar is maintained as close to normal as possible. The American Diabetes Association recommends that if your pre–meal glucose levels are consistently above 130 mg/dL or your hemoglobin A_{1c} (HbA$_{1c}$) is more than 7%, you should talk to your doctor. A change in your diabetes therapy may be needed. If your blood tests consistently show below–normal glucose levels, you should also let your doctor know. Proper control of your diabetes requires close and constant cooperation with your doctor. Despite diabetes, you can lead an active and healthy life if you eat a balanced diet, exercise regularly, and take your insulin injections as prescribed by your doctor.

Always keep an extra supply of insulin as well as a spare syringe and needle on hand. Always wear diabetic identification so that appropriate treatment can be given if complications occur away from home.

70/30 HUMAN INSULIN
Description

Humulin is synthesized in a special non-disease-producing laboratory strain of *Escherichia coli* bacteria that has been genetically altered to produce human insulin. Humulin 70/30 is a mixture of 70% Human Insulin Isophane Suspension and 30% Human Insulin Injection (rDNA ori-

gin). It is an intermediate-acting insulin combined with the more rapid onset of action of Regular human insulin. The duration of activity may last up to 24 hours following injection. The time course of action of any insulin may vary considerably in different individuals or at different times in the same individual. As with all insulin preparations, the duration of action of Humulin 70/30 is dependent on dose, site of injection, blood supply, temperature, and physical activity. Humulin 70/30 is a sterile suspension and is for subcutaneous injection only. It should not be used intravenously or intramuscularly. The concentration of Humulin 70/30 is 100 units/mL (U-100).

Identification

Human insulin from Eli Lilly and Company has the trademark Humulin. Your doctor has prescribed the type of insulin that he/she believes is best for you.

DO NOT USE ANY OTHER INSULIN EXCEPT ON YOUR DOCTOR'S ADVICE AND DIRECTION.

Always check the carton and the bottle label for the name and letter designation of the insulin you receive from your pharmacy to make sure it is the same as prescribed by your doctor.

Always check the appearance of your bottle of Humulin 70/30 before withdrawing each dose. Before each injection the Humulin 70/30 bottle must be carefully shaken or rotated several times to completely mix the insulin. Humulin 70/30 suspension should look uniformly cloudy or milky after mixing. If not, repeat the above steps until contents are mixed.

Do not use Humulin 70/30:

- if the insulin substance (the white material) remains at the bottom of the bottle after mixing or
- if there are clumps in the insulin after mixing, or
- if solid white particles stick to the bottom or wall of the bottle, giving a frosted appearance.

If you see anything unusual in the appearance of Humulin 70/30 suspension in your bottle or notice your insulin requirements changing, talk to your doctor.

Storage

Not in-use (unopened): Humulin 70/30 bottles not in-use should be stored in a refrigerator, but not in the freezer.

In-use (opened): The Humulin 70/30 bottle you are currently using can be kept unrefrigerated as long as it is kept as cool as possible [below 86°F (30°C)] away from heat and light.

Do not use Humulin 70/30 after the expiration date stamped on the label or if it has been frozen.

INSTRUCTIONS FOR INSULIN VIAL USE

NEVER SHARE NEEDLES AND SYRINGES

Correct Syringe Type

Doses of insulin are measured in **units**. U-100 insulin contains 100 units/mL (1 mL=1 cc). With Humulin 70/30, it is important to use a syringe that is marked for U-100 insulin preparations. Failure to use the proper syringe can lead to a mistake in dosage, causing serious problems for you, such as a blood glucose level that is too low or too high.

Syringe Use

To help avoid contamination and possible infection, follow these instructions exactly.

Disposable syringes and needles should be used only once and then discarded by placing the used needle in a puncture-resistant disposable container. Properly dispose of the puncture-resistant container as directed by your Health Care Professional.

Preparing the Dose

1. Wash your hands.
2. Carefully shake or rotate the bottle of insulin several times to completely mix the insulin.
3. Inspect the insulin. Humulin 70/30 suspension should look uniformly cloudy or milky. Do not use Humulin 70/30 if you notice anything unusual in its appearance.
4. If using a new Humulin 70/30 bottle, flip off the plastic protective cap, but **do not** remove the stopper. Wipe the top of the bottle with an alcohol swab.
5. Draw an amount of air into the syringe that is equal to the Humulin 70/30 dose. Put the needle through rubber top of the Humulin 70/30 bottle and inject the air into the bottle.
6. Turn the Humulin 70/30 bottle and syringe upside down. Hold the bottle and syringe firmly in one hand and shake gently.

7. Making sure the tip of the needle is in the Humulin 70/30 suspension, withdraw the correct dose of Humulin 70/30 into the syringe.
8. Before removing the needle from the Humulin 70/30 bottle, check the syringe for air bubbles. If bubbles are present, hold the syringe straight up and tap its side until the bubbles float to the top. Push the bubbles out with the plunger and then withdraw the correct dose.
9. Remove the needle from the bottle and lay the syringe down so that the needle does not touch anything.

Injection Instructions

1. To avoid tissue damage, choose a site for each injection that is at least 1/2 inch from the previous injection site. The usual sites of injection are abdomen, thighs, and arms.
2. Cleanse the skin with alcohol where the injection is to be made.
3. With one hand, stabilize the skin by spreading it or pinching up a large area.
4. Insert the needle as instructed by your doctor.
5. Push the plunger in as far as it will go.
6. Pull the needle out and apply gentle pressure over the injection site for several seconds. **Do not rub the area.**
7. Place the used needle in a puncture-resistant disposable container and properly dispose of the puncture-resistant container as directed by your Health Care Professional.

DOSAGE

Your doctor has told you which insulin to use, how much, and when and how often to inject it. Because each patient's diabetes is different, this schedule has been individualized for you.

Your usual dose of Humulin 70/30 may be affected by changes in your diet, activity, or work schedule. Carefully follow your doctor's instructions to allow for these changes. Other things that may affect your Humulin 70/30 dose are:

Illness

Illness, especially with nausea and vomiting, may cause your insulin requirements to change. Even if you are not eating, you will still require insulin. You and your doctor should establish a sick day plan for you to use in case of illness. When you are sick, test your blood glucose frequently. If instructed by your doctor, test your ketones and report the results to your doctor.

Pregnancy

Good control of diabetes is especially important for you and your unborn baby. Pregnancy may make managing your diabetes more difficult. If you are planning to have a baby, are pregnant, or are nursing a baby, talk to your doctor.

Medication

Insulin requirements may be increased if you are taking other drugs with blood-glucose-raising activity, such as oral contraceptives, corticosteroids, or thyroid replacement therapy. Insulin requirements may be reduced in the presence of drugs that lower blood glucose or affect how your body responds to insulin, such as oral antidiabetic agents, salicylates (for example, aspirin), sulfa antibiotics, alcohol, certain antidepressants and some kidney and blood pressure medicines. Your Health Care Professional may be aware of other medications that may affect your diabetes control. Therefore, always discuss any medications you are taking with your doctor.

Exercise

Exercise may lower your body's need for insulin during and for some time after the physical activity. Exercise may also speed up the effect of an insulin dose, especially if the exercise involves the area of injection site (for example, the leg should not be used for injection just prior to running). Discuss with your doctor how you should adjust your insulin regimen to accommodate exercise.

Travel

When traveling across more than 2 time zones, you should talk to your doctor concerning adjustments in your insulin schedule.

COMMON PROBLEMS OF DIABETES

Hypoglycemia (Low Blood Sugar)

Hypoglycemia (too little glucose in the blood) is one of the most frequent adverse events experienced by insulin users. It can be brought about by:

1. **Missing or delaying meals.**
2. Taking too much insulin.

Continued on next page

Humulin 70/30—Cont.

3. Exercising or working more than usual.
4. An infection or illness associated with diarrhea or vomiting.
5. A change in the body's need for insulin.
6. Diseases of the adrenal, pituitary, or thyroid gland, or progression of kidney or liver disease.
7. Interactions with certain drugs, such as oral antidiabetic agents, salicylates (for example, aspirin), sulfa antibiotics, certain antidepressants and some kidney and blood pressure medicines.
8. Consumption of alcoholic beverages.

Symptoms of mild to moderate hypoglycemia may occur suddenly and can include:

• sweating	• drowsiness
• dizziness	• sleep disturbances
• palpitation	• anxiety
• tremor	• blurred vision
• hunger	• slurred speech
• restlessness	• depressed mood
• tingling in the hands, feet, lips, or tongue	• irritability
• lightheadedness	• abnormal behavior
• inability to concentrate	• unsteady movement
• headache	• personality changes

Signs of severe hypoglycemia can include:

• disorientation	• seizures
• unconsciousness	• death

Therefore, it is important that assistance be obtained immediately.

Early warning symptoms of hypoglycemia may be different or less pronounced under certain conditions, such as long duration of diabetes, diabetic nerve disease, use of medications such as beta-blockers, changing insulin preparations, or intensified control (3 or more insulin injections per day) of diabetes.

A few patients who have experienced hypoglycemic reactions after transfer from animal–source insulin to human insulin have reported that the early warning symptoms of hypoglycemia were less pronounced or different from those experienced with their previous insulin.

Without recognition of early warning symptoms, you may not be able to take steps to avoid more serious hypoglycemia. Be alert for all of the various types of symptoms that may indicate hypoglycemia. Patients who experience hypoglycemia without early warning symptoms should monitor their blood glucose frequently, especially prior to activities such as driving. If the blood glucose is below your normal fasting glucose, you should consider eating or drinking sugar–containing foods to treat your hypoglycemia.

Mild to moderate hypoglycemia may be treated by eating foods or drinks that contain sugar. Patients should always carry a quick source of sugar, such as hard candy or glucose tablets. More severe hypoglycemia may require the assistance of another person. Patients who are unable to take sugar orally or who are unconscious require an injection of glucagon or should be treated with intravenous administration of glucose at a medical facility.

You should learn to recognize your own symptoms of hypoglycemia. If you are uncertain about these symptoms, you should monitor your blood glucose frequently to help you learn to recognize the symptoms that you experience with hypoglycemia.

If you have frequent episodes of hypoglycemia or experience difficulty in recognizing the symptoms, you should talk to your doctor to discuss possible changes in therapy, meal plans, and/or exercise programs to help you avoid hypoglycemia.

Hyperglycemia (High Blood Sugar) and Diabetic Ketoacidosis (DKA)

Hyperglycemia (too much glucose in the blood) may develop if your body has too little insulin.

Hyperglycemia can be brought about by any of the following:
1. Omitting your insulin or taking less than your doctor has prescribed.
2. Eating significantly more than your meal plan suggests.
3. Developing a fever, infection, or other significant stressful situation.

In patients with type 1 or insulin-dependent diabetes, prolonged hyperglycemia can result in DKA (a life-threatening emergency). The first symptoms of DKA usually come on gradually, over a period of hours or days, and include a drowsy feeling, flushed face, thirst, loss of appetite, and fruity odor on the breath. With DKA, blood and urine tests show large amounts of glucose and ketones. Heavy breathing and a rapid pulse are more severe symptoms. If uncorrected, prolonged hyperglycemia or DKA can lead to nausea, vomiting, stomach pain, dehydration, loss of consciousness, or death. Therefore, it is important that you obtain medical assistance immediately.

Lipodystrophy

Rarely, administration of insulin subcutaneously can result in lipoatrophy (seen as an apparent depression of the skin) or lipohypertrophy (seen as a raised area of the skin). If you notice either of these conditions, talk to your doctor. A change in your injection technique may help alleviate the problem.

Allergy

Local Allergy — Patients occasionally experience redness, swelling, and itching at the site of injection. This condition, called local allergy, usually clears up in a few days to a few weeks. In some instances, this condition may be related to factors other than insulin, such as irritants in the skin cleansing agent or poor injection technique. If you have local reactions, talk to your doctor.

Systemic Allergy — Less common, but potentially more serious, is generalized allergy to insulin, which may cause rash over the whole body, shortness of breath, wheezing, reduction in blood pressure, fast pulse, or sweating. Severe cases of generalized allergy may be life threatening. If you think you are having a generalized allergic reaction to insulin, call your doctor immediately.

ADDITIONAL INFORMATION

Information about diabetes may be obtained from your diabetes educator.

Additional information about diabetes and Humulin can be obtained by calling The Lilly Answers Center at 1-800-LillyRx (1-800-545-5979) or by visiting www.Lilly-Diabetes.com.

Patient Information revised August 22, 2007

Vials manufactured by
Eli Lilly and Company, Indianapolis, IN 46285, USA or Lilly France, F-67640 Fegersheim, France
for Eli Lilly and Company, Indianapolis, IN 46285, USA
Copyright © 1992, 2007, Eli Lilly and Company. All rights reserved.
PV 5722 AMP

INFORMATION FOR THE PATIENT

3 ML PREFILLED INSULIN DELIVERY DEVICE
HUMULIN® 70/30 Pen
70% HUMAN INSULIN
ISOPHANE SUSPENSION
AND
30% HUMAN INSULIN INJECTION
(rDNA ORIGIN)
100 UNITS PER ML (U-100)
WARNINGS
THIS LILLY HUMAN INSULIN PRODUCT DIFFERS FROM ANIMAL-SOURCE INSULINS BECAUSE IT IS STRUCTURALLY IDENTICAL TO THE INSULIN PRODUCED BY YOUR BODY'S PANCREAS AND BECAUSE OF ITS UNIQUE MANUFACTURING PROCESS.

ANY CHANGE OF INSULIN SHOULD BE MADE CAUTIOUSLY AND ONLY UNDER MEDICAL SUPERVISION. CHANGES IN STRENGTH, MANUFACTURER, TYPE (E.G., REGULAR, NPH, ANALOG), SPECIES, OR METHOD OF MANUFACTURE MAY RESULT IN THE NEED FOR A CHANGE IN DOSAGE.

SOME PATIENTS TAKING HUMULIN® (HUMAN INSULIN, rDNA ORIGIN) MAY REQUIRE A CHANGE IN DOSAGE FROM THAT USED WITH OTHER INSULINS. IF AN ADJUST-

MENT IS NEEDED, IT MAY OCCUR WITH THE FIRST DOSE OR DURING THE FIRST SEVERAL WEEKS OR MONTHS.
TO OBTAIN AN ACCURATE DOSE, CAREFULLY READ AND FOLLOW THE INSULIN DELIVERY DEVICE USER MANUAL AND THIS "INFORMATION FOR THE PATIENT" INSERT BEFORE USING THIS PRODUCT.
THE PEN MUST BE PRIMED TO A STREAM OF INSULIN (NOT JUST A FEW DROPS) BEFORE EACH INJECTION, YOU SHOULD PRIME THE PEN, A NECESSARY STEP TO MAKE SURE THE PEN IS READY TO DOSE. YOU MAY NEED TO PRIME A NEW PEN UP TO SIX TIMES BEFORE A STREAM OF INSULIN APPEARS.
THE PEN IS IMPORTANT TO CONFIRM THAT INSULIN COMES OUT WHEN YOU PUSH THE INJECTION BUTTON AND TO REMOVE AIR THAT MAY COLLECT IN THE INSULIN CARTRIDGE DURING NORMAL USE. IF YOU DO NOT PRIME, YOU MAY RECEIVE TOO MUCH OR TOO LITTLE INSULIN (*see also* INSTRUCTIONS FOR INSULIN PEN USE section).

DIABETES

Insulin is a hormone produced by the pancreas, a large gland that lies near the stomach. This hormone is necessary for the body's correct use of food, especially sugar. Diabetes occurs when the pancreas does not make enough insulin to meet your body's needs.

To control your diabetes, your doctor has prescribed injections of insulin products to keep your blood glucose at a near-normal level. You have been instructed to test your blood and/or your urine regularly for glucose. Studies have shown that some chronic complications of diabetes such as eye disease, kidney disease, and nerve disease can be significantly reduced if the blood sugar is maintained as close to normal as possible. The American Diabetes Association recommends that if your pre-meal glucose levels are consistently above 130 mg/dL or your hemoglobin A_{1c} (HbA_{1c}) is more than 7%, you should talk to your doctor. A change in your diabetes therapy may be needed. If your blood tests consistently show below-normal glucose levels, you should also let your doctor know. Proper control of your diabetes requires close and constant cooperation with your doctor. Despite diabetes, you can lead an active and healthy life if you eat a balanced diet, exercise regularly, and take your insulin injections as prescribed by your doctor.

Always keep an extra supply of insulin as well as a spare syringe and needle on hand. Always wear diabetic identification so that appropriate treatment can be given if complications occur away from home.

70/30 HUMAN INSULIN

Description

Humulin is synthesized in a special non-disease-producing laboratory strain of *Escherichia coli* bacteria that has been genetically altered to produce human insulin. Humulin 70/30 is a mixture of 70% Human Insulin Isophane Suspension and 30% Human Insulin Injection, (rDNA origin). It is an intermediate-acting insulin combined with the more rapid onset of action of Regular human insulin. The duration of activity may last up to 24 hours following injection. The time course of action of any insulin may vary considerably in different individuals or at different times in the same individual. As with all insulin preparations, the duration of action of Humulin 70/30 is dependent on dose, site of injection, blood supply, temperature, and physical activity. Humulin 70/30 is a sterile suspension and is for subcutaneous injection only. It should not be used intravenously or intramuscularly. The concentration of Humulin 70/30 is 100 units/mL (U-100).

Identification

Human insulin from Eli Lilly and Company has the trademark Humulin.
Your doctor has prescribed the type of insulin that he/she believes is best for you.
DO NOT USE ANY OTHER INSULIN EXCEPT ON YOUR DOCTOR'S ADVICE AND DIRECTION.
The Humulin 70/30 Pen is available in boxes of 5 prefilled insulin delivery devices ("insulin Pens"). The Humulin 70/30 Pen is not designed to allow any other insulin to be mixed in its cartridge, or for the cartridge to be removed.
Always check the carton and the Pen label for the name and letter designation of the insulin you receive from your pharmacy to make sure it is the same as prescribed by your doctor.

Always check the appearance of Humulin 70/30 suspension in your insulin Pen before using. A cartridge of Humulin 70/30 contains a small glass bead to assist in mixing. Roll the Pen back and forth between the palms 10 times (see Figure 1). Holding Gently turn the Pen by one end, invert it 180° slowly up and down 10 times to allow until the small glass bead to travel the full length with each inversion insulin is evenly mixed (see Figure 2). Humulin 70/30 suspension should look uniformly cloudy or milky after mixing. If not evenly mixed, repeat the above steps until contents are mixed. Pens containing Humulin 70/30 suspension should be examined frequently.

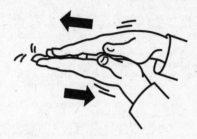

Figure 1

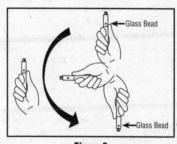

Figure 2

Do not use Humulin 70/30:
• if the insulin substance (the white material) remains visibly separated from the liquid after mixing or
• if there are clumps in the insulin after mixing, or
• if solid white particles stick to the walls of the cartridge, giving a frosted appearance.
If you see anything unusual in the appearance of the Humulin 70/30 suspension in your Pen or notice your insulin requirements changing, talk to your doctor.
Never attempt to remove the cartridge from the Humulin 70/30 Pen. Inspect the cartridge through the clear cartridge holder.

Storage

Not in-use (unopened): Humulin 70/30 Pens not in-use should be stored in a refrigerator, but not in the freezer.
In-use (opened): Humulin 70/30 Pens in-use should **NOT** be refrigerated but should be kept at room temperature [below 86°F (30°C)] away from direct heat and light. The Humulin 70/30 Pen you are currently using must be discarded **10 days** after the first use, even if it still contains Humulin 70/30.
Do not use Humulin 70/30 after the expiration date stamped on the label or if it has been frozen.

INSTRUCTIONS FOR INSULIN PEN USE

It is important to read, understand, and follow the instructions in the Insulin Delivery Device User Manual before using. Failure to follow instructions may result in getting too much or too little insulin. The needle must be changed and the Pen must be primed to a stream of insulin (not just a few drops) before each injection to make sure the Pen is ready to dose. You may need to prime a new Pen up to six times before a stream of insulin appears. Performing these steps before each injection is important to confirm that in-

Continued on next page

Humulin 70/30—Cont.

sulin comes out when you push the injection button, and to remove air that may collect in the insulin cartridge during normal use.

Every time you inject:
• **Use a new needle.**
• **Prime to a stream of insulin (not just a few drops) to make sure the Pen is ready to dose.**
• **Make sure you got your full dose.**
NEVER SHARE INSULIN PENS, CARTRIDGES, OR NEEDLES.

PREPARING FOR INJECTION
1. Wash your hands.
2. To avoid tissue damage, choose a site for each injection that is at least 1/2 inch from the previous injection site. The usual sites of injection are abdomen, thighs, and arms.
3. Follow the instructions in your Insulin Delivery Device User Manual to prepare for injection.
4. After injecting the dose, pull the needle out and apply gentle pressure over the injection site for several seconds. **Do not rub the area.**
5. After the injection, remove the needle from the Humulin 70/30 Pen. **Do not reuse needles.**
6. Place the used needle in a puncture-resistant disposable container and properly dispose of the puncture-resistant container as directed by your Health Care Professional.

DOSAGE
Your doctor has told you which insulin to use, how much, and when and how often to inject it. Because each patient's diabetes is different, this schedule has been individualized for you.

Your usual dose of Humulin 70/30 may be affected by changes in your diet, activity, or work schedule. Carefully follow your doctor's instructions to allow for these changes. Other things that may affect your Humulin 70/30 dose are:

Illness
Illness, especially with nausea and vomiting, may cause your insulin requirements to change. Even if you are not eating, you will still require insulin. You and your doctor should establish a sick day plan for you to use in case of illness. When you are sick, test your blood glucose frequently. If instructed by your doctor, test your ketones and report the results to your doctor.

Pregnancy
Good control of diabetes is especially important for you and your unborn baby. Pregnancy may make managing your diabetes more difficult. If you are planning to have a baby, are pregnant, or are nursing a baby, talk to your doctor.

Medication
Insulin requirements may be increased if you are taking other drugs with blood-glucose-raising activity, such as oral contraceptives, corticosteroids, or thyroid replacement therapy. Insulin requirements may be reduced in the presence of drugs that lower blood glucose or affect how your body responds to insulin, such as oral antidiabetic agents, salicylates (for example, aspirin), sulfa antibiotics, alcohol, certain antidepressants and some kidney and blood pressure medicines. Your Health Care Professional may be aware of other medications that may affect your diabetes control. Therefore, always discuss any medications you are taking with your doctor.

Exercise
Exercise may lower your body's need for insulin during and for some time after the physical activity. Exercise may also speed up the effect of an insulin dose, especially if the exercise involves the area of injection site (for example, the leg should not be used for injection just prior to running). Discuss with your doctor how you should adjust your insulin regimen to accommodate exercise.

Travel
When traveling across more than 2 time zones, you should talk to your doctor concerning adjustments in your insulin schedule.

COMMON PROBLEMS OF DIABETES
Hypoglycemia (Low Blood Sugar)
Hypoglycemia (too little glucose in the blood) is one of the most frequent adverse events experienced by insulin users. It can be brought about by:
1. **Missing or delaying meals.**
2. Taking too much insulin.

3. Exercising or working more than usual.
4. An infection or illness associated with diarrhea or vomiting.
5. A change in the body's need for insulin.
6. Diseases of the adrenal, pituitary, or thyroid gland, or progression of kidney or liver disease.
7. Interactions with certain drugs, such as oral antidiabetic agents, salicylates (for example, aspirin), sulfa antibiotics, certain antidepressants and some kidney and blood pressure medicines.
8. Consumption of alcoholic beverages.

Symptoms of mild to moderate hypoglycemia may occur suddenly and can include:

• sweating	• drowsiness
• dizziness	• sleep disturbances
• palpitation	• anxiety
• tremor	• blurred vision
• hunger	• slurred speech
• restlessness	• depressed mood
• tingling in the hands, feet, lips, or tongue	• irritability
• lightheadedness	• abnormal behavior
• inability to concentrate	• unsteady movement
• headache	• personality changes

Signs of severe hypoglycemia can include:

• disorientation	• seizures
• unconsciousness	• death

Therefore, it is important that assistance be obtained immediately.

Early warning symptoms of hypoglycemia may be different or less pronounced under certain conditions, such as long duration of diabetes, diabetic nerve disease, use of medications such as beta-blockers, changing insulin preparations, or intensified control (3 or more insulin injections per day) of diabetes.

A few patients who have experienced hypoglycemic reactions after transfer from animal-source insulin to human insulin have reported that the early warning symptoms of hypoglycemia were less pronounced or different from those experienced with their previous insulin.

Without recognition of early warning symptoms, you may not be able to take steps to avoid more serious hypoglycemia. Be alert for all of the various types of symptoms that may indicate hypoglycemia. Patients who experience hypoglycemia without early warning symptoms should monitor their blood glucose frequently, especially prior to activities such as driving. If the blood glucose is below your normal fasting glucose, you should consider eating or drinking sugar-containing foods to treat your hypoglycemia.

Mild to moderate hypoglycemia may be treated by eating foods or drinks that contain sugar. Patients should always carry a quick source of sugar, such as hard candy or glucose tablets. More severe hypoglycemia may require the assistance of another person. Patients who are unable to take sugar orally or who are unconscious require an injection of glucagon or should be treated with intravenous administration of glucose at a medical facility.

You should learn to recognize your own symptoms of hypoglycemia. If you are uncertain about these symptoms, you should monitor your blood glucose frequently to help you learn to recognize the symptoms that you experience with hypoglycemia.

If you have frequent episodes of hypoglycemia or experience difficulty in recognizing the symptoms, you should talk to your doctor to discuss possible changes in therapy, meal plans, and/or exercise programs to help you avoid hypoglycemia.

Hyperglycemia (High Blood Sugar) and Diabetic Ketoacidosis (DKA)
Hyperglycemia (too much glucose in the blood) may develop if your body has too little insulin.

Hyperglycemia can be brought about by any of the following:
1. Omitting your insulin or taking less than your doctor has prescribed.

2. Eating significantly more than your meal plan suggests.

3. Developing a fever, infection, or other significant stressful situation.

In patients with type 1 or insulin-dependent diabetes, prolonged hyperglycemia can result in DKA (a life-threatening emergency). The first symptoms of DKA usually come on gradually, over a period of hours or days, and include a drowsy feeling, flushed face, thirst, loss of appetite, and fruity odor on the breath. With DKA, blood and urine tests show large amounts of glucose and ketones. Heavy breathing and a rapid pulse are more severe symptoms. If uncorrected, prolonged hyperglycemia or DKA can lead to nausea, vomiting, stomach pain, dehydration, loss of consciousness, or death. Therefore, it is important that you obtain medical assistance immediately.

Lipodystrophy

Rarely, administration of insulin subcutaneously can result in lipoatrophy (seen as an apparent depression of the skin) or lipohypertrophy (seen as a raised area of the skin). If you notice either of these conditions, talk to your doctor. A change in your injection technique may help alleviate the problem.

Allergy

Local Allergy — Patients occasionally experience redness, swelling, and itching at the site of injection. This condition, called local allergy, usually clears up in a few days to a few weeks. In some instances, this condition may be related to factors other than insulin, such as irritants in the skin cleansing agent or poor injection technique. If you have local reactions, talk to your doctor.

Systemic Allergy — Less common, but potentially more serious, is generalized allergy to insulin, which may cause rash over the whole body, shortness of breath, wheezing, reduction in blood pressure, fast pulse, or sweating. Severe cases of generalized allergy may be life threatening. If you think you are having a generalized allergic reaction to insulin, call your doctor immediately.

ADDITIONAL INFORMATION

Information about diabetes may be obtained from your diabetes educator.

Additional information about diabetes and Humulin can be obtained by calling The Lilly Answers Center at 1-800-LillyRx (1-800-545-5979) or by visiting www.LillyDiabetes.com.

Patient Information revised March 16, 2009

Pens manufactured by

Eli Lilly and Company, Indianapolis, IN 46285, USA or Lilly France, F-67640 Fegersheim, France

for Eli Lilly and Company, Indianapolis, IN 46285, USA

Copyright © 1998, 2009, Eli Lilly and Company. All rights reserved.

PA 9147 FSAMP

HUMULIN® N   OTC

[hū ′mŭ-lĭn ĕn]

NPH

HUMAN INSULIN (rDNA ORIGIN)

ISOPHANE SUSPENSION

100 UNITS PER ML (U-100)

INFORMATION FOR THE PATIENT

10 mL Vial (1000 Units per vial)

WARNINGS

THIS LILLY HUMAN INSULIN PRODUCT DIFFERS FROM ANIMAL-SOURCE INSULINS BECAUSE IT IS STRUCTURALLY IDENTICAL TO THE INSULIN PRODUCED BY YOUR BODY'S PANCREAS AND BECAUSE OF ITS UNIQUE MANUFACTURING PROCESS.

ANY CHANGE OF INSULIN SHOULD BE MADE CAUTIOUSLY AND ONLY UNDER MEDICAL SUPERVISION. CHANGES IN STRENGTH, MANUFACTURER, TYPE (E.G., REGULAR, NPH, ANALOG), SPECIES, OR METHOD OF MANUFACTURE MAY RESULT IN THE NEED FOR A CHANGE IN DOSAGE.

SOME PATIENTS TAKING HUMULIN® (HUMAN INSULIN, rDNA ORIGIN) MAY REQUIRE A CHANGE IN DOSAGE FROM THAT USED WITH OTHER INSULINS. IF AN ADJUSTMENT IS NEEDED, IT MAY OCCUR WITH THE FIRST DOSE OR DURING THE FIRST SEVERAL WEEKS OR MONTHS.

DIABETES

Insulin is a hormone produced by the pancreas, a large gland that lies near the stomach. This hormone is necessary for the body's correct use of food, especially sugar. Diabetes occurs when the pancreas does not make enough insulin to meet your body's needs.

To control your diabetes, your doctor has prescribed injections of insulin products to keep your blood glucose at a near-normal level. You have been instructed to test your blood and/or your urine regularly for glucose. Studies have shown that some chronic complications of diabetes such as eye disease, kidney disease, and nerve disease can be significantly reduced if the blood sugar is maintained as close to normal as possible. The American Diabetes Association recommends that if your pre-meal glucose levels are consistently above 130 mg/dL or your hemoglobin A_{1c} (HbA_{1c}) is more than 7%, you should talk to your doctor. A change in your diabetes therapy may be needed. If your blood tests consistently show below-normal glucose levels, you should also let your doctor know. Proper control of your diabetes requires close and constant cooperation with your doctor. Despite diabetes, you can lead an active and healthy life if you eat a balanced diet, exercise regularly, and take your insulin injections as prescribed by your doctor.

Always keep an extra supply of insulin as well as a spare syringe and needle on hand. Always wear diabetic identification so that appropriate treatment can be given if complications occur away from home.

NPH HUMAN INSULIN

Description

Humulin is synthesized in a special non-disease-producing laboratory strain of *Escherichia coli* bacteria that has been genetically altered to produce human insulin. Humulin N [Human insulin (rDNA origin) isophane suspension] is a crystalline suspension of human insulin with protamine and zinc providing an intermediate-acting insulin with a slower onset of action and a longer duration of activity (up to 24 hours) than that of Regular human insulin. The time course of action of any insulin may vary considerably in different individuals or at different times in the same individual. As with all insulin preparations, the duration of action of Humulin N is dependent on dose, site of injection, blood supply, temperature, and physical activity. Humulin N is a sterile suspension and is for subcutaneous injection only. It should not be used intravenously or intramuscularly. The concentration of Humulin N is 100 units/mL (U-100).

Identification

Human insulin from Eli Lilly and Company has the trademark Humulin. Your doctor has prescribed the type of insulin that he/she believes is best for you.

DO NOT USE ANY OTHER INSULIN EXCEPT ON YOUR DOCTOR'S ADVICE AND DIRECTION.

Always check the carton and the bottle label for the name and letter designation of the insulin you receive from your pharmacy to make sure it is the same as prescribed by your doctor.

Always check the appearance of your bottle of Humulin N before withdrawing each dose. Before each injection the Humulin N bottle must be carefully shaken or rotated several times to completely mix the insulin. Humulin N suspension should look uniformly cloudy or milky after mixing. If not, repeat the above steps until contents are mixed. Do not use Humulin N:

• if the insulin substance (the white material) remains at the bottom of the bottle after mixing or

• if there are clumps in the insulin after mixing, or

• if solid white particles stick to the bottom or wall of the bottle, giving a frosted appearance.

If you see anything unusual in the appearance of Humulin N suspension in your bottle or notice your insulin requirements changing, talk to your doctor.

Storage

Not in-use (unopened): Humulin N bottles not in-use should be stored in a refrigerator, but not in the freezer.

In-use (opened): The Humulin N bottle you are currently using can be kept unrefrigerated as long as it is kept as cool as possible [below 86°F (30°C)] away from heat and light.

Do not use Humulin N after the expiration date stamped on the label or if it has been frozen.

Continued on next page

Humulin N Pen—Cont.

INSTRUCTIONS FOR INSULIN VIAL USE
NEVER SHARE NEEDLES AND SYRINGES.

Correct Syringe Type
Doses of insulin are measured in **units**. U-100 insulin contains 100 units/mL (1 mL=1 cc). With Humulin N, it is important to use a syringe that is marked for U-100 insulin preparations. Failure to use the proper syringe can lead to a mistake in dosage, causing serious problems for you, such as a blood glucose level that is too low or too high.

Syringe Use
To help avoid contamination and possible infection, follow these instructions exactly.

Disposable syringes and needles should be used only once and then discarded by placing the used needle in a puncture-resistant disposable container. Properly dispose of the puncture-resistant container as directed by your Health Care Professional.

Preparing the Dose
1. Wash your hands.
2. Carefully shake or rotate the bottle of insulin several times to completely mix the insulin.
3. Inspect the insulin. Humulin N suspension should look uniformly cloudy or milky. Do not use Humulin N if you notice anything unusual in its appearance.
4. If using a new Humulin N bottle, flip off the plastic protective cap, but **do not** remove the stopper. Wipe the top of the bottle with an alcohol swab.
5. If you are mixing insulins, refer to the "Mixing Humulin N and Regular Human Insulin"section below.
6. Draw an amount of air into the syringe that is equal to the Humulin N dose. Put the needle through rubber top of the Humulin N bottle and inject the air into the bottle.
7. Turn the Humulin N bottle and syringe upside down. Hold the bottle and syringe firmly in one hand and shake gently.
8. Making sure the tip of the needle is in the Humulin N suspension, withdraw the correct dose of Humulin N into the syringe.
9. Before removing the needle from the Humulin N bottle, check the syringe for air bubbles. If bubbles are present, hold the syringe straight up and tap its side until the bubbles float to the top. Push the bubbles out with the plunger and then withdraw the correct dose.
10. Remove the needle from the bottle and lay the syringe down so that the needle does not touch anything.
11. If you do not need to mix your Humulin N with Regular human insulin, go to the "Injection Instructions"section below and follow the directions.

Mixing Humulin N and Regular Human Insulin (Humulin R)
1. Humulin N should be mixed with Humulin R only on the advice of your doctor.
2. Draw an amount of air into the syringe that is equal to the amount of Humulin N you are taking. Insert the needle into the Humulin N bottle and inject the air. Withdraw the needle.
3. Draw an amount of air into the syringe that is equal to the amount of Humulin R you are taking. Insert the needle into the Humulin R bottle and inject the air, but **do not** withdraw the needle.
4. Turn the Humulin R bottle and syringe upside down.
5. Making sure the tip of the needle is in the Humulin R solution, withdraw the correct dose of Humulin R into the syringe.
6. Before removing the needle from the Humulin R bottle, check the syringe for air bubbles. If bubbles are present, hold the syringe straight up and tap its side until the bubbles float to the top. Push the bubbles out with the plunger and then withdraw the correct dose.
7. Remove the syringe with the needle from the Humulin R bottle and insert it into the Humulin N bottle. Turn the Humulin N bottle and syringe upside down. Hold the bottle and syringe firmly in one hand and shake gently. Making sure the tip of the needle is in the Humulin N, withdraw the correct dose of Humulin N.
8. Remove the needle from the bottle and lay the syringe down so that the needle does not touch anything.
9. Follow the directions under "Injection Instructions" section below.

Follow your doctor's instructions on whether to mix your insulins ahead of time or just before giving your injection. It is important to be consistent in your method.

Syringes from different manufacturers may vary in the amount of space between the bottom line and the needle. Because of this, do not change:
• the sequence of mixing, or
• the model and brand of syringe or needle that your doctor has prescribed.

Injection Instructions
1. To avoid tissue damage, choose a site for each injection that is at least 1/2 inch from the previous injection site. The usual sites of injection are abdomen, thighs, and arms.
2. Cleanse the skin with alcohol where the injection is to be made.
3. With one hand, stabilize the skin by spreading it or pinching up a large area.
4. Insert the needle as instructed by your doctor.
5. Push the plunger in as far as it will go.
6. Pull the needle out and apply gentle pressure over the injection site for several seconds. **Do not rub the area**.
7. Place the used needle in a puncture-resistant disposable container and properly dispose of the puncture-resistant container as directed by your Health Care Professional.

DOSAGE
Your doctor has told you which insulin to use, how much, and when and how often to inject it. Because each patient's diabetes is different, this schedule has been individualized for you.

Your usual dose of Humulin N may be affected by changes in your diet, activity, or work schedule. Carefully follow your doctor's instructions to allow for these changes. Other things that may affect your Humulin N dose are:

Illness
Illness, especially with nausea and vomiting, may cause your insulin requirements to change. Even if you are not eating, you will still require insulin. You and your doctor should establish a sick day plan for you to use in case of illness. When you are sick, test your blood glucose frequently. If instructed by your doctor, test your ketones and report the results to your doctor.

Pregnancy
Good control of diabetes is especially important for you and your unborn baby. Pregnancy may make managing your diabetes more difficult. If you are planning to have a baby, are pregnant, or are nursing a baby, talk to your doctor.

Medication
Insulin requirements may be increased if you are taking other drugs with blood-glucose-raising activity, such as oral contraceptives, corticosteroids, or thyroid replacement therapy. Insulin requirements may be reduced in the presence of drugs that lower blood glucose or affect how your body responds to insulin, such as oral antidiabetic agents, salicylates (for example, aspirin), sulfa antibiotics, alcohol, certain antidepressants and some kidney and blood pressure medicines. Your Health Care Professional may be aware of other medications that may affect your diabetes control. Therefore, always discuss any medications you are taking with your doctor.

Exercise
Exercise may lower your body's need for insulin during and for some time after the physical activity. Exercise may also speed up the effect of an insulin dose, especially if the exercise involves the area of injection site (for example, the leg should not be used for injection just prior to running). Discuss with your doctor how you should adjust your insulin regimen to accommodate exercise.

Travel
When traveling across more than 2 time zones, you should talk to your doctor concerning adjustments in your insulin schedule.

COMMON PROBLEMS OF DIABETES
Hypoglycemia (Low Blood Sugar)
Hypoglycemia (too little glucose in the blood) is one of the most frequent adverse events experienced by insulin users. It can be brought about by:
1. **Missing or delaying meals.**
2. Taking too much insulin.
3. Exercising or working more than usual.

4. An infection or illness associated with diarrhea or vomiting.
5. A change in the body's need for insulin.
6. Diseases of the adrenal, pituitary, or thyroid gland, or progression of kidney or liver disease.
7. Interactions with certain drugs, such as oral antidiabetic agents, salicylates (for example, aspirin), sulfa antibiotics, certain antidepressants and some kidney and blood pressure medicines.
8. Consumption of alcoholic beverages.

Symptoms of mild to moderate hypoglycemia may occur suddenly and can include:

• sweating	• drowsiness
• dizziness	• sleep disturbances
• palpitation	• anxiety
• tremor	• blurred vision
• hunger	• slurred speech
• restlessness	• depressed mood
• tingling in the hands, feet, lips, or tongue	• irritability
	• abnormal behavior
• lightheadedness	• unsteady movement
• inability to concentrate	• personality changes
• headache	

Signs of severe hypoglycemia can include:

• disorientation	• seizures
• unconsciousness	• death

Therefore, it is important that assistance be obtained immediately.

Early warning symptoms of hypoglycemia may be different or less pronounced under certain conditions, such as long duration of diabetes, diabetic nerve disease, use of medications such as beta–blockers, changing insulin preparations, or intensified control (3 or more insulin injections per day) of diabetes.

A few patients who have experienced hypoglycemic reactions after transfer from animal–source insulin to human insulin have reported that the early warning symptoms of hypoglycemia were less pronounced or different from those experienced with their previous insulin.

Without recognition of early warning symptoms, you may not be able to take steps to avoid more serious hypoglycemia. Be alert for all of the various types of symptoms that may indicate hypoglycemia. Patients who experience hypoglycemia without early warning symptoms should monitor their blood glucose frequently, especially prior to activities such as driving. If the blood glucose is below your normal fasting glucose, you should consider eating or drinking sugar–containing foods to treat your hypoglycemia.

Mild to moderate hypoglycemia may be treated by eating foods or drinks that contain sugar. Patients should always carry a quick source of sugar, such as hard candy or glucose tablets. More severe hypoglycemia may require the assistance of another person. Patients who are unable to take sugar orally or who are unconscious require an injection of glucagon or should be treated with intravenous administration of glucose at a medical facility.

You should learn to recognize your own symptoms of hypoglycemia. If you are uncertain about these symptoms, you should monitor your blood glucose frequently to help you learn to recognize the symptoms that you experience with hypoglycemia.

If you have frequent episodes of hypoglycemia or experience difficulty in recognizing the symptoms, you should talk to your doctor to discuss possible changes in therapy, meal plans, and/or exercise programs to help you avoid hypoglycemia.

Hyperglycemia (High Blood Sugar) and Diabetic Ketoacidosis (DKA)

Hyperglycemia (too much glucose in the blood) may develop if your body has too little insulin.

Hyperglycemia can be brought about by any of the following:

1. Omitting your insulin or taking less than your doctor has prescribed.
2. Eating significantly more than your meal plan suggests.

3. Developing a fever, infection, or other significant stressful situation.

In patients with type 1 or insulin-dependent diabetes, prolonged hyperglycemia can result in DKA (a life-threatening emergency). The first symptoms of DKA usually come on gradually, over a period of hours or days, and include a drowsy feeling, flushed face, thirst, loss of appetite, and fruity odor on the breath. With DKA, blood and urine tests show large amounts of glucose and ketones. Heavy breathing and a rapid pulse are more severe symptoms. If uncorrected, prolonged hyperglycemia or DKA can lead to nausea, vomiting, stomach pain, dehydration, loss of consciousness, or death. Therefore, it is important that you obtain medical assistance immediately.

Lipodystrophy

Rarely, administration of insulin subcutaneously can result in lipoatrophy (seen as an apparent depression of the skin) or lipohypertrophy (seen as a raised area of the skin). If you notice either of these conditions, talk to your doctor. A change in your injection technique may help alleviate the problem.

Allergy

Local Allergy—Patients occasionally experience redness, swelling, and itching at the site of injection. This condition, called local allergy, usually clears up in a few days to a few weeks. In some instances, this condition may be related to factors other than insulin, such as irritants in the skin cleansing agent or poor injection technique. If you have local reactions, talk to your doctor.

Systemic Allergy—Less common, but potentially more serious, is generalized allergy to insulin, which may cause rash over the whole body, shortness of breath, wheezing, reduction in blood pressure, fast pulse, or sweating. Severe cases of generalized allergy may be life threatening. If you think you are having a generalized allergic reaction to insulin, call your doctor immediately.

ADDITIONAL INFORMATION

Information about diabetes may be obtained from your diabetes educator.

Additional information about diabetes and Humulin can be obtained by calling The Lilly Answers Center at 1-800-LillyRx · (1-800-545-5979) or by visiting www.LillyDiabetes.com.

Patient Information revised August 22, 2007

Vials manufactured by

Eli Lilly and Company, Indianapolis, IN 46285, USA or Lilly France, F-67640 Fegersheim, France

for Eli Lilly and Company, Indianapolis, IN 46285, USA

Copyright © 1997, 2007, Eli Lilly and Company. All rights reserved.

PV 5712 AMP

INFORMATION FOR THE PATIENT

3 ML PREFILLED INSULIN DELIVERY DEVICE

HUMULIN® N Pen

NPH

HUMAN INSULIN

(rDNA ORIGIN) ISOPHANE SUSPENSION

100 UNITS PER ML (U-100)

WARNINGS

THIS LILLY HUMAN INSULIN PRODUCT DIFFERS FROM ANIMAL–SOURCE INSULINS BECAUSE IT IS STRUCTURALLY IDENTICAL TO THE INSULIN PRODUCED BY YOUR BODY'S PANCREAS AND BECAUSE OF ITS UNIQUE MANUFACTURING PROCESS.

ANY CHANGE OF INSULIN SHOULD BE MADE CAUTIOUSLY AND ONLY UNDER MEDICAL SUPERVISION. CHANGES IN STRENGTH, MANUFACTURER, TYPE (E.G., REGULAR, NPH, ANALOG), SPECIES, OR METHOD OF MANUFACTURE MAY RESULT IN THE NEED FOR A CHANGE IN DOSAGE.

SOME PATIENTS TAKING HUMULIN® (HUMAN INSULIN, rDNA ORIGIN) MAY REQUIRE A CHANGE IN DOSAGE FROM THAT USED WITH OTHER INSULINS. IF AN ADJUSTMENT IS NEEDED, IT MAY OCCUR WITH THE FIRST DOSE OR DURING THE FIRST SEVERAL WEEKS OR MONTHS.

TO OBTAIN AN ACCURATE DOSE, CAREFULLY READ AND FOLLOW THE INSULIN DELIVERY DEVICE USER MANUAL AND THIS "INFORMATION FOR THE PATIENT" INSERT BE-

Continued on next page

Humulin N Pen—Cont.

FORE USING THIS PRODUCT. THE PEN MUST BE PRIMED TO A STREAM OF INSULIN (NOT JUST A FEW DROPS) BEFORE EACH INJECTION TO MAKE SURE THE PEN IS READY TO DOSE. YOU MAY NEED TO PRIME A NEW PEN UP TO SIX TIMES BEFORE A STREAM OF INSULIN APPEARS.

PRIMING THE PEN IS IMPORTANT TO CONFIRM THAT INSULIN COMES OUT WHEN YOU PUSH THE INJECTION BUTTON AND TO REMOVE AIR THAT MAY COLLECT IN THE INSULIN CARTRIDGE DURING NORMAL USE. IF YOU DO NOT PRIME, YOU MAY RECEIVE TOO MUCH OR TOO LITTLE INSULIN *(see also* INSTRUCTIONS FOR INSULIN PEN USE section).

DIABETES

Insulin is a hormone produced by the pancreas, a large gland that lies near the stomach. This hormone is necessary for the body's correct use of food, especially sugar. Diabetes occurs when the pancreas does not make enough insulin to meet your body's needs.

To control your diabetes, your doctor has prescribed injections of insulin products to keep your blood glucose at a near–normal level. You have been instructed to test your blood and/or your urine regularly for glucose. Studies have shown that some chronic complications of diabetes such as eye disease, kidney disease, and nerve disease can be significantly reduced if the blood sugar is maintained as close to normal as possible. The American Diabetes Association recommends that if your pre-meal glucose levels are consistently above 130 mg/dL or your hemoglobin A_{1c} (HbA_{1c}) is more than 7%, you should talk to your doctor. A change in your diabetes therapy may be needed. If your blood tests consistently show below-normal glucose levels, you should also let your doctor know. Proper control of your diabetes requires close and constant cooperation with your doctor. Despite diabetes, you can lead an active and healthy life if you eat a balanced diet, exercise regularly, and take your insulin injections as prescribed by your doctor.

Always keep an extra supply of insulin as well as a spare syringe and needle on hand. Always wear diabetic identification so that appropriate treatment can be given if complications occur away from home.

NPH HUMAN INSULIN

Description

Humulin is synthesized in a special non-disease-producing laboratory strain of *Escherichia coli* bacteria that has been genetically altered to produce human insulin. Humulin N [Human insulin (rDNA origin) isophane suspension] is a crystalline suspension of human insulin with protamine and zinc providing an intermediate-acting insulin with a slower onset of action and a longer duration of activity (up to 24 hours) than that of Regular human insulin. The time course of action of any insulin may vary considerably in different individuals or at different times in the same individual. As with all insulin preparations, the duration of action of Humulin N is dependent on dose, site of injection, blood supply, temperature, and physical activity. Humulin N is a sterile suspension and is for subcutaneous injection only. It should not be used intravenously or intramuscularly. The concentration of Humulin N is 100 units/mL (U-100).

Identification

Human insulin from Eli Lilly and Company has the trademark Humulin. Your doctor has prescribed the type of insulin that he/she believes is best for you.

DO NOT USE ANY OTHER INSULIN EXCEPT ON YOUR DOCTOR'S ADVICE AND DIRECTION.

The Humulin N Pen is available in boxes of 5 prefilled insulin delivery devices ("insulin Pens"). The Humulin N Pen is not designed to allow any other insulin to be mixed in its cartridge, or for the cartridge to be removed.

Always check the carton and the Pen label for the name and letter designation of the insulin you receive from your pharmacy to make sure it is the same as prescribed by your doctor.

Always check the appearance of Humulin N suspension in your insulin Pen before using. A cartridge of Humulin N contains a small glass bead to assist in mixing. Roll the Pen back and forth between the palms 10 times (see Figure 1). Gently turn the Pen up and down 10 times until the insulin

is evenly mixed (see Figure 2). If not evenly mixed, repeat the above steps until contents are mixed. Pens containing Humulin N suspension should be examined frequently.

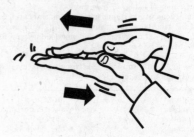

Figure 1.

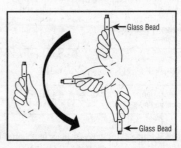

Figure 2.

Do not use Humulin N:
- if the insulin substance (the white material) remains visibly separated from the liquid after mixing or
- if there are clumps in the insulin after mixing, or
- if solid white particles stick to the walls of the cartridge, giving a frosted appearance.

If you see anything unusual in the appearance of the Humulin N suspension in your Pen or notice your insulin requirements changing, talk to your doctor.

Never attempt to remove the cartridge from the Humulin N Pen. Inspect the cartridge through the clear cartridge holder.

Storage

Not in-use (unopened): Humulin N Pens not in-use should be stored in a refrigerator, but not in the freezer.

In-use (opened): Humulin N Pens in-use should **NOT** be refrigerated but should be kept at room temperature [below 86°F (30°C)] away from direct heat and light. The Humulin N Pen you are currently using must be discarded **2 weeks** after the first use, even if it still contains Humulin N.

Do not use Humulin N after the expiration date stamped on the label or if it has been frozen.

INSTRUCTIONS FOR INSULIN PEN USE

It is important to read, understand, and follow the instructions in the Insulin Delivery Device User Manual before using. Failure to follow instructions may result in getting too much or too little insulin. The needle must be changed and the Pen must be primed to a stream of insulin (not just a few drops) before each injection to make sure the Pen is ready to dose. You may need to prime a new Pen up to six times before a stream of insulin appears. Performing these steps before each injection is important to confirm that insulin comes out when you push the injection button, and to remove air that may collect in the insulin cartridge during normal use.

Every time you inject:
- Use a new needle.
- Prime to a stream of insulin (not just a few drops) to make sure the Pen is ready to dose.
- Make sure you got your full dose.

NEVER SHARE INSULIN PENS, CARTRIDGES, OR NEEDLES.

PREPARING FOR INJECTION

1. Wash your hands.
2. To avoid tissue damage, choose a site for each injection that is at least 1/2 inch from the previous injection site.

The usual sites of injection are abdomen, thighs, and arms.

3. Follow the instructions in your Insulin Delivery Device User Manual to prepare for injection.

4. After injecting the dose, pull the needle out and apply gentle pressure over the injection site for several seconds. **Do not rub the area.**

5. After the injection, remove the needle from the Humulin N Pen. **Do not reuse needles.**

6. Place the used needle in a puncture-resistant disposable container and properly dispose of the puncture-resistant container as directed by your Health Care Professional.

DOSAGE

Your doctor has told you which insulin to use, how much, and when and how often to inject it. Because each patient's diabetes is different, this schedule has been individualized for you.

Your usual dose of Humulin N may be affected by changes in your diet, activity, or work schedule. Carefully follow your doctor's instructions to allow for these changes. Other things that may affect your Humulin N dose are:

Illness

Illness, especially with nausea and vomiting, may cause your insulin requirements to change. Even if you are not eating, you will still require insulin. You and your doctor should establish a sick day plan for you to use in case of illness. When you are sick, test your blood glucose frequently. If instructed by your doctor, test your ketones and report the results to your doctor.

Pregnancy

Good control of diabetes is especially important for you and your unborn baby. Pregnancy may make managing your diabetes more difficult. If you are planning to have a baby, are pregnant, or are nursing a baby, talk to your doctor.

Medication

Insulin requirements may be increased if you are taking other drugs with blood-glucose-raising activity, such as oral contraceptives, corticosteroids, or thyroid replacement therapy. Insulin requirements may be reduced in the presence of drugs that lower blood glucose or affect how your body responds to insulin, such as oral antidiabetic agents, salicylates (for example, aspirin), sulfa antibiotics, alcohol, certain antidepressants and some kidney and blood pressure medicines. Your Health Care Professional may be aware of other medications that may affect your diabetes control. Therefore, always discuss any medications you are taking with your doctor.

Exercise

Exercise may lower your body's need for insulin during and for some time after the physical activity. Exercise may also speed up the effect of an insulin dose, especially if the exercise involves the area of injection site (for example, the leg should not be used for injection just prior to running). Discuss with your doctor how you should adjust your insulin regimen to accommodate exercise.

Travel

When traveling across more than 2 time zones, you should talk to your doctor concerning adjustments in your insulin schedule.

COMMON PROBLEMS OF DIABETES

Hypoglycemia (Low Blood Sugar)

Hypoglycemia (too little glucose in the blood) is one of the most frequent adverse events experienced by insulin users. It can be brought about by:

1. **Missing or delaying meals.**
2. Taking too much insulin.
3. Exercising or working more than usual.
4. An infection or illness associated with diarrhea or vomiting.
5. A change in the body's need for insulin.
6. Diseases of the adrenal, pituitary, or thyroid gland, or progression of kidney or liver disease.
7. Interactions with certain drugs, such as oral antidiabetic agents, salicylates (for example, aspirin), sulfa antibiotics, certain antidepressants and some kidney and blood pressure medicines.
8. Consumption of alcoholic beverages.

Symptoms of mild to moderate hypoglycemia may occur suddenly and can include:

- sweating
- dizziness
- palpitation
- tremor
- hunger
- restlessness
- tingling in the hands, feet, lips, or tongue
- lightheadedness
- inability to concentrate
- headache
- drowsiness
- sleep disturbances
- anxiety
- blurred vision
- slurred speech
- depressed mood
- irritability
- abnormal behavior
- unsteady movement
- personality changes

Signs of severe hypoglycemia can include:

- disorientation
- unconsciousness
- seizures
- death

Therefore, it is important that assistance be obtained immediately.

Early warning symptoms of hypoglycemia may be different or less pronounced under certain conditions, such as long duration of diabetes, diabetic nerve disease, use of medications such as beta-blockers, changing insulin preparations, or intensified control (3 or more insulin injections per day) of diabetes.

A few patients who have experienced hypoglycemic reactions after transfer from animal-source insulin to human insulin have reported that the early warning symptoms of hypoglycemia were less pronounced or different from those experienced with their previous insulin.

Without recognition of early warning symptoms, you may not be able to take steps to avoid more serious hypoglycemia. Be alert for all of the various types of symptoms that may indicate hypoglycemia. Patients who experience hypoglycemia without early warning symptoms should monitor their blood glucose frequently, especially prior to activities such as driving. If the blood glucose is below your normal fasting glucose, you should consider eating or drinking sugar-containing foods to treat your hypoglycemia.

Mild to moderate hypoglycemia may be treated by eating foods or drinks that contain sugar. Patients should always carry a quick source of sugar, such as hard candy or glucose tablets. More severe hypoglycemia may require the assistance of another person. Patients who are unable to take sugar orally or who are unconscious require an injection of glucagon or should be treated with intravenous administration of glucose at a medical facility.

You should learn to recognize your own symptoms of hypoglycemia. If you are uncertain about these symptoms, you should monitor your blood glucose frequently to help you learn to recognize the symptoms that you experience with hypoglycemia.

If you have frequent episodes of hypoglycemia or experience difficulty in recognizing the symptoms, you should talk to your doctor to discuss possible changes in therapy, meal plans, and/or exercise programs to help you avoid hypoglycemia.

Hyperglycemia (High Blood Sugar) and Diabetic Ketoacidosis (DKA)

Hyperglycemia (too much glucose in the blood) may develop if your body has too little insulin.

Hyperglycemia can be brought about by any of the following:

1. Omitting your insulin or taking less than your doctor has prescribed.
2. Eating significantly more than your meal plan suggests.
3. Developing a fever, infection, or other significant stressful situation.

In patients with type 1 or insulin-dependent diabetes, prolonged hyperglycemia can result in DKA (a life-threatening emergency). The first symptoms of DKA usually come on gradually, over a period of hours or days, and include a drowsy feeling, flushed face, thirst, loss of appetite, and fruity odor on the breath. With DKA, blood and urine tests show large amounts of glucose and ketones. Heavy breathing and a rapid pulse are more severe symptoms. If uncor-

Continued on next page

Humulin N Pen—Cont.

rected, prolonged hyperglycemia or DKA can lead to nausea, vomiting, stomach pain, dehydration, loss of consciousness, or death. Therefore, it is important that you obtain medical assistance immediately.

Lipodystrophy

Rarely, administration of insulin subcutaneously can result in lipoatrophy (seen as an apparent depression of the skin) or lipohypertrophy (seen as a raised area of the skin). If you notice either of these conditions, talk to your doctor. A change in your injection technique may help alleviate the problem.

Allergy

Local Allergy—Patients occasionally experience redness, swelling, and itching at the site of injection. This condition, called local allergy, usually clears up in a few days to a few weeks. In some instances, this condition may be related to factors other than insulin, such as irritants in the skin cleansing agent or poor injection technique. If you have local reactions, talk to your doctor.

Systemic Allergy—Less common, but potentially more serious, is generalized allergy to insulin, which may cause rash over the whole body, shortness of breath, wheezing, reduction in blood pressure, fast pulse, or sweating. Severe cases of generalized allergy may be life threatening. If you think you are having a generalized allergic reaction to insulin, call your doctor immediately.

ADDITIONAL INFORMATION

Information about diabetes may be obtained from your diabetes educator.

Additional information about diabetes and Humulin can be obtained by calling The Lilly Answers Center at 1-800-LillyRx (1-800-545-5979) or by visiting www.LillyDiabetes.com.

Patient Information revised March 16, 2009

Pens manufactured by

Eli Lilly and Company, Indianapolis, IN 46285, USA or Lilly France, F-67640 Fegersheim, France

for Eli Lilly and Company, Indianapolis, IN 46285, USA

Copyright © 1998, 2009, Eli Lilly and Company. All rights reserved.

PA 9135 FSAMP

HUMULIN® R REGULAR   OTC

[hū' mŭ-lĭn-ŭ]

INSULIN HUMAN INJECTION, USP (rDNA origin)
100 UNITS PER ML (U-100)

INFORMATION FOR THE PATIENT
10 mL Vial (100 Units per vial)

WARNINGS

THIS LILLY HUMAN INSULIN PRODUCT DIFFERS FROM ANIMAL-SOURCE INSULINS BECAUSE IT IS STRUCTURALLY IDENTICAL TO THE INSULIN PRODUCED BY YOUR BODY'S PANCREAS AND BECAUSE OF ITS UNIQUE MANUFACTURING PROCESS.

ANY CHANGE OF INSULIN SHOULD BE MADE CAUTIOUSLY AND ONLY UNDER MEDICAL SUPERVISION. CHANGES IN STRENGTH, MANUFACTURER, TYPE (E.G., REGULAR, NPH, ANALOG), SPECIES, OR METHOD OF MANUFACTURE MAY RESULT IN THE NEED FOR A CHANGE IN DOSAGE.

SOME PATIENTS TAKING HUMULIN® (HUMAN INSULIN, rDNA ORIGIN) MAY REQUIRE A CHANGE IN DOSAGE FROM THAT USED WITH OTHER INSULINS. IF AN ADJUSTMENT IS NEEDED, IT MAY OCCUR WITH THE FIRST DOSE OR DURING THE FIRST SEVERAL WEEKS OR MONTHS.

DIABETES

Insulin is a hormone produced by the pancreas, a large gland that lies near the stomach. This hormone is necessary for the body's correct use of food, especially sugar. Diabetes occurs when the pancreas does not make enough insulin to meet your body's needs.

To control your diabetes, your doctor has prescribed injections of insulin products to keep your blood glucose at a near-normal level. You have been instructed to test your blood and/or your urine regularly for glucose. Studies have

shown that some chronic complications of diabetes such as eye disease, kidney disease, and nerve disease can be significantly reduced if the blood sugar is maintained as close to normal as possible. The American Diabetes Association recommends that if your pre-meal glucose levels are consistently above 130 mg/dL or your hemoglobin A_{1c} (HbA_{1c}) is more than 7%, you should talk to your doctor. A change in your diabetes therapy may be needed. If your blood tests consistently show below-normal glucose levels, you should also let your doctor know. Proper control of your diabetes requires close and constant cooperation with your doctor. Despite diabetes, you can lead an active and healthy life if you eat a balanced diet, exercise regularly, and take your insulin injections as prescribed by your doctor.

Always keep an extra supply of insulin as well as a spare syringe and needle on hand. Always wear diabetic identification so that appropriate treatment can be given if complications occur away from home.

REGULAR HUMAN INSULIN

Description

Humulin is synthesized in a special non-disease-producing laboratory strain of *Escherichia coli* bacteria that has been genetically altered to produce human insulin. Humulin R [Regular insulin human injection, USP (rDNA origin)] consists of zinc-insulin crystals dissolved in a clear fluid. Humulin R has had nothing added to change the speed or length of its action. It takes effect rapidly and has a relatively short duration of activity (4 to 12 hours) as compared with other insulins. The time course of action of any insulin may vary considerably in different individuals or at different times in the same individual. As with all insulin preparations, the duration of action of Humulin R is dependent on dose, site of injection, blood supply, temperature, and physical activity. Humulin R is a sterile solution and is for subcutaneous injection. It should not be used intramuscularly. The concentration of Humulin R is 100 units/mL (U-100).

Identification

Human insulin from Eli Lilly and Company has the trademark Humulin. Your doctor has prescribed the type of insulin that he/she believes is best for you.

DO NOT USE ANY OTHER INSULIN EXCEPT ON YOUR DOCTOR'S ADVICE AND DIRECTION.

Always check the carton and the bottle label for the name and letter designation of the insulin you receive from your pharmacy to make sure it is the same as prescribed by your doctor.

Always check the appearance of your bottle of Humulin R before withdrawing each dose. Humulin R is a clear and colorless liquid with a water-like appearance and consistency. Do not use Humulin R:

• if it appears cloudy, thickened, or slightly colored, or
• if solid particles are visible.

If you see anything unusual in the appearance of Humulin R solution in your bottle or notice your insulin requirements changing, talk to your doctor.

Storage

Not in-use (unopened): Humulin R bottles not in-use should be stored in a refrigerator, but not in the freezer.

In-use (opened): The Humulin R bottle you are currently using can be kept unrefrigerated as long as it is kept as cool as possible [below 86°F (30°C)] away from heat and light.

Do not use Humulin R after the expiration date stamped on the label or if it has been frozen.

INSTRUCTIONS FOR INSULIN VIAL USE
NEVER SHARE NEEDLES AND SYRINGES.

Correct Syringe Type

Doses of insulin are measured in **units**. U-100 insulin contains 100 units/mL (1 mL=1 cc). With Humulin R, it is important to use a syringe that is marked for U-100 insulin preparations. Failure to use the proper syringe can lead to a mistake in dosage, causing serious problems for you, such as a blood glucose level that is too low or too high.

Syringe Use

To help avoid contamination and possible infection, follow these instructions exactly.

Disposable syringes and needles should be used only once and then discarded by placing the used needle in a puncture-resistant disposable container. Properly dispose of the puncture-resistant container as directed by your Health Care Professional.

Preparing the Dose

1. Wash your hands.
2. Inspect the insulin. Humulin R solution should look clear and colorless. Do not use Humulin R if it appears cloudy, thickened, or slightly colored, or if you see particles in the solution. Do not use Humulin R if you notice anything unusual in its appearance.
3. If using a new Humulin R bottle, flip off the plastic protective cap, but **do not** remove the stopper. Wipe the top of the bottle with an alcohol swab.
4. If you are mixing insulins, refer to the "Mixing Humulin R with Longer-Acting Human Insulins" section below.
5. Draw an amount of air into the syringe that is equal to the Humulin R dose. Put the needle through rubber top of the Humulin R bottle and inject the air into the bottle.
6. Turn the Humulin R bottle and syringe upside down. Hold the bottle and syringe firmly in one hand.
7. Making sure the tip of the needle is in the Humulin R solution, withdraw the correct dose of Humulin R into the syringe.
8. Before removing the needle from the Humulin R bottle, check the syringe for air bubbles. If bubbles are present, hold the syringe straight up and tap its side until the bubbles float to the top. Push the bubbles out with the plunger and then withdraw the correct dose.
9. Remove the needle from the bottle and lay the syringe down so that the needle does not touch anything.
10. If you do not need to mix your Humulin R with a longer-acting insulin, go to the "Injection Instructions" section below and follow the directions.

Mixing Humulin R with Longer-Acting Human Insulins

1. Humulin R should be mixed with longer-acting human insulins only on the advice of your doctor.
2. Draw an amount of air into the syringe that is equal to the amount of longer-acting insulin you are taking. Insert the needle into the longer-acting insulin bottle and inject the air. Withdraw the needle.
3. Draw an amount of air into the syringe that is equal to the amount of Humulin R you are taking. Insert the needle into the Humulin R bottle and inject the air, but **do not** withdraw the needle.
4. Turn the Humulin R bottle and syringe upside down.
5. Making sure the tip of the needle is in the Humulin R solution, withdraw the correct dose of Humulin R into the syringe.
6. Before removing the needle from the Humulin R bottle, check the syringe for air bubbles. If bubbles are present, hold the syringe straight up and tap its side until the bubbles float to the top. Push the bubbles out with the plunger and then withdraw the correct dose.
7. Remove the syringe with the needle from the Humulin R bottle and insert it into the longer-acting insulin bottle. Turn the longer-acting insulin bottle and syringe upside down. Hold the bottle and syringe firmly in one hand and shake gently. Making sure the tip of the needle is in the longer-acting insulin, withdraw the correct dose of longer-acting insulin.
8. Remove the needle from the bottle and lay the syringe down so that the needle does not touch anything.
9. Follow the directions under "Injection Instructions" section below.

Follow your doctor's instructions on whether to mix your insulins ahead of time or just before giving your injection. It is important to be consistent in your method.

Syringes from different manufacturers may vary in the amount of space between the bottom line and the needle. Because of this, do not change:
- the sequence of mixing, or
- the model and brand of syringe or needle that your doctor has prescribed.

Injection Instructions

1. To avoid tissue damage, choose a site for each injection that is at least 1/2 inch from the previous injection site. The usual sites of injection are abdomen, thighs, and arms.
2. Cleanse the skin with alcohol where the injection is to be made.
3. With one hand, stabilize the skin by spreading it or pinching up a large area.
4. Insert the needle as instructed by your doctor.

5. Push the plunger in as far as it will go.
6. Pull the needle out and apply gentle pressure over the injection site for several seconds. **Do not rub the area.**
7. Place the used needle in a puncture-resistant disposable container and properly dispose of the puncture-resistant container as directed by your Health Care Professional.

DOSAGE

Your doctor has told you which insulin to use, how much, and when and how often to inject it. Because each patient's diabetes is different, this schedule has been individualized for you.

Your usual dose of Humulin R may be affected by changes in your diet, activity, or work schedule. Carefully follow your doctor's instructions to allow for these changes. Other things that may affect your Humulin R dose are:

Illness

Illness, especially with nausea and vomiting, may cause your insulin requirements to change. Even if you are not eating, you will still require insulin. You and your doctor should establish a sick day plan for you to use in case of illness. When you are sick, test your blood glucose frequently. If instructed by your doctor, test your ketones and report the results to your doctor.

Pregnancy

Good control of diabetes is especially important for you and your unborn baby. Pregnancy may make managing your diabetes more difficult. If you are planning to have a baby, are pregnant, or are nursing a baby, talk to your doctor.

Medication

Insulin requirements may be increased if you are taking other drugs with blood-glucose-raising activity, such as oral contraceptives, corticosteroids, or thyroid replacement therapy. Insulin requirements may be reduced in the presence of drugs that lower blood glucose or affect how your body responds to insulin, such as oral antidiabetic agents, salicylates (for example, aspirin), sulfa antibiotics, alcohol, certain antidepressants and some kidney and blood pressure medicines. Your Health Care Professional may be aware of other medications that may affect your diabetes control. Therefore, always discuss any medications you are taking with your doctor.

Exercise

Exercise may lower your body's need for insulin during and for some time after the physical activity. Exercise may also speed up the effect of an insulin dose, especially if the exercise involves the area of injection site (for example, the leg should not be used for injection just prior to running). Discuss with your doctor how you should adjust your insulin regimen to accommodate exercise.

Travel

When traveling across more than 2 time zones, you should talk to your doctor concerning adjustments in your insulin schedule.

COMMON PROBLEMS OF DIABETES

Hypoglycemia (Low Blood Sugar)

Hypoglycemia (too little glucose in the blood) is one of the most frequent adverse events experienced by insulin users. It can be brought about by:

1. **Missing or delaying meals.**
2. Taking too much insulin.
3. Exercising or working more than usual.
4. An infection or illness associated with diarrhea or vomiting.
5. A change in the body's need for insulin.
6. Diseases of the adrenal, pituitary, or thyroid gland, or progression of kidney or liver disease.
7. Interactions with certain drugs, such as oral antidiabetic agents, salicylates (for example, aspirin), sulfa antibiotics, certain antidepressants and some kidney and blood pressure medicines.
8. Consumption of alcoholic beverages.

Symptoms of mild to moderate hypoglycemia may occur suddenly and can include:

- sweating
- dizziness
- palpitation
- tremor
- hunger

Continued on next page

Humulin R Regular—Cont.

- restlessness
- tingling in the hands, feet, lips, or tongue
- lightheadedness
- inability to concentrate
- headache
- drowsiness
- sleep disturbances
- anxiety
- blurred vision
- slurred speech
- depressed mood
- irritability
- abnormal behavior
- unsteady movement
- personality changes

Signs of severe hypoglycemia can include:

- disorientation
- unconsciousness
- seizures
- death

Therefore, it is important that assistance be obtained immediately.

Early warning symptoms of hypoglycemia may be different or less pronounced under certain conditions, such as long duration of diabetes, diabetic nerve disease, use of medications such as beta–blockers, changing insulin preparations, or intensified control (3 or more insulin injections per day) of diabetes.

A few patients who have experienced hypoglycemic reactions after transfer from animal-source insulin to human insulin have reported that the early warning symptoms of hypoglycemia were less pronounced or different from those experienced with their previous insulin.

Without recognition of early warning symptoms, you may not be able to take steps to avoid more serious hypoglycemia. Be alert for all of the various types of symptoms that may indicate hypoglycemia. Patients who experience hypoglycemia without early warning symptoms should monitor their blood glucose frequently, especially prior to activities such as driving. If the blood glucose is below your normal fasting glucose, you should consider eating or drinking sugar-containing foods to treat your hypoglycemia.

Mild to moderate hypoglycemia may be treated by eating foods or drinks that contain sugar. Patients should always carry a quick source of sugar, such as hard candy or glucose tablets. More severe hypoglycemia may require the assistance of another person. Patients who are unable to take sugar orally or who are unconscious require an injection of glucagon or should be treated with intravenous administration of glucose at a medical facility.

You should learn to recognize your own symptoms of hypoglycemia. If you are uncertain about these symptoms, you should monitor your blood glucose frequently to help you learn to recognize the symptoms that you experience with hypoglycemia.

If you have frequent episodes of hypoglycemia or experience difficulty in recognizing the symptoms, you should talk to your doctor to discuss possible changes in therapy, meal plans, and/or exercise programs to help you avoid hypoglycemia.

Hyperglycemia (High Blood Sugar) and Diabetic Ketoacidosis (DKA)

Hyperglycemia (too much glucose in the blood) may develop if your body has too little insulin. Hyperglycemia can be brought about by any of the following:

1. Omitting your insulin or taking less than your doctor has prescribed.
2. Eating significantly more than your meal plan suggests.
3. Developing a fever, infection, or other significant stressful situation.

In patients with type 1 or insulin-dependent diabetes, prolonged hyperglycemia can result in DKA (a life-threatening emergency). The first symptoms of DKA usually come on gradually, over a period of hours or days, and include a drowsy feeling, flushed face, thirst, loss of appetite, and fruity odor on the breath. With DKA, blood and urine tests show large amounts of glucose and ketones. Heavy breathing and a rapid pulse are more severe symptoms. If uncorrected, prolonged hyperglycemia or DKA can lead to nausea, vomiting, stomach pain, dehydration, loss of consciousness, or death. Therefore, it is important that you obtain medical assistance immediately.

Lipodystrophy

Rarely, administration of insulin subcutaneously can result in lipoatrophy (seen as an apparent depression of the skin) or lipohypertrophy (seen as a raised area of the skin). If you notice either of these conditions, talk to your doctor. A change in your injection technique may help alleviate the problem.

Allergy

Local Allergy—Patients occasionally experience redness, swelling, and itching at the site of injection. This condition, called local allergy, usually clears up in a few days to a few weeks. In some instances, this condition may be related to factors other than insulin, such as irritants in the skin cleansing agent or poor injection technique. If you have local reactions, talk to your doctor.

Systemic Allergy—Less common, but potentially more serious, is generalized allergy to insulin, which may cause rash over the whole body, shortness of breath, wheezing, reduction in blood pressure, fast pulse, or sweating. Severe cases of generalized allergy may be life threatening. If you think you are having a generalized allergic reaction to insulin, call your doctor immediately.

ADDITIONAL INFORMATION

Information about diabetes may be obtained from your diabetes educator.

Additional information about diabetes and Humulin can be obtained by calling The Lilly Answers Center at 1-800-LillyRx (1-800-545-5979) or by visiting www.LillyDiabetes.com.

Patient Information revised August 22, 2007

Vials manufactured by
Eli Lilly and Company, Indianapolis, IN 46285, USA or Hospira, Inc., Lake Forest, IL 60045, USA or
Lilly France, F-67640 Fegersheim, France
for Eli Lilly and Company, Indianapolis, IN 46285, USA
Copyright © 1997, 2007, Eli Lilly and Company. All rights reserved.
PV 5692 AMP

McNeil Consumer Healthcare
Division of McNeil-PPC, Inc.
FORT WASHINGTON, PA 19034

Direct Inquiries to:
Consumer Relationship Center
Fort Washington, PA 19034
800-962-5357

BENADRYL® ALLERGY ULTRATAB TABLETS   OTC

Active ingredient (in each tablet)   *Purpose*
Diphenhydramine HCl 25 mg .... Antihistamine

Uses
- temporarily relieves these symptoms due to hay fever or other upper respiratory allergies:
  - runny nose • sneezing • itchy, watery eyes • itching of the nose or throat
- temporarily relieves these symptoms due to the common cold:
  - runny nose • sneezing

Warnings

Do not use with any other product containing diphenhydramine, even one used on skin.

Ask a doctor before use if you have
- a breathing problem such as emphysema or chronic bronchitis

- glaucoma
- trouble urinating due to an enlarged prostate gland

Ask a doctor or pharmacist before use if you are taking sedatives or tranquilizers

When using this product
- marked drowsiness may occur
- avoid alcoholic drinks
- alcohol, sedatives, and tranquilizers may increase drowsiness
- be careful when driving a motor vehicle or operating machinery
- excitability may occur, especially in children

If pregnant or breast-feeding, ask a health professional before use.

Keep out of reach of children. In case of overdose, get medical help or contact a Poison Control Center right away. (1-800-222-1222)

Directions
- take every 4 to 6 hours
- do not take more than 6 times in 24 hours

adults and children 12 years and over	1 to 2 tablets
children 6 to under 12 years	1 tablet
children under 6 years	do not use this product in children under 6 years of age

Other information
- each tablet contains: **calcium 15 mg**
- store between 20–25°C (68–77°). Avoid high humidity. Protect from light.

Inactive ingredients carnauba wax, crospovidone D&C red # 27 aluminum lake, dibasic calcium phosphate dihydrate, hypromellose, magnesium stearate, microcrystalline cellulose, polyethylene glycol, polysorbate 80, pregelatinized starch, stearic acid, titanium dioxide

---

CHILDREN'S BENADRYL® ALLERGY LIQUID   OTC

Active ingredient (in each 5 mL)*   **Purpose**
Diphenhydramine HCl 12.5 mg .... Antihistamine
*5 mL = one teaspoon

Uses
- temporarily relieves these symptoms due to hay fever or other upper respiratory allergies:
  - runny nose • sneezing • itchy, watery eyes • itching of the nose or throat

Warnings
Do not use
- to make a child sleepy
- with any other product containing diphenhydramine, even one used on skin

Ask a doctor before use if the child has
- a breathing problem such as chronic bronchitis
- glaucoma
- a sodium-restricted diet

Ask a doctor or pharmacist before use if the child is taking sedatives or tranquilizers

When using this product
- marked drowsiness may occur
- sedatives and tranquilizers may increase drowsiness
- excitability may occur, especially in children

Keep out of reach of children. In case of overdose, get medical help or contact a Poison Control Center right away. (1-800-222-1222)

Directions
- find right dose on chart
- use only enclosed dosing cup designed for use with this product. Do not use any other dosing device.
- take every 4 to 6 hours
- do not take more than 6 doses in 24 hours

children under 2 years	do not use
children 2 to 5 years	do not use unless directed by a doctor
children 6 to 11 years	1 to 2 teaspoonfuls (12.5 mg to 25 mg)

Attention: use only enclosed dosing cup designed for use with this product. Do not use any other dosing device.

Other information
- each teaspoon contains: **sodium 14 mg**
- store between 20–25°C (68–77°F). Protect from light. Store in outer carton until contents used.

Inactive ingredients anhydrous citric acid, D&C red # 33, FD&C red # 40, flavors, glycerin, monoammonium glycyrrhizinate, poloxamer 407, purified water, sodium benzoate, sodium chloride, sodium citrate, sucrose

---

IMODIUM® A–D LIQUID, CAPLETS, AND EZ CHEWS   OTC
(loperamide hydrochloride)

Description
Each 7.5 mL (1½ teaspoonful) of IMODIUM® A-D liquid contains loperamide hydrochloride 1 mg. IMODIUM® A-D liquid is stable, and has a mint flavor.
Each caplet of IMODIUM® A-D contains 2 mg of loperamide hydrochloride and is scored and colored green.
Each EZ Chew tablet of IMODIUM® AD contains 2mg of loperamide hydrochloride.

Actions
IMODIUM® A-D contains a clinically proven antidiarrheal medication. Loperamide HCl acts by slowing intestinal motility and by affecting water and electrolyte movement through the bowel.

Use
controls symptoms of diarrhea, including Travelers' Diarrhea.

Warnings
Allergy alert: Do not use if you have ever had a rash or other allergic reaction to loperamide HCl
Do not use if you have bloody or black stool
Ask a doctor before use if you have
- fever • mucus in the stool • a history of liver disease
Ask a doctor or pharmacist before use if you are taking antibiotics
When using this product tiredness, drowsiness or dizziness may occur. Be careful when driving or operating machinery.
Stop use and ask a doctor if
- symptoms get worse • diarrhea lasts for more than 2 days
- you get abdominal swelling or bulging.
These may be signs of a serious condition
If pregnant or breast feeding, ask a health professional before use.
Keep out of reach of children. In case of overdose, get medical help or contact a Poison Control Center right away. (1-800-222-1222)

Directions
Imodium A-D Caplets and EZ Chews
- **drink plenty of clear fluids to help prevent dehydration caused by diarrhea**
- take only on an empty stomach (1 hour before or 2 hours after a meal) (EZ Chews only)
- find right dose on chart. If possible, use weight to dose; otherwise, use age.

adults and children 12 years and over	2 caplets or chewable tablets after the first loose stool; 1 caplet or chewable tablet after each subsequent loose stool; but no more than 4 caplets or chewable tablets in 24 hours

Continued on next page

Imodium A-D—Cont.

children 9–11 years (60–95 lbs)	1 caplet or chewable tablet after the first loose stool; ½ caplet or chewable tablet after each subsequent loose stool; but no more than 3 caplets or chewable tablets in 24 hours
children 6–8 years (48–59 lbs)	1 caplet or chewable tablet after the first loose stool; ½ caplet or chewable tablet after each subsequent loose stool; but no more than 2 caplets or chewable tablets in 24 hours
children under 6 years (up to 47 lbs)	ask a doctor

Imodium A-D Liquid
- **drink plenty of clear fluids to help prevent dehydration caused by diarrhea**
- find right dose on chart. If possible, use weight to dose; otherwise use age.
- shake well before using
- only use attached measuring cup to dose product

adults and children 12 years and over	30 mL (6 tsp) after the first loose stool; 15 mL (3 tsp) after each subsequent loose stool; but no more than 60 mL (12 tsp) in 24 hours
children 9–11 years (60–95 lbs)	15 mL (3 tsp) after first loose stool; 7.5 mL (1½ tsp) after each subsequent loose stool; but no more than 45 mL (9 tsp) in 24 hours
children 6–8 years (48–59 lbs)	15 mL (3 tsp) after first loose stool; 7.5 mL (1½ tsp) after each subsequent loose stool; but no more than 30 mL (6 tsp) in 24 hours
children under 6 years (up to 47 lbs)	ask a doctor

Imodium A-D Liquid Professional Dosage Schedule for children 2–5 years old (24–47 lbs): 1½ teaspoonful after first loose bowel movement, followed by 1½ teaspoonful after each subsequent loose bowel movement. Do not exceed 4½ teaspoonsful a day.

Other information:

Liquid:	• each 30 mL (6 tsp) contains: **sodium 16 mg**
	• store between 20–25°C (68–77°F)
Caplets:	• each caplet contains: **calcium 10 mg**
	• store between 20–25°C (68–77°F)
EZ Chews:	• store between 20–25°C (68–77°F)

Professional Information:
Overdosage information
Overdosage of loperamide HCl in man may result in constipation, CNS depression and nausea. A slurry of activated charcoal administered promptly after ingestion of loperamide hydrochloride can reduce the amount of drug which is absorbed. If vomiting occurs spontaneously upon ingestion, a slurry of 100 grams of activated charcoal should be administered orally as soon as fluids can be retained. If vomiting has not occurred, and CNS depression is evident, gastric lavage should be performed followed by administration of 100 gms of the activated charcoal slurry through the gastric tube. In the event of overdosage, patients should be monitored for signs of CNS depression for at least 24 hours. Children may be more sensitive to central nervous system effects than adults. If CNS depression is observed, naloxone

may be administered. If responsive to naloxone, vital signs must be monitored carefully for recurrence of symptoms of drug overdose for at least 24 hours after the last dose of naloxone.

Inactive ingredients:
Liquid: carboxymethylcellulose sodium, citric acid, D&C yellow #10, FD&C blue #1, glycerin, flavor, microcrystalline cellulose, propylene glycol, purified water, simethicone emulsion, sodium benzoate, sucralose, titanium dioxide, xanthan gum
Caplets: colloidal silicon dioxide, dibasic calcium phosphate, D&C yellow # 10 aluminum lake, FD&C blue # 1 aluminum lake, magnesium stearate, microcrystalline cellulose
EZ Chews: acesulfame potassium, basic polymethacrylate, cellulose acetate, confectioner's sugar, crospovidone, D&C yellow #10 aluminum lake, dextrose excipient, FD&C blue #1 aluminum lake, flavors, magnesium stearate, microcrystalline cellulose, sucralose

How Supplied:
Liquid: Mint flavored liquid 4 fl. oz. and 8 fl. oz. tamper-evident bottles with child resistant safety caps and special dosage cups. Mint flavored liquid 4 fl. oz. for children.
Caplets: Green scored caplets in 6s, 12s, 18, 24s, 48s and 72s blister packaging which is tamper evident and child resistant, 2s in a tamper resistant pouch.
EZ Chews: Chewable Coolmint Flavored Tablets of 20, 40 and 60.

IMODIUM® MULTI-SYMPTOM RELIEF   OTC
Caplets & Chewable Tablets

Description
Each easy to swallow caplet and mint-flavored chewable tablet of *Imodium® Multi-Symptom Relief* contains loperamide HCl 2 mg/simethicone 125 mg.

Actions
Imodium® Multi-Symptom Relief combines original prescription strength Imodium® to control the symptoms of diarrhea plus simethicone to relieve bloating, pressure and cramps commonly referred to as gas. Loperamide HCl acts by slowing intestinal motility and by affecting water and electrolyte movement through the bowel. Simethicone acts in the stomach and intestines by altering the surface tension of gas bubbles enabling them to coalesce, thereby freeing and eliminating the gas more easily by belching or passing flatus.

Use relieves symptoms of diarrhea plus bloating, pressure, and cramps, commonly referred to as gas

Warnings
Allergy alert: Do not use if you have ever had a rash or other allergic reaction to loperamide HCl
Do not use if you have bloody or black stool
Ask a doctor before use if you have
• fever • mucus in the stool • a history of liver disease
Ask a doctor or pharmacist before use if you are taking antibiotics
When using this product tiredness, drowsiness or dizziness may occur. Be careful when driving or operating machinery.
Stop use and ask a doctor if
• symptoms get worse • diarrhea lasts for more than 2 days
• you get abdominal swelling or bulging.
These may be signs of a serious condition.
If pregnant or breast-feeding, ask a health professional before use.
Keep out of reach of children. In case of overdose, get medical help or contact a Poison Control Center right away. (1-800-222-1222)

Directions
- **drink plenty of clear fluids to help prevent dehydration caused by diarrhea**
- take only on an empty stomach (1 hour before or 2 hours after a meal) (caplets only)
- find right dose on chart. If possible, use weight to dose; otherwise use age

adults and children 12 years and over	2 caplets or chew 2 tablets and take with water (for chewables) after the first loose stool; 1 caplet/tablet and take with water (for chewables) after each subsequent loose stool; but no more than 4 caplets/tablets in 24 hours
children 9–11 years (60–95 lbs)	1 caplet or chew 1 tablet and take with water (for chewables) after the first loose stool; ½ caplet/tablet and take with water (for chewables) after each subsequent loose stool; but no more than 3 caplets/tablets in 24 hours
children 6–8 years (48–59 lbs)	1 caplet or chew 1 tablet and take with water (for chewables) after the first loose stool; ½ caplet/tablet and take with water (for chewables) after each subsequent loose stool; but no more than 2 caplets/tablets in 24 hours
children under 6 years (up to 47 lbs)	ask a doctor

Other information:
Caplets:
- each caplet contains: **calcium 165 mg, sodium 4 mg**
- store between 20–25°C (68–77°F). Protect from light.

Chewable Tablets:
- each tablet contains: **calcium 50 mg**
- store between 20–25°C (68–77°F)

Professional Information:
Overdosage information

Overdosage of loperamide HCl in man may result in constipation, CNS depression and nausea. A slurry of activated charcoal administered promptly after ingestion of loperamide hydrochloride can reduce the amount of drug which is absorbed. If vomiting occurs spontaneously upon ingestion, a slurry of 100 grams of activated charcoal should be administered orally as soon as fluids can be retained. If vomiting has not occurred, and CNS depression is evident, gastric lavage should be performed followed by administration of 100 gms of the activated charcoal slurry through the gastric tube. In the event of overdosage, patients should be monitored for signs of CNS depression for at least 24 hours. Children may be more sensitive to central nervous system effects than adults. If CNS depression is observed, naloxone may be administered. If responsive to naloxone, vital signs must be monitored carefully for recurrence of symptoms of drug overdose for at least 24 hours after the last dose of naloxone. No treatment is necessary for the simethicone ingestion in this circumstance.

Inactive ingredients:
Caplets: acesulfame potassium, croscarmellose sodium dibasic calcium phosphate, flavor, microcrystalline cellulose, stearic acid
Chewable Tablets: cellulose acetate, confectioner's sugar, D&C Yellow # 10 aluminum lake, dextrates, FD&C Blue # 1 aluminum lake, flavors, microcrystalline cellulose, polymethacrylates, saccharin sodium, sorbitol, stearic acid, tribasic calcium phosphate

How Supplied
Mint Chewable Tablets in 18's, and blister packaging which is tamper evident and child resistant. Each Imodium® Multi-Symptom Relief tablet is round, light green in color and has "IMODIUM" embossed on one side and "2/125" on the other side. Imodium® Multi-Symptom Relief Caplets are available in blister packs of 12's and 18's and bottles of 30's, 42's. Each Imodium® Multi-Symptom Relief Caplet is oval, white color and has "IMO" embossed on one side and "2/125" on the other side.

CHILDREN'S MOTRIN® Dosing Chart

[See table on next page]

MOTRIN® IB
(Ibuprofen)
Tablets and Caplets   OTC

Description
Each *MOTRIN® IB Tablet and Caplet* contains ibuprofen 200 mg (NSAID)*
*Nonsteroidal anti-inflammatory drug

Uses
- temporarily relieves minor aches and pains due to:
  - headache • muscular aches • minor pain of arthritis • toothache • backache • the common cold • menstrual cramps
- temporarily reduces fever

Directions
- **do not take more than directed**
- **the smallest effective dose should be used**
- do not take longer than 10 days, unless directed by a doctor (see Warnings)

adults and children 12 years and older	• take 1 tablet or caplet every 4 to 6 hours while symptoms persist • if pain or fever does not respond to 1 tablet or caplet, 2 tablets or caplets may be used • do not exceed 6 tablets or caplets in 24 hours, unless directed by a doctor
children under 12 years	• ask a doctor

Warnings
Allergy alert: Ibuprofen may cause a severe allergic reaction, especially in people allergic to aspirin. Symptoms may include:
- hives • facial swelling • asthma (wheezing) • shock
- skin reddening • rash • blisters

If an allergic reaction occurs, stop use and seek medical help right away.

Stomach bleeding warning: This product contains an NSAID, which may cause severe stomach bleeding. The chance is higher if you:
- are age 60 or older
- have had stomach ulcers or bleeding problems
- take a blood thinning (anticoagulant) or steroid drug
- take other drugs containing prescription or nonprescription NSAID (aspirin, ibuprofen, naproxen, or others)
- have 3 or more alcoholic drinks every day while using this product
- take more or for a longer time than directed

Do not use
- if you have ever had an allergic reaction to any other pain reliever/fever reducer
- right before or after heart surgery

Ask a doctor before use if
- you have problems or serious side effects from taking pain relievers or fever reducers
- you have asthma
- you have a history of stomach problems. Such as heartburn
- the stomach bleeding warning applies to you
- you have liver cirrhosis
- you have high blood pressure
- you have heart or kidney disease
- you have taken a diuretic

Ask a doctor or pharmacist before use if you are
- taking aspirin for heart attack or stroke, because ibuprofen may decrease this benefit of aspirin
- under a doctor's care for any serious condition
- taking any other drug

When using this product
- take with food or milk if stomach upset occurs
- the risk of heart attack or stroke may increase if you use more than directed or for longer than directed

Continued on next page

Table 2. Children's Motrin Dosing Chart

PRODUCT FORM	INGREDIENTS	0-5 mos*	6-11 mos	12-23 mos	2-3 yrs	4-5 yrs	6-8 yrs	9-10 yrs	11 yrs	
AGE GROUP*		0-5 mos*	6-11 mos	12-23 mos	2-3 yrs	4-5 yrs	6-8 yrs	9-10 yrs	11 yrs	
WEIGHT	(if possible use weight to dose; otherwise use age)	6-11 lbs	12-17 lbs	18-23 lbs	24-35 lbs	36-47 lbs	48-59 lbs	60-71 lbs	72-95 lbs	**Maximum doses/ 24 hrs**
PRODUCT FORM	**INGREDIENTS**	Dose to be administered based on weight or age† Please advise caregivers to use the enclosed Dosage device when administering medication								
Infants' Drops	**Per 1.25 mL**									
Infants' Motrin Concentrated Drops	Ibuprofen 50 mg	—	1.25 mL	1.875 mL	—	—	—	—	—	4 times in 24 hrs
Children's Liquid	**Per 5 mL = 1 teaspoonful (TSP)**									
Children's Motrin Suspension	Ibuprofen 100 mg	—	—	—	1 TSP or 5 mL	1 ½ TSP or 7.5 mL	2 TSP or 10 mL	2 ½ TSP or 12.5 mL	3 TSP or 15 mL	4 times in 24 hrs
Junior Strength Tablets & Caplets	**Per tablet/ caplet**									
Junior Strength Motrin Chewable Tablets	Ibuprofen 100 mg	—	—	—	1 tablet	1 ½ tablets	2 tablets	2 ½ tablets	3 tablets	4 times in 24 hrs
Junior Strength Motrin Caplets	Ibuprofen 100 mg	—	—	—	—	—	2 caplets	2 ½ caplets	3 caplets	4 times in 24 hrs

These products do not contain directions or complete warnings for adult use.
† Do not give more than directed. If needed, repeat dose every 6-8 hours; except for Children's Motrin Cold which is every 6 hours.
* Under 6 mos, ask a doctor.
- Do not give longer than 10 days, unless directed by a doctor (see WARNINGS).
- Infants' drops: Shake well before using. Dispense liquid slowly into the child's mouth, toward the inner cheek.
- Infants' Motrin Drops are more concentrated than Children's Motrin Liquids. The Infants' Concentrated Drops have been specifically designed for use only with enclosed dosing device. Do not use any other dosing device with this product.
- Children's Motrin Liquids are less concentrated than Infants' Motrin Drops. The Children's Motrin Liquids have been specifically designed for use with the enclosed measuring cup. Use only enclosed measuring cup to dose this product. Shake well before using.
- Children's Motrin Suspensions (including cold)—replace original bottle cap to maintain child resistance

Stop use and ask a doctor if
- you experience any of the following signs of stomach bleeding
- feel faint, vomit blood, or have bloody or black stools.
- have stomach pain that does not get better
- pain gets worse or lasts more than 10 days
- fever gets worse or lasts more than 3 days
- redness or swelling is present in the painful area
- any new symptoms appear

If pregnant or breast-feeding, ask a health professional before use. It is especially important not to use ibuprofen during the last 3 months of pregnancy unless definitely directed to do so by a doctor because it may cause problems in the unborn child or complications during delivery.

Keep out of reach of children. In case of overdose, get medical help or contact a Poison Control Center right away. (1-800-222-1222)

Other information:
- store between 20–25°C (68–77°F)

Professional Information:
Overdosage information **FOR ADULT MOTRIN®**
IBUPROFEN
The *toxicity of ibuprofen* overdose is dependent upon the amount of drug ingested and the time elapsed since ingestion, though individual response may vary, which makes it necessary to evaluate each case individually. Although uncommon, serious toxicity and death have been reported in the medical literature with ibuprofen overdosage. The most frequently reported symptoms of ibuprofen overdose include abdominal pain, nausea, vomiting, lethargy and drowsiness. Other central nervous system symptoms include headache, tinnitus, CNS depression and seizures. Metabolic acidosis, coma, acute renal failure and apnea (primarily in very young children) may rarely occur. Cardiovascular toxicity, including hypotension, bradycardia, tachycardia and atrial fibrillation, also have been reported. The *treatment of acute ibuprofen overdose* is primarily supportive. Management of hypotension, acidosis and gastrointestinal bleeding may be necessary. In cases of acute overdose, the stomach should be emptied through ipecac-induced emesis or lavage. Emesis is most effective if initiated within 30 minutes of ingestion. Orally administered activated charcoal may help in reducing the absorption and reabsorption of ibuprofen. In children, the estimated amount of ibuprofen ingested per body weight may be helpful to predict the potential for development of toxicity although each case must be evaluated. Ingestion of less than 100 mg/kg is unlikely to produce toxicity. Children ingesting 100 to 200 mg/kg may be managed with induced emesis and a minimal observation time of four hours. Children ingesting 200 to 400 mg/kg of ibuprofen should have immediate gastric emptying and at least four hours observation in a health care facility. Children ingesting greater than 400 mg/kg require immediate medical referral, careful observation and appropriate supportive therapy. Ipecac-induced emesis is not recommended in overdoses greater than 400 mg/kg because of the risk of convulsions and the potential for aspiration of gastric contents. In adult patients the history of the dose reportedly ingested does not appear to be predictive of toxicity. The need for referral and follow-up must be judged by the circumstances at the time of the overdose ingestion. Symptomatic adults should be admitted to a health care facility for observation.

Inactive ingredients:
Tablets and Caplets: carnauba wax, colloidal silicon dioxide, corn starch, FD&C yellow #6, hypromellose, iron oxide, magnesium stearate, polydextrose, polyethylene glycol, pregelatinized starch, propylene glycol, shellac, stearic acid, titanium dioxide

How Supplied
Tablets: (orange, printed "MOTRIN IB" in black) in tamper evident packaging of 24, 50, 100, and 165.
Caplets: (orange, printed "MOTRIN IB" in black) in tamper evident packaging of 6 ct, 8 ct and 24, 50, 100, 165, 225, and 300

INFANTS' MOTRIN® ibuprofen   **OTC**
Concentrated Drops

CHILDREN'S MOTRIN® ibuprofen
Oral Suspension

JUNIOR STRENGTH MOTRIN® ibuprofen
Caplets and Chewable Tablets

Product information for all dosages of Children's MOTRIN have been combined under this heading

Description
Infants' MOTRIN® Concentrated Drops are available in an alcohol-free, berry-flavored suspension and a non-staining, dye-free, berry-flavored suspension. Each 1.25 mL contains ibuprofen 50 mg. *Children's MOTRIN® Oral Suspension* is available as an alcohol-free, berry, dye-free berry, bubblegum, grape or tropical punch flavored suspension. Each 5 mL (teaspoon) of *Children's MOTRIN® Oral Suspension* contains ibuprofen 100 mg. *Junior Strength MOTRIN® Chewable Tablets* and *Junior Strength MOTRIN® Caplets* contain ibuprofen 100 mg. *Junior Strength MOTRIN® Chewable Tablets* are available in orange or grape flavors. *Junior Strength MOTRIN® Caplets* are available as easy-to-swallow caplets (capsule-shaped tablet).

Uses temporarily:
- reduces fever
- relieves minor aches and pains due to the common cold, flu, sore throat, headaches and toothaches

Directions
See Table 2: Children's Motrin Dosing Chart on pg. 1900

Warnings
Allergy alert: Ibuprofen may cause a severe allergic reaction, especially in people allergic to aspirin. Symptoms may include:
- hives • facial swelling • asthma (wheezing) • shock
- skin reddening • rash • blisters

If an allergic reaction occurs, stop use and seek medical help right away.

Stomach bleeding warning: This product contains a nonsteroidal anti-inflammatory drug (NSAID), which may cause severe stomach bleeding. The chance is higher if the child:
- has had stomach ulcers or bleeding problems
- takes a blood thinning (anticoagulant) or steroid drug
- takes other drugs containing an NSAID (aspirin, ibuprofen, naproxen, or others)
- takes more or for a longer time than directed

Sore throat warning: Severe or persistent sore throat or sore throat accompanied by high fever, headache, nausea, and vomiting may be serious. Consult doctor promptly. Do not use more than 2 days or administer to children under 3 years of age unless directed by doctor.

Do not use
- if the child has ever had an allergic reaction to any other pain reliever/fever reducer
- right before or after heart surgery

Ask a doctor before use if
- stomach bleeding warnings applies to your child
- child has a history of stomach problems, such as heartburn
- child has problems or serious side effects from taking pain relievers or fever reducers
- child has not been drinking fluids
- child has lost a lot of fluid due to vomiting or diarrhea
- child has high blood pressure, heart disease, liver cirrhosis, or kidney disease
- child has asthma
- child is taking a diuretic

Ask a doctor or pharmacist before use if the child is
- under a doctor's care for any serious condition
- taking any other drug

When using this product
- mouth or throat burning may occur; give with food or water (*Junior Strength MOTRIN® Chewable Tablets* only)
- take with food or milk if stomach upset occurs
- the risk of heart attack or stroke may increase if you use more than directed or for longer than directed

Continued on next page

Motrin Infants'—Cont.

Stop use and ask a doctor if
- child experiences any of the following signs of stomach bleeding
  - feels faint • vomits blood • has bloody or black stools • has stomach pain that does not get better
- stomach pain or upset gets worse or lasts
- the child does not get any relief within first day (24 hours) of treatment
- fever or pain gets worse or lasts more than 3 days
- redness or swelling is present in the painful area
- any new symptoms appear

Keep out of reach of children. In case of overdose, get medical help or contact a Poison Control Center right away (1-800-222-1222).

Other information: *Infants', Children's and Junior Strength MOTRIN® products:*
- store between 20–25°C (68–77°F)

Children's MOTRIN® Suspension Liquid:
- each teaspoon contains: **sodium 2 mg**

Junior Strength MOTRIN® Chewable Tablets:
- phenylketonurics: contains phenylalanine 2.8 mg per tablet

Professional Information:
Overdosage information for all infants', children's & junior strength MOTRIN® products
Ibuprofen: The *toxicity of ibuprofen* overdose is dependent upon the amount of drug ingested and the time elapsed since ingestion, though individual response may vary, which makes it necessary to evaluate each case individually. Although uncommon, serious toxicity and death have been reported in the medical literature with ibuprofen overdosage. The most frequently reported symptoms of ibuprofen overdose include abdominal pain, nausea, vomiting, lethargy and drowsiness. Other central nervous system symptoms include headache, tinnitus, CNS depression and seizures. Metabolic acidosis, coma, acute renal failure and apnea (primarily in very young children) may rarely occur. Cardiovascular toxicity, including hypotension, bradycardia, tachycardia and atrial fibrillation, also have been reported.
The *treatment of acute ibuprofen overdose* is primarily supportive. Management of hypotension, acidosis and gastrointestinal bleeding may be necessary. In cases of acute overdose, the stomach should be emptied through ipecac-induced emesis or lavage. Emesis is most effective if initiated within 30 minutes of ingestion. Orally administered activated charcoal may help in reducing the absorption and reabsorption of ibuprofen. In children, the estimated amount of ibuprofen ingested per body weight may be helpful to predict the potential for development of toxicity although each case must be evaluated. Ingestion of less than 100 mg/kg is unlikely to produce toxicity. Children ingesting 100 to 200 mg/kg may be managed with induced emesis and a minimal observation time of four hours. Children ingesting 200 to 400 mg/kg of ibuprofen should have immediate gastric emptying and at least four hours observation in a health care facility. Children ingesting greater than 400 mg/kg require immediate medical referral, careful observation and appropriate supportive therapy. Ipecac-induced emesis is not recommended in overdoses greater than 400 mg/kg because of the risk of convulsions and the potential for aspiration of gastric contents.
In adult patients the history of the dose reportedly ingested does not appear to be predictive of toxicity. The need for referral and follow-up must be judged by the circumstances at the time of the overdose ingestion. Symptomatic adults should be admitted to a health care facility for observation.
For additional emergency information, please contact your local poison control center.

Inactive ingredients
Infants' MOTRIN® Concentrated Drops: Berry-Flavored: anhydrous citric acid, caramel, ethyl alcohol, FD&C red #40, flavors, glycerin, polysorbate 80, pregelatinized starch, purified water, sodium benzoate, sorbitol solution, sucrose, xanthan gum. **Dye-Free Berry-Flavored:** anhydrous citric acid, caramel, ethyl alcohol, flavors, glycerin, polysorbate 80, pregelatinized starch, purified water, sodium benzoate, sorbitol solution, sucrose, xanthan gum.
Children's MOTRIN® Oral Suspension: Berry-Flavored: acesulfame potassium, anhydrous citric acid, D&C yellow #10,

FD&C red #40, flavors, glycerin, polysorbate 80, pregelatinized starch, purified water, sodium benzoate, xanthan gum. **Dye-Free Berry-Flavored:** acesulfame potassium, anhydrous citric acid, flavors, glycerin, polysorbate 80, pregelatinized starch, purified water, sodium benzoate, sucrose, xanthan gum. **Bubble Gum-Flavored:** acesulfame potassium, anhydrous citric acid, FD&C red #40, flavors, glycerin, polysorbate 80, pregelatinized starch, purified water, sodium benzoate, sucrose, xanthan gum. **Grape-Flavored:** acesulfame potassium, anhydrous citric acid, D&C red #33, FD&C blue #1, FD&C red #40, flavors, glycerin, polysorbate 80, pregelatinized starch, purified water, sodium benzoate, sucrose, xanthan gum. **Tropical Punch Flavored:** acesulfame potassium, anhydrous citric acid, FD&C Red #40, flavors, glycerin, polysorbate 80, pregelatinized starch, purified water, sodium benzoate, sucralose, sucrose, xanthan gum.
Junior Strength MOTRIN® Chewable Tablets: **Orange-Flavored:** acesulfame potassium, anhydrous citric acid, aspartame, FD&C yellow #6 aluminum lake, flavor, fumaric acid, hydroxyethyl cellulose, hypromellose, magnesium stearate, mannitol, microcrystalline cellulose, povidone, sodium lauryl sulfate, sodium starch glycolate. **Grape-Flavored:** acesulfame potassium, anhydrous citric acid, aspartame, D&C red #7 calcium lake, D&C red #30 aluminum lake, FD&C blue #1 aluminum lake, flavor, fumaric acid, hydroxyethyl cellulose, hypromellose, magnesium stearate, mannitol, microcrystalline cellulose, povidone, sodium lauryl sulfate, sodium starch glycolate. **Easy-To-Swallow Caplets:** carnauba wax, colloidal silicon dioxide, corn starch, D&C yellow #10 aluminum lake, FD&C yellow #6 aluminum lake, hypromellose, microcrystalline cellulose, polydextrose, polyethylene glycol, pregelatinized starch, shellac, sodium starch glycolate, titanium dioxide, triacetin

How Supplied
Infants' MOTRIN® Concentrated Drops: Berry-flavored, pink-colored liquid and Berry-Flavored, Dye-Free, white-colored liquid in ½ fl. oz. bottles w/calibrated plastic syringe. Dye-Free Berry also available in 1 oz. size
Children's MOTRIN® Oral Suspension: Berry-flavored, pink-colored; (2 and 4 fl. oz) Berry-Flavored, Dye-Free white-colored, Bubble Gum-flavored, pink-colored, Grape-flavored, purple-colored, and Tropical Punch flavored liquid in tamper evident bottles (4 fl. oz.)
Junior Strength MOTRIN® Chewable Tablets: Orange-flavored, orange-colored chewable tablets or Grape-flavored, purple-colored chewable tablets in 24 count bottles.
Junior Strength MOTRIN® Caplets: Easy-to-swallow caplets (capsule shaped tablets) in 24 count bottles.

EXTRA STRENGTH ROLAIDS®   OTC
SOFTCHEWS VANILLA CREME

Active ingredient (in each chew)	**Purpose**
Calcium carbonate 1177 mg	Antacid

Uses relieves:
- heartburn
- sour stomach
- acid indigestion
- upset stomach due to these symptoms

Warnings
Ask a doctor or pharmacist before use if you are now taking a prescription drug. Antacids may interact with certain prescription drugs.
Do not take more than 6 chews in a 24-hour period, or use the maximum dosage for more than 2 weeks, except under the advice and supervision of a physician. **Keep out of reach of children.**

Directions chew and swallow 2 to 3 chews, hourly if needed
Other information
- each chew contains: **calcium 485 mg, magnesium 5 mg, potassium 10 mg, sodium 8 mg**
- **contains milk**
- Store between 20–25°C (68–77°F) in a dry place

Inactive ingredients corn starch, corn syrup, corn syrup solids, flavoring, glycerin, hydrogenated coconut oil, nonfat dry milk, sodium chloride, soy lecithin, and sucrose

ST. JOSEPH 81 mg Aspirin   OTC
ST. JOSEPH 81 mg Adult Low Strength Aspirin
Chewable & Enteric Coated Tablets

Description
Each St. Joseph Adult Low Strength Aspirin tablet contains
81 mg of aspirin.

Uses
temporarily relieves minor aches and pains

Directions
• drink a full glass of water with each dose

adults and children 12 years and over	• take 4 to 8 tablets every 4 hours while symptoms last • do not exceed 48 tablets in 24 hours or as directed by a doctor
children under 12 years	do not use unless directed by a doctor

Warnings
Reye's syndrome: Children and teenagers who have or are
recovering from chicken pox or flu-like symptoms should not
use this product. When using this product, if changes in behavior with nausea and vomiting occur, consult a doctor because these symptoms could be an early sign of Reye's syndrome, a rare but serious illness.
Allergy alert: Aspirin may cause a severe allergic reaction
which may include:
  • hives • facial swelling • asthma (wheezing) • shock
Alcohol warning: If you consume 3 or more alcoholic
drinks every day, ask your doctor whether you should take
aspirin or other pain relievers or fever reducers. Aspirin
may cause stomach bleeding.
Do not use
  • if you have ever had an allergic reaction to any pain
    reliever or fever reducer
  • for at least 7 days after tonsillectomy or oral surgery
    unless directed by a doctor *(chewable tablet only)*
Ask a doctor before use if you have
  • asthma • ulcers • bleeding problems • stomach prob-
    lems that last or come back such as heartburn, upset
    stomach or pain
Ask a doctor or pharmacist before use if you are taking a
prescription drug for:
  • anticoagulation (blood thinning) • gout • diabetes
  • arthritis
Stop use and ask a doctor if
  • allergic reaction occurs. Seek medical help right away.
  • ringing in the ears or loss of hearing occurs
  • pain gets worse or lasts more than 10 days
  • new symptoms occur
  • redness or swelling is present
These could be signs of a serious condition.
If pregnant or breast-feeding, ask a health professional before use. It is especially important not to use aspirin during
the last three months of pregnancy unless definitely directed to do so by a doctor because it may cause problems in
the unborn child or complications during delivery.
Keep out of reach of children. In case of overdose, get medical help or contact a Poison Control Center right away.
(1-800-222-1222)
Other information:
• store between 20–25°C (68–77°F). Avoid high humidity.

Inactive ingredients:
*St. Joseph 81 mg Adult Low
Strength Aspirin Chewable Tablets:* corn starch, FD&C yellow #6 aluminum lake, flavor, mannitol, saccharin, silicon
dioxide, stearic acid.
Enteric Coated Tablets: colloidal silicon dioxide, FD&C red
#40 dye, FD&C yellow #6 dye, glyceryl monostearate, iron
oxide, magnesium stearate, methacrylic acid copolymer dis-
persion, microcrystalline cellulose, pregelatinized starch,
propylene glycol, shellac, simethicone emulsion, stearic
acid, triethyl citrate.

How Supplied
St. Joseph Adult Low Strength Aspirin Chewable Tablets
are round, orange flavored, orange colored tablets that are
debossed with the "SJ" logo. Available in: tamper evident
bottles of 38 and 108 (Tri-Pack).

*St. Joseph Adult Low Strength Aspirin Enteric Coated Tab-
lets* are round, pink-coated tablets that are printed with the
"StJ" logo. Available in: tamper evident bottles of 36, 100,
180 and 300.

Comprehensive Prescribing Information
Description
St. Joseph Adult Low Strength Aspirin Chewable & Enteric
Coated Tablets (acetylsalicylic acid) are available in 81 mg
for oral administration. Aspirin is an odorless white, needle-
like crystalline or powdery substance. When exposed to
moisture, aspirin hydrolyzes into salicylic and acetic acids,
and gives off a vinegary-odor. It is highly lipid soluble and
slightly soluble in water.

Clinical Pharmacology
Mechanism of Action: Aspirin is a more potent inhibitor of
both prostaglandin synthesis and platelet aggregation than
other salicylic acid derivatives. The differences in activity
between aspirin and salicylic acid are thought to be due to
the acetyl group on the aspirin molecule. This acetyl group
is responsible for the inactivation of cyclo-oxygenase via
acetylation.
Pharmacokinetics: Absorption: In general, immediate release aspirin is well and completely absorbed from the gastrointestinal (GI) tract. Following absorption, aspirin is hydrolyzed to salicylic acid with peak plasma levels of salicylic
acid occurring within 1–2 hours of dosing (see Pharmacokinetics—Metabolism). The rate of absorption from the GI
tract is dependent upon the dosage form, the presence or
absence of food, gastric pH (the presence or absence of GI
antacids or buffering agents), and other physiologic factors.
Enteric coated aspirin products are erratically absorbed
from the GI tract.
Distribution: Salicylic acid is widely distributed to all tissues and fluids in the body including the central nervous
system (CNS), breast milk, and fetal tissues. The highest
concentrations are found in the plasma, liver, renal cortex,
heart, and lungs. The protein binding of salicylate is
concentration-dependent, i.e., nonlinear. At low concentrations (<100 micrograms/milliliter µg/mL), approximately
90 percent of plasma salicylate is bound to albumin while at
higher concentrations (400 µg/mL), only about 75 percent is
bound. The early signs of salicylic overdose (salicylism), including tinnitus (ringing in the ears), occur at plasma concentrations approximating 200 µg/mL. Severe toxic effects
are associated with levels 400 µg/mL. (See Adverse Reactions and Overdosage.)
Metabolism: Aspirin is rapidly hydrolyzed in the plasma
to salicylic acid such that plasma levels of aspirin are essentially undetectable 1–2 hours after dosing. Salicylic acid is
primarily conjugated in the liver to form salicyluric acid, a
phenolic glucuronide, an acyl glucuronide, and a number of
minor metabolites. Salicylic acid has a plasma half-life of
approximately 6 hours. Salicylate metabolism is saturable
and total body clearance decreases at higher serum concentrations due to the limited ability of the liver to form both
salicyluric acid and phenolic glucuronide. Following toxic
doses (10–20 grams (g)), the plasma half-life may be increased to over 20 hours.
Elimination: The elimination of salicylic acid follows zero
order pharmacokinetics; (i.e., the rate of drug elimination is
constant in relation to plasma concentration). Renal excretion of unchanged drug depends upon urine pH. As urinary
pH rises above 6.5, the renal clearance of free salicylate increases from <5 percent to 80 percent. Alkalinization of the
urine is a key concept in the management of salicylate overdose. (See Overdosage.) Following therapeutic doses, approximately 10 percent is found excreted in the urine as salicylic acid, 75 percent as salicyluric acid, and 10 percent
phenolic and 5 percent acyl glucuronides of salicylic acid.
Pharmacodynamics: Aspirin affects platelet aggregation
by irreversibly inhibiting prostaglandin cyclo-oxygenase.
The effect lasts for the life of the platelet and prevents the
formation of the platelet aggregating factor thromboxane
A2. Nonacetylated salicylates do not inhibit this enzyme
and have no effect on platelet aggregation. At somewhat
higher doses, aspirin reversibly inhibits the formation of
prostaglandin I2 (prostacyclin), which is an arterial vasodilator and inhibits platelet aggregation.
At higher doses, aspirin is an effective anti-inflammatory
agent, partially due to inhibition of inflammatory mediators

Continued on next page

St. Joseph Aspirin—Cont.

via cyclo-oxygenase inhibition in peripheral tissues. In vitro studies suggest that other mediators of inflammation may also be suppressed by aspirin administration, although the precise mechanism of action has not been elucidated. It is this nonspecific suppression of cyclo-oxygenase activity in peripheral tissues following large doses that leads to its primary side effect of gastric irritation. (See Adverse Reactions.)

Clinical Studies

Ischemic Stroke and Transient Ischemic Attack (TIA): In clinical trials of subjects with TIA's due to fibrin platelet emboli or ischemic stroke, aspirin has been shown to significantly reduce the risk of the combined endpoint of stroke or death and the combined endpoint of TIA, stroke, or death by about 13–18 percent.

Suspected Acute Myocardial Infarction (MI): In a large, multi-center study of aspirin, streptokinase, and the combination of aspirin and streptokinase in 17,187 patients with suspected acute MI, aspirin treatment produced a 23-percent reduction in the risk of vascular mortality. Aspirin was also shown to have an additional benefit in patients given a thrombolytic agent.

Prevention of Recurrent MI and Unstable Angina Pectoris: These indications are supported by the results of six large, randomized, multi-center, placebo-controlled trials of predominantly male post-MI subjects and one randomized placebo-controlled study of men with unstable angina pectoris. Aspirin therapy in MI subjects was associated with a significant reduction (about 20 percent) in the risk of the combined endpoint of subsequent death and/or nonfatal reinfarction in these patients. In aspirin-treated unstable angina patients, the event rate was reduced to 5 percent from the 10 percent rate in the placebo group.

Chronic Stable Angina Pectoris: In a randomized, multi-center, double-blind trial designed to assess the role of aspirin for prevention of MI in patients with chronic stable angina pectoris, aspirin significantly reduced the primary combined endpoint of nonfatal MI, fatal MI, and sudden death by 34 percent. The secondary endpoint for vascular events (first occurrence of MI, stroke, or vascular death) was also significantly reduced (32 percent).

Revascularization Procedures: Most patients who undergo coronary artery revascularization procedures have already had symptomatic coronary artery disease for which aspirin is indicated. Similarly, patients with lesions of the carotid bifurcation sufficient to require carotid endarterectomy are likely to have had a precedent event. Aspirin is recommended for patients who undergo revascularization procedures if there is a preexisting condition for which aspirin is already indicated.

Rheumatologic Diseases: In clinical studies in patients with rheumatoid arthritis, juvenile rheumatoid arthritis, ankylosing spondylitis and osteoarthritis, aspirin has been shown to be effective in controlling various indices of clinical disease activity.

Animal Toxicology

The acute oral 50 percent lethal dose in rats is about 1.5 g/kilogram (kg) and in mice 1.1 g/kg. Renal papillary necrosis and decreased urinary concentrating ability occur in rodents chronically administered high doses. Dose-dependent gastric mucosal injury occurs in rats and humans. Mammals may develop aspirin toxicosis associated with GI symptoms, circulatory effects, and central nervous system depression. (See Overdosage.)

Indications and Usage

Vascular Indications (Ischemic Stroke, TIA, Acute MI, Prevention of Recurrent MI, Unstable Angina Pectoris, and Chronic Stable Angina Pectoris): Aspirin is indicated to: (1) Reduce the combined risk of death and nonfatal stroke in patients who have had ischemic stroke or transient ischemia of the brain due to fibrin platelet emboli, (2) reduce the risk of vascular mortality in patients with a suspected acute MI, (3) reduce the combined risk of death and nonfatal MI in patients with a previous MI or unstable angina pectoris, and (4) reduce the combined risk of MI and sudden death in patients with chronic stable angina pectoris.

Revascularization Procedures (Coronary Artery Bypass Graft (CABG), Percutaneous Transminase Coronary Angioplasty (PTCA), and Carotid Endarterectomy): Aspirin is indicated in patients who have undergone revascularization procedures (i.e., CABG, PTCA, or carotid endarterectomy) when there is a preexisting condition for which aspirin is already indicated.

Rheumatologic Disease Indications (Rheumatoid Arthritis, Juvenile Rheumatoid Arthritis, Spondyloarthropathies, Osteoarthritis, and the Arthritis and Pleurisy of Systemic Lupus Erythematosus (SLE)): Aspirin is indicated for the relief of the signs and symptoms of rheumatoid arthritis, juvenile rheumatoid arthritis, osteoarthritis, spondyloarthopathies, and arthritis and pleurisy associated with SLE.

Contraindications

Allergy: Aspirin is contraindicated in patients with known allergy to nonsteroidal anti-inflammatory drug products and in patients with the syndrome of asthma, rhinitis, and nasal polyps. Aspirin may cause severe urticaria, angioedema, or bronchospasm (asthma).

Reye's Syndrome: Aspirin should not be used in children or teenagers for viral infections, with or without fever, because of the risk of Reye's syndrome with concomitant use of aspirin in certain viral illnesses.

Warnings

Alcohol Warning: Patients who consume three or more alcoholic drinks every day should be counseled about the bleeding risks involved with chronic, heavy alcohol use while taking aspirin.

Coagulation Abnormalities: Even low doses of aspirin can inhibit platelet function leading to an increase in bleeding time. This can adversely affect patients with inherited (hemophilia) or acquired (liver disease or vitamin K deficiency) bleeding disorders.

GI Side Effects: GI side effects include stomach pain, heartburn, nausea, vomiting, and gross GI bleeding. Although minor upper GI symptoms, such as dyspepsia, are common and can occur anytime during therapy, physicians should remain alert for signs of ulceration and bleeding, even in the absence of previous GI symptoms. Physicians should inform patients about the signs and symptoms of GI side effects and what steps to take if they occur.

Peptic Ulcer Disease: Patients with a history of active peptic ulcer disease should avoid using aspirin, which can cause gastric mucosal irritation and bleeding.

Precautions

General: Renal Failure: Avoid aspirin in patients with severe renal failure (glomerular filtration rate less than 10 mL/minute)

Hepatic Insufficiency: Avoid aspirin in patients with severe hepatic insufficiency.

Sodium Restricted Diets: Patients with sodium-retaining states, such as congestive heart failure or renal failure, should avoid sodium-containing buffered aspirin preparations because of their high sodium content.

Laboratory Tests: Aspirin has been associated with elevated hepatic enzymes, blood urea nitrogen, serum creatinine, hyperkalemia, proteinuria, and prolonged bleeding time.

Drug Interactions: Angiotensin Converting Enzyme (ACE) Inhibitors: The hyponatremic and hypotensive effects of ACE inhibitors may be diminished by the concomitant administration of aspirin due to its indirect effect on the renin-angiotensin conversion pathway.

Acetazolamide: Concurrent use of aspirin and acetazolamide can lead to high serum concentrations of acetazolamide (and toxicity) due to competition at the renal tubule for secretion.

Anticoagulant Therapy (Heparin and Warfarin): Patients on anticoagulation therapy are at increased risk for bleeding because of drug-drug interactions and the effect on platelets. Aspirin can displace warfarin from protein binding sites, leading to prolongation of both the prothrombin time and the bleeding time. Aspirin can increase the anticoagulant activity of heparin, increasing bleeding risk.

Anticonvulsants: Salicylate can displace protein-bound phenytoin and valproic acid, leading to a decrease in the total concentration of phenytoin and an increase in serum valproic acid levels.

Beta Blockers: The hypotensive effects of beta blockers may be diminished by the concomitant administration of aspirin due to inhibition of renal prostaglandins, leading to decreased renal blood flow, and salt and fluid retention.

Diuretics: The effectiveness of diuretics in patients with underlying renal or cardiovascular disease may be dimin-

ished by the concomitant administration of aspirin due to inhibition of renal prostaglandins, leading to decreased renal blood flow and salt and fluid retention.

Methotrexate: Salicylate can inhibit renal clearance of methotrexate, leading to bone marrow toxicity, especially in the elderly or renal impaired.

Nonsteroidal Anti-Inflammatory Drugs (NSAID's): The concurrent use of aspirin with other NSAID's should be avoided because this may increase bleeding or lead to decreased renal function.

Oral Hypoglycemics: Moderate doses of aspirin may increase the effectiveness of oral hypoglycemic drugs, leading to hypoglycemia.

Uricosuric Agents (Probenecid and Sulfinpyrazone): Salicylates antagonize the uricosuric action of uricosuric agents.

Carcinogenesis, Mutagenesis, Impairment of Fertility: Administration of aspirin for 68 weeks at 0.5 percent in the feed of rats was not carcinogenic. In the Ames Salmonella assay, aspirin was not mutagenic; however, aspirin did induce chromosome aberrations in cultured human fibroblasts. Aspirin inhibits ovulation in rats. (See Pregnancy.)

Pregnancy: Pregnant women should only take aspirin if clearly needed. Because of the known effects of NSAID's on the fetal cardiovascular system (closure of the ductus arteriosus), use during the third trimester of pregnancy should be avoided. Salicylate products have also been associated with alterations in maternal and neonatal hemostasis mechanisms, decreased birth weight, and with perinatal mortality.

Labor and Delivery: Aspirin should be avoided 1 week prior to and during labor and delivery because it can result in excessive blood loss at delivery. Prolonged gestation and labor due to prostaglandin inhibition have been reported.

Nursing Mothers: Nursing mothers should avoid using aspirin because salicylate is excreted in breast milk. Use of high doses may lead to rashes, platelet abnormalities, and bleeding in nursing infants.

Pediatric Use: Pediatric dosing recommendations for juvenile rheumatoid arthritis are based on well-controlled clinical studies. An initial dose of 90–130 mg/kg/day in divided doses, with an increase as needed for anti-inflammatory efficacy (target plasma salicylate levels of 150–300 µg/mL) are effective. At high doses (i.e., plasma levels of greater than 200 µg/mL), the incidence of toxicity increases.

Adverse Reactions

Many adverse reactions due to aspirin ingestion are dose-related. The following is a list of adverse reactions that have been reported in the literature. (See Warnings.)

Body as a Whole: Fever, hypothermia, thirst.

Cardiovascular: Dysrhythmias, hypotension, tachycardia.

Central Nervous System: Agitation, cerebral edema, coma, confusion, dizziness, headache, subdural or intracranial hemorrhage, lethargy, seizures.

Fluid and Electrolyte: Dehydration, hyperkalemia, metabolic acidosis, respiratory alkalosis.

Gastrointestinal: Dyspepsia, GI bleeding, ulceration and perforation, nausea, vomiting, transient elevations of hepatic enzymes, hepatitis, Reye's Syndrome, pancreatitis.

Hematologic: Prolonged prothrombin time, disseminated intravascular coagulation, coagulopathy, thrombocytopenia.

Hypersensitivity: Acute anaphylaxis, angioedema, asthma, bronchospasm, laryngeal edema, urticaria.

Musculoskeletal: Rhabdomyolysis.

Metabolism: Hypoglycemia (in children), hyperglycemia.

Reproductive: Prolonged pregnancy and labor, stillbirths, lower birth weight infants, antepartum and postpartum bleeding.

Special Senses: Hearing loss, tinnitus. Patients with high frequency hearing loss may have difficulty perceiving tinnitus. In these patients, tinnitus cannot be used as a clinical indicator of salicylism.

Urogenital: Interstitial nephritis, papillary necrosis, proteinuria, renal insufficiency and failure.

Drug Abuse and Dependence

Aspirin is nonnarcotic. There is no known potential for addiction associated with the use of aspirin.

Overdosage

Salicylate toxicity may result from acute ingestion (overdose) or chronic intoxication. The early signs of salicylic overdose (salicylism), including tinnitus (ringing in the ears), occur at plasma concentrations approaching 200 µg/

mL. Plasma concentrations of aspirin above 300 µg/mL are clearly toxic. Severe toxic effects are associated with levels above 400 µg/mL (See Clinical Pharmacology.) A single lethal dose of aspirin in adults is not known with certainty but death may be expected at 30 g. For real or suspected overdose, a Poison Control Center should be contacted immediately. Careful medical management is essential.

Signs and Symptoms: In acute overdose, severe acid-base and electrolyte disturbances may occur and are complicated by hyperthermia and dehydration. Respiratory alkalosis occurs early while hyperventilation is present, but is quickly followed by metabolic acidosis.

Treatment: Treatment consists primarily of supporting vital functions, increasing salicylate elimination, and correcting the acid-base disturbance. Gastric emptying and/or lavage is recommended as soon as possible after ingestion, even if the patient has vomited spontaneously. After lavage and/or emesis, administration of activated charcoal, as a slurry, is beneficial, if less than 3 hours have passed since ingestion. Charcoal adsorption should not be employed prior to emesis and lavage. Severity of aspirin intoxication is determined by measuring the blood salicylate level. Acid-base status should be closely followed with serial blood gas and serum pH measurements. Fluid and electrolyte balance should also be maintained. In severe cases, hyperthermia and hypovolemia are the major immediate threats to life. Children should be sponged with tepid water. Replacement fluids should be administered intravenously and augmented with correction of acidosis. Plasma electrolytes and pH should be monitored to promote alkaline diuresis of salicylate if renal function is normal. Infusion of glucose may be required to control hypoglycemia. Hemodialysis and peritoneal dialysis can be performed to reduce the body drug content. In patients with renal insufficiency or in cases of life-threatening intoxication, dialysis is usually required. Exchange transfusion may be indicated in infants and young children.

Dosage and Administration

Each dose of aspirin should be taken with a full glass of water unless the patient is fluid restricted. Anti-inflammatory and analgesic dosages should be individualized.

Ischemic Stroke and TIA: 50–325 mg once a day. Continue therapy indefinitely

Suspected Acute MI: The initial dose of 160–162.5 mg is administered as soon as an MI is suspected. The maintenance dose of 160–162.5 mg a day is continued for 30 days post-infarction. After 30 days, consider further therapy based on dosage and administration for prevention of recurrent MI.

Prevention of Recurrent MI: 75–325 mg once a day. Continue therapy indefinitely.

Unstable Angina Pectoris: 75–325 mg once a day. Continue therapy indefinitely.

Chronic Stable Angina Pectoris: 75–325 mg once a day. Continue therapy indefinitely.

CABG: 325 mg daily starting 6 hours post-procedure. Continue therapy for 1 year post-procedure.

PTCA: The initial dose of 325 mg daily should be given 2 hours pre-surgery. Maintenance dose is 160–325 mg daily. Continue therapy indefinitely.

Carotid Endarterectomy: Doses of 80 mg once daily to 650 mg twice daily, started presurgery, are recommended. Continue therapy indefinitely.

Rheumatoid Arthritis: The initial dose is 3 g a day in divided doses. Increase as needed for anti-inflammatory efficacy with target plasma salicylate levels of 150–300 µg/mL. At high doses (i.e., plasma levels of greater than 200 µg/mL), the incidence of toxicity increases.

Juvenile Rheumatoid Arthritis: Initial dose is 90–130 mg/kg/day in divided doses. Increase as needed for anti-inflammatory efficacy with target plasma salicylate levels of 150–300 µg/mL. At high doses (i.e., plasma levels of greater than 200 µg/mL), the incidence of toxicity increases.

Spondyloarthropathies: Up to 4 g per day in divided doses.

Osteoarthritis: Up to 3 g per day in divided doses.

Arthritis and Pleurisy of SLE: The initial dose is 3 g a day in divided doses. Increase as needed for anti-inflammatory

Continued on next page

St. Joseph Aspirin—Cont.

efficacy with target plasma salicylate levels of 150–300 µg/mL. At high doses (i.e., plasma levels of greater than 200 µg/mL), the incidence of toxicity increases.

CHILDREN'S SUDAFED® NASAL DECONGESTANT LIQUID
OTC

Active ingredient   Purpose
(in each 5 mL*)
Pseudoephedrine HCl 15 mg .... Nasal decongestant

*5 mL = one teaspoonful

Uses
- temporarily relieves nasal congestion due to the common cold, hay fever or other upper respiratory allergies
- temporarily relieves sinus congestion and pressure
- promotes nasal and/or sinus drainage

Warnings

Do not use in a child who is taking a prescription monoamine oxidase inhibitor (MAOI) (certain drugs for depression, psychiatric or emotional conditions, or Parkinson's disease), or for 2 weeks after stopping the MAOI drug. If you do not know if your child's prescription drug contains an MAOI, ask a doctor or pharmacist before giving this product.

Ask a doctor before use if the child has
- heart disease • high blood pressure • thyroid disease
- diabetes

When using this product do not exceed recommended dose

Stop use and ask a doctor if
- nervousness, dizziness, or sleeplessness occur
- symptoms do not improve within 7 days or occur with a fever

Keep out of reach of children. In case of overdose, get medical help or contact a Poison Control Center right away. (1-800-222-1222)

Directions
- find right dose on chart
- use only enclosed dosing cup designed for use with this product. Do not use any other dosing device.
- if needed, repeat dose every 4 to 6 hours
- do not use more than 4 times in 24 hours

under 4 years	do not use
4 to 5 years	one (1) teaspoonful
6 to 11 years	two (2) teaspoonfuls

ATTENTION: use only enclosed dosing cup designed for use with this product. Do not use any other dosing device.

Other information
- each teaspoonful contains: **sodium 5 mg**
- store between 20–25°C (68–77°F)

Inactive ingredients anhydrous citric acid, edetate disodium, FD&C blue # 1, FD&C red # 40, flavor, glycerin, menthol, poloxamer 407, polyethylene glycol, povidone K-90, purified water, saccharin sodium, sodium benzoate, sodium citrate, sorbitol solution

---

CHILDREN'S SUDAFED PE® NASAL DECONGESTANT LIQUID
OTC

Active ingredient (in each 5 mL*)   **Purpose**
Phenylephrine HCl 2.5 mg .... Nasal decongestant
*5 mL = one teaspoonful

Use temporarily relieves nasal congestion due to the common cold, hay fever or other upper respiratory allergies

Warnings

Do not use in a child who is taking a prescription monoamine oxidase inhibitor (MAOI) (certain drugs for depres-

sion, psychiatric, or emotional conditions, or Parkinson's disease), or for 2 weeks after stopping the MAOI drug. If you do not know if your child's prescription drug contains an MAOI, ask a doctor or pharmacist before giving this product.

Ask a doctor before use if the child has
- heart disease
- high blood pressure
- thyroid disease
- diabetes
- a sodium-restricted diet

When using this product do not exceed recommended dose

Stop use and ask a doctor if
- nervousness, dizziness, or sleeplessness occur
- symptoms do not improve within 7 days or occur with a fever

Keep out of reach of children. In case of overdose, get medical help or contact a Poison Control Center right away. (1-800-222-1222)

Directions
- find right dose on chart
- use only enclosed dosing cup designed for use with this product. Do not use any other dosing device.
- if needed, repeat every 4 hours
- do not use more than 6 times in 24 hours

under 4 years	do not use
4 to 5 years	one (1) teaspoonful
6 to 11 years	two (2) teaspoonfuls

Other information
- each teaspoonful contains: **sodium 14 mg**
- store between 20°-25°C (68°-77°F). Protect from light. Store in outer container until contents are used.

Inactive ingredients carboxymethylcellulose sodium, citric acid, edetate disodium, FD&C red # 40, flavors, glycerin, sodium benzoate, sodium citrate, sorbitol, sucralose, water

---

SUDAFED® NASAL DECONGESTANT TABLETS
OTC

Active ingredient (in each tablet)   **Purpose**
Pseudoephedrine HCl 30 mg .... Nasal decongestant

Uses
- temporarily relieves nasal congestion due to the common cold, hay fever or other upper respiratory allergies
- temporarily relieves sinus congestion and pressure

Warnings

Do not use if you are now taking a prescription monoamine oxidase inhibitor (MAOI) (certain drugs for depression, psychiatric or emotional conditions, or Parkinson's disease), or for 2 weeks after stopping the MAOI drug. If you do not know if your prescription drug contains an MAOI, ask a doctor or pharmacist before taking this product.

Ask a doctor before use if you have
- heart disease
- high blood pressure
- thyroid disease
- diabetes
- trouble urinating due to an enlarged prostate gland

When using this product do not exceed recommended dose

Stop use and ask a doctor if
- nervousness, dizziness, or sleeplessness occur
- symptoms do not improve within 7 days or occur with a fever

If pregnant or breast-feeding, ask a health professional before use.

Keep out of reach of children. In case of overdose, get medical help or contact a Poison Control Center right away. (1-800-222-1222)

Directions

adults and children 12 years and over	• take 2 tablets every 4 to 6 hours

	• do not take more than 8 tablets in 24 hours
children ages 6 to 12 years	• take 1 tablet every 4 to 6 hours • do not take more than 4 tablets in 24 hours
children under 6 years	do not use this product in children under 6 years of age

Other information
• store between 20–25°C (68–77°F)

Inactive ingredients carnauba wax, colloidal silicon dioxide, D&C yellow #10 aluminum lake, FD&C red #40 aluminum lake, FD&C yellow #6 aluminum lake, iron oxide, magnesium stearate, microcrystalline cellulose, polyethylene glycol, polyvinyl alcohol, pregelatinized starch, shellac, sodium starch glycolate, talc, titanium dioxide

---

SUDAFED® 24 HOUR NON-DROWSY   OTC
NASAL DECONGESTANT TABLETS

Active ingredient (in each tablet)   Purpose
Pseudoephedrine HCl 240 mg .... Nasal decongestant

Uses
• temporarily relieves nasal congestion due to the common cold, hay fever or other upper respiratory allergies
• reduces swelling of nasal passages
• relieves sinus pressure

Warnings
Do not use if you are now taking a prescription monoamine oxidase inhibitor (MAOI) (certain drugs for depression, psychiatric or emotional conditions, or Parkinson's disease), or for 2 weeks after stopping the MAOI drug. If you do not know if your prescription drug contains an MAOI, ask a doctor or pharmacist before taking this product.

Ask a doctor before use if you have
• heart disease
• high blood pressure
• thyroid disease
• diabetes
• trouble urinating due to an enlarged prostate gland
• had obstruction or narrowing of the bowel. Rarely, tablets of this kind may cause bowel obstruction (blockage), usually in people with severe narrowing of the bowel (esophagus, stomach or intestine).

When using this product do not exceed recommended dosage

Stop use and ask a doctor if
• nervousness, dizziness, or sleeplessness occur
• symptoms do not improve within 7 days or occur with a fever
• you experience persistent abdominal pain or vomiting

If pregnant or breast-feeding, ask a health professional before use.

Keep out of reach of children. In case of overdose, get medical help or contact a Poison Control Center right away. (1-800-222-1222)

Directions
• adults and children 12 years and over: **swallow one** whole tablet with water every 24 hours
  • **do not exceed one tablet in 24 hours**
  • **do not divide, crush, chew or dissolve the tablet**
  • the tablet does not completely dissolve and may be seen in the stool (this is normal)
children under 12 years: do not use this product in children under 12 years of age

Other information
• each tablet contains: **sodium 10 mg**
• store at 15° to 25°C (59° to 77°F) in a dry place

Inactive ingredients cellulose, cellulose acetate, hydroxypropyl cellulose, hypromellose, magnesium stearate, polyethlene glycol, polysorbate 80, povidone, sodium chloride, and titanium dioxide

SUDAFED OM™ SINUS COLD   OTC
MOISTURIZING NASAL SPRAY
SUDAFED OM™ SINUS CONGESTION
MOISTURIZING NASAL SPRAY

Active ingredient (in each spray)   Purpose
Oxymetazoline HCl 0.05% .... Nasal decongestant

Uses
• temporarily relieves nasal congestion due to:
  •the common cold •hay fever •upper respiratory allergies
• helps clear nasal passages; shrinks swollen membranes
• temporarily restores freer breathing through the nose
• helps decongest sinus openings and passages; temporarily relieves sinus congestion and pressure

Warnings
Ask a doctor before use if you have
• heart disease
• thyroid disease
• diabetes
• high blood pressure
• trouble urinating due to an enlarged prostate gland

When using this product
• do not exceed recommended dosage
• use of this container by more than one person may cause infection
• temporary discomfort such as burning, stinging, sneezing, or increased nasal discharge may occur
• frequent or prolonged use may cause nasal congestion to recur or worsen

Stop use and ask a doctor if
• symptoms persist for more than 3 days

If pregnant or breast-feeding, ask a health professional before use.

Keep out of reach of children. In case of overdose, get medical help or contact a Poison Control Center right away. (1-800-222-1222)

Directions
adults and children 6 years to under 12 years of age (with adult supervision): 2 or 3 sprays in each nostril, not more often than every 10 to 12 hours. Do not exceed 2 doses in any 24 hour period.

children under 6 years: do not use

Other information
• store between 20-25°C (68-77°F)

Inactive ingredients
Sudafed OM Sinus Congestion Moisturizing Nasal Spray: benzalkonium chloride solution, dibasic sodium phosphate, edetate disodium, glycerin, hypromellose, monobasic sodium phosphate, polyethylene glycol, propylene glycol, purified water

---

SUDAFED PE® NASAL DECONGESTANT   OTC

Drug Facts

Active ingredient (in each tablet)   Purpose
Phenylephrine HCl 10 mg .... Nasal decongestant

Uses
• temporarily relieves nasal congestion due to the common cold, hay fever or other upper respiratory allergies
• temporarily relieves sinus congestion and pressure

Warnings
Do not use if you are now taking a prescription monoamine oxidase inhibitor (MAOI) (certain drugs for depression, psychiatric or emotional conditions, or Parkinson's disease), or for 2 weeks after stopping the MAOI drug. If you do not know if your prescription drug contains an MAOI, ask a doctor or pharmacist before taking this product.

Ask a doctor before use if you have
• heart disease
• high blood pressure
• thyroid disease
• diabetes
• trouble urinating due to an enlarged prostate gland

When using this product do not exceed recommended dose

Continued on next page

Sudafed PE—Cont.

Stop use and ask a doctor if
• nervousness, dizziness, or sleeplessness occur
• symptoms do not improve within 7 days or occur with a fever
If pregnant or breast-feeding, ask a health professional before use.
Keep out of reach of children. In case of overdose, get medical help or contact a Poison Control Center right away. (1-800-222-1222)

Directions

adults and children 12 years of age and over	• take 1 tablet every 4 hours • do not take more than 6 tablets in 24 hours
children under 12 years	• do not use this product in children under 12 years of age

Other information
• store between 20-25° C (68-77° F)
Inactive ingredients carnauba wax, corn starch, D & C yellow # 10 alumium lake, FD&C red # 40 aluminum lake, FD&C yellow # 6 aluminum lake, magnesium stearate, microcrystalline cellulose, polyethylene glycol, polyvinyl alcohol, powdered cellulose, pregelatinized sodium starch glycolate, talc, titanium dioxide.

SUDAFED® 12 HOUR NASAL DECONGESTANT NON-DROWSY CAPLETS
OTC

Active ingredient (in each tablet) — **Purpose**
Pseudoephedrine HCl 120 mg .... Nasal decongestant

Uses
• temporarily relieves nasal congestion due to the common cold, hay fever or other upper respiratory allergies
• temporarily relieves sinus congestion and pressure

Warnings
Do not use if you are now taking a prescription monoamine oxidase inhibitor (MAOI) (certain drugs for depression, psychiatric or emotional conditions, or Parkinson's disease), or for 2 weeks after stopping the MAOI drug. If you do not know if your prescription drug contains an MAOI, ask a doctor or pharmacist before taking this product.
Ask a doctor before use if you have
• heart disease
• high blood pressure
• thyroid disease
• diabetes
• trouble urinating due to an enlarged prostate gland
When using this product do not exceed recommended dosage
Stop use and ask a doctor if
• nervousness, dizziness, or sleeplessness occur
• symptoms do not improve within 7 days or occur with a fever
If pregnant or breast-feeding, ask a health professional before use.
Keep out of reach of children. In case of overdose, get medical help or contact a Poison Control Center right away. (1-800-222-1222)

Directions
• adults and children 12 years and over: take one tablet every 12 hours do not to exceed 2 tablets in 24 hours
• children under 12 years of age: do not use this product in children under 12 years of age
Other information
• store at 59° to 77°F in a dry place
• protect from light
Inactive ingredients candelilla wax, hypromellose, magnesium stearate, microcrystalline cellulose, polyethylene glycol, povidone, and titanium dioxide. Printed with edible blue ink.

CONCENTRATED TYLENOL®
acetaminophen Infants' Drops
OTC

CHILDREN'S TYLENOL®
acetaminophen Suspension Liquid and Meltaways

JR. TYLENOL®
acetaminophen Meltaways

Product information for all dosages of Children's TYLENOL have been combined under this heading

Description
Concentrated TYLENOL® Infants' Drops are stable, alcohol-free, grape-flavored and purple in color, cherry-flavored and red in color or dye-free cherry flavored. Each 0.8 mL contains 80 mg acetaminophen. *Concentrated TYLENOL® Infants' Drops* features the SAFE-TY-LOCK™ Bottle. The SAFE-TY-LOCK™ Bottle has a unique safety barrier inside the bottle which helps make administration easier. The integrated dropper promotes proper administration. The innovative design eliminates excess product on dropper. The star-shaped barrier inside the bottle minimizes spills and discourages pouring into a spoon. *Children's TYLENOL® Suspension Liquid* is stable, alcohol-free, cherry blast-flavored and red in color, bubble-gum yum-flavored and pink in color, grape splash-flavored and purple in color, or very berry strawberry-flavored and red in color. Each 5 mL (one teaspoonful) contains 160 mg acetaminophen. Each *Children's TYLENOL® Meltaways* contains 80 mg acetaminophen in a grape punch or bubble-gum burst flavor. Each *Jr. TYLENOL® Meltaways* contains 160 mg acetaminophen in grape punch or bubblegum burst flavor.

Actions
Acetaminophen is a clinically proven analgesic/antipyretic. Acetaminophen is thought to produce analgesia by elevation of the pain threshold and antipyresis through action on the hypothalamic heat-regulating center. Acetaminophen is equal to aspirin in analgesic and antipyretic effectiveness and it is unlikely to produce many of the side effects associated with aspirin and aspirin-containing products.

Uses
Concentrated TYLENOL® Infants' Drops: temporarily:
• reduces fever
• relieves minor aches and pains due to: • the common cold • flu • headache • sore throat • toothache
Children's TYLENOL® Suspension Liquid and Children's TYLENOL® Meltaways: temporarily relieves minor aches and pains due to: • the common cold • flu • headache • sore throat • toothache
Jr. TYLENOL® Meltaways: temporarily relieves minor aches and pains due to:
• the common cold • flu • headache
• temporarily reduces fever

Directions
• this product does not contain directions or complete warnings for adult use
See Table 1: Children's Tylenol Dosing Chart on pg. 1880

Warnings
Liver warning: This product contains acetaminophen. Severe liver damage may occur if your child takes
• more than 5 doses in 24 hours, which is the maximum daily amount
• with other drugs containing acetaminophen
Do not use
• with any other drug containing acetaminophen (prescription or nonprescription). If you are not sure whether a drug contains acetaminophen, ask a doctor or pharmacist.
• if your child is allergic to acetaminophen or any of the inactive ingredients in this product.
Sore throat warning: if sore throat is severe, persists for more than 2 days, is accompanied or followed by fever, headache, rash, nausea, or vomiting, consult a doctor promptly (excluding *Jr. TYLENOL® Meltaways*).
Ask a doctor before use if your child has liver disease
Ask a doctor or pharmacist before use if you child is taking the blood thinning drug warfarin
When using this product do not exceed recommended dose (see overdose warning)

Stop use and ask a doctor if
- pain gets worse or lasts more than 5 days
- fever gets worse or lasts more than 3 days
- new symptoms occur
- redness or swelling is present

These could be signs of a serious condition

Keep out of reach of children.

Overdose warning: Taking more than the recommended dose (overdose) may cause liver damage. In case of overdose, get medical help or contact a Poison Control Center right away. (1-800-222-1222) Quick medical attention is critical for adults as well as for children even if you do not notice any signs or symptoms.

Other Information:

Concentrated TYLENOL® Infants' Drops:
- store between 20–25°C (68–77°F)

Children's TYLENOL® Suspension Liquid:
- each teaspoon contains: **sodium 2mg** (excludes Dye-Free Cherry)
- store between 20–25°C (68–77°F)

Children's TYLENOL® Meltaways:
- store between 20–25°C (68–77°F). Avoid high humidity. (Grape Punch: Protect from light).

Jr. TYLENOL® Meltaways:
- store between 20–25°C (68–77°F). Avoid high humidity. (Grape Punch: Protect from light).

PROFESSIONAL INFORMATION:
OVERDOSAGE INFORMATION for all Infants', Children's & Jr. Tylenol® Products

Acetaminophen:

Acetaminophen in massive overdosage may cause hepatic toxicity in some patients. In adults and adolescents (≥ 12 years of age), hepatic toxicity may occur following ingestion of greater than 7.5 to 10 grams over a period of 8 hours or less. Fatalities are infrequent (less than 3–4% of untreated cases) and have rarely been reported with overdoses of less than 15 grams. In children (<12 years of age), an acute overdosage of less than 150 mg/kg has not been associated with hepatic toxicity. Early symptoms following a potentially hepatotoxic overdose may include: nausea, vomiting, diaphoresis and general malaise. Clinical and laboratory evidence of hepatic toxicity may not be apparent until 48 to 72 hours postingestion. In adults and adolescents, any individual presenting with an unknown amount of acetaminophen ingested or with a questionable or unreliable history about the time of ingestion should have a plasma acetaminophen level drawn and be treated with *N*-acetylcysteine. For full prescribing information, refer to the *N*-acetylcysteine package insert. Do not await results of assays for plasma acetaminophen levels before initiating treatment with *N*-acetylcysteine. The following additional procedures are recommended: Promptly initiate gastric decontamination of the stomach. A plasma acetaminophen assay should be obtained as early as possible, but no sooner than four hours following ingestion. If an acetaminophen *extended release* product is involved, it may be appropriate to obtain an additional plasma acetaminophen level 4–6 hours following the initial acetaminophen level. If either acetaminophen level plots above the treatment line on the acetaminophen overdose nomogram, *N*-acetylcysteine treatment should be continued for a full course of therapy. Liver function studies should be obtained initially and repeated at 24-hour intervals. Serious toxicity or fatalities have been extremely infrequent following an acute acetaminophen overdose in young children, possibly because of differences in the way they metabolize acetaminophen. In children, the maximum potential amount ingested can be more easily estimated. If more than 150 mg/kg or an unknown amount was ingested, obtain a plasma acetaminophen level as soon as possible, but no sooner than 4 hours following ingestion. If an acetaminophen *extended release* product is involved, it may be appropriate to obtain an additional plasma acetaminophen level 4–6 hours following the initial acetaminophen level. If either acetaminophen level plots above the treatment line on the acetaminophen overdose nomogram, *N*-acetylcysteine treatment should be initiated and continued for a full course of therapy. If an assay cannot be obtained and the estimated acetaminophen ingestion exceeds 150 mg/kg, dosing with *N*-acetylcysteine should be initiated and continued for a full course of therapy. For addi-

tional emergency information, call your regional poison center or call the Rocky Mountain Poison Center toll-free, (1-800-525-6115).

Our pediatric Tylenol® combination products contain active ingredients in addition to acetaminophen. The following is basic overdose information regarding those ingredients.

Chlorpheniramine: Chlorpheniramine toxicity should be treated as you would an anthihistamine/anticholinergic overdose and is likely to be present within a few hours after acute ingestion.

Dextromethorphan: Acute dextromethorphan overdose usually does not result in serious signs and symptoms unless massive amounts have been ingested. Signs and symptoms of a substantial overdose may include nausea and vomiting, visual disturbances, CNS disturbances and urinary retention.

Diphenhydramine: Diphenhydramine toxicity should be treated as you would an antihistamine/anticholinergic overdose and is likely to be present within a few hours after acute ingestion.

Phenylephrine: Symptoms from phenylephrine overdose most often consist of hypertension, anxiety, nervousness, restlessness, tachycardia, bradycardia, headache, dizziness and/or palpitations. Symptoms usually are transient and typically require no treatment.

For additional emergency information, please contact your local poison control center.

Inactive Ingredients:

Concentrated TYLENOL® Infants' Drops: **Cherry-**anhydrous citric acid, FD&C red #40, flavors, glycerin, high fructose corn syrup, microcrystalline cellulose and carboxymethylcellulose sodium, purified water, sodium benzoate, sorbitol solution, xanthan gum **Grape-**anhydrous citric acid, D&C red #33, FD&C blue #1, flavors, glycerin, high fructose corn syrup, microcrystalline cellulose and carboxymethylcellulose sodium, purified water, sodium benzoate, sorbitol solution, xanthan gum

Cherry (Dye-Free) Flavored: anhydrous citric acid, butylparaben, flavors, glycerin, microcrystalline cellulose and carboxymethylcellulose sodium, propylene glycol propyparaben, purified water, sorbitol solution, sucralose, xanthan gum

Children's TYLENOL® Suspension Liquids

Cherry Blast-anhydrous citric acid, butylparaben, FD&C red #40, flavors, glycerin, high fructose corn syrup, microcrystalline cellulose and carboxymethylcellulose sodium, propylene glycol, purified water, sodium benzoate, sorbitol solution, sucralose, xanthan gum

Bubble Gum-butylparaben, carboxymethylcellulose sodium, cellulose, citric acid, corn syrup, D&C red #33, FD&C red #40, flavors, glycerin, propylene glycol, purified water, sodium benzoate, sorbitol, sucralose, xanthan gum

Grape-butylparaben, carboxymethylcellulose sodium, cellulose, citric acid, corn syrup, D&C red #33, FD&C blue #1, flavors, glycerin, propylene glycol, purified water, sodium benzoate, sorbitol, sucralose, xanthan gum

Strawberry-anhydrous citric acid, butylparaben, FD&C red #40, flavors, glycerin, high fructose corn syrup, microcrystalline cellulose and carboxymethylcellulose, sodium, propylene glycol, purified water, sodium benzoate, sorbitol solution, sucralose, xanthan gum

Cherry (Dye-Free) Flavored: anhydrous citric acid, butylparaben, flavors, glycerin, microcrystalline cellulose and carboxymethylcellulose sodium, propylene glycol propyparaben, purified water, sorbitol solution, sucralose, xanthan gum

Children's Tylenol Meltaways

Grape-Punch-Flavored: cellulose acetate, citric acid, crospovidone, dextrose, D&C red #7, D&C red #30, FD&C blue #1, flavors, magnesium stearate, povidone, sucralose.

Ch. Ty. Meltaway BB Burst-anhydrous citric acid, cellulose acetate, crospovidone, D&C red #7, calcium lake, dextrose excipient, flavor, magnesium stearate, sucralose

Jr. TYLENOL® Meltaways Bubblegum Burst Flavored: cellulose acetate, citric acid, crospovidone, D&C red #7, dextrose, flavors, magnesium stearate, povidone, sucralose.

Continued on next page

Children's Tylenol® Dosing Chart

Attention: use only enclosed dosing cup specifically designed for use with this product. Do not use any other dosing device.

PRODUCT FORM	INGREDIENTS	0–3 mos* / 6–11 lbs*	4–11 mos* / 12–17 lbs*	12–23 mos* / 18–23 lbs*	2–3 yrs / 24–35 lbs	4–5 yrs / 36–47 lbs	6–8 yrs / 48–59 lbs	9–10 yrs / 60–71 lbs	11 yrs / 72–95 lbs	12 yrs / 96 lbs and over	Maximum Doses/ 24 hrs
		shake well before using • find right dose on chart below. If possible, use weight to dose; otherwise, use age. • Dose to be administered based on weight or age • If needed, repeat dose every 4 hours									
Infants' Drops	**Per dropperful (0.8 mL)**										
Concentrated Tylenol Infants' Drops	Acetaminophen 80 mg	(0.4 mL)*	(0.8 mL)*	1.2 mL (0.8 + 0.4 mL)*	1.6 mL (0.8 + 0.8 mL)	—	—	—	—	—	5 times in 24 hrs
Children's Liquids	**Per 5 mL = 1 teaspoonful (TSP)**										
Children's Tylenol Suspension	Acetaminophen 160 mg	—	½ TSP*	¾ TSP*	1 TSP	1½ TSP	2 TSP	2½ TSP	3 TSP	—	5 times in 24 hrs
Children's Tylenol Plus Cold & Allergy Suspension	Acetaminophen 160 mg, Diphenhydramine HCl 12.5 mg, Phenylephrine HCl 2.5 mg	Do not use			Do not use unless directed by a doctor		2 TSP	2 TSP	2 TSP	—	5 times in 24 hrs
Children's Tylenol Plus Cold & Stuffy Nose Suspension	Acetaminophen 160 mg, Chlorpheniramine maleate 1 mg, Dextromethorphan HBr 5 mg	Do not use			Do not use unless directed by a doctor		2 TSP	2 TSP	2 TSP	—	5 times in 24 hrs
Children's Tylenol Plus Cough and Runny Nose Suspension	Acetaminophen 160 mg, Chlorpheniramine maleate 1 mg, Dextromethorphan HBr 5 mg	Do not use			Do not use unless directed by a doctor		2 TSP	2 TSP	2 TSP	—	5 times in 24 hrs

Product	Active Ingredients								5 times in 24 hrs
Children's Tylenol Plus Cough and Sore Throat Suspension	Acetaminophen 160 mg Dextromethorphan HBr 5 mg	Do not use		1 TSP	2 TSP	2 TSP	2 TSP	—	5 times in 24 hrs
Children's Tylenol Plus Multi-Symptom Cold Suspension	Acetaminophen 160 mg Chlorpheniramine maleate 1 mg Dextromethorphan HBr 5 mg Phenylephrine HCl 2.5 mg	Do not use		Do not use unless directed by a doctor	2 TSP	2 TSP	2 TSP	—	5 times in 24 hrs
Children's Tylenol Plus Cold & Cough Suspension	Acetaminophen 160 mg Dextromethorphan HBr 5 mg Phenylephrine HCl 2.5 mg	Do not use		1 TSP	2 TSP	2 TSP	2 TSP	—	5 times in 24 hrs
Children's Tylenol Plus Flu	Acetaminophen 160 mg Chlorpheniramine maleate 1 mg Dextromethorphan HBr 5 mg Phenylephrine HCl 2.5 mg	Do not use		Do not use unless directed by a doctor	2 TSP	2 TSP	2 TSP	—	5 times in 24 hrs
Children's Tylenol Plus Cold Suspension	Acetaminophen 160 mg Chlorpheniramine maleate 1 mg Phenylephrine HCl 2.5 mg	Do not use		Do not use unless directed by a doctor	2 TSP	2 TSP	2 TSP	—	5 times in 24 hrs
Children's Tylenol Tablets	**Per tablet**								
Children's Tylenol Meltaway Tablets	Acetaminophen 80 mg	Ask a doctor	2 tablets	3 tablets	4 tablets	5 tablets	6 tablets	—	5 times in 24 hrs
Junior Tylenol Meltaway Tablets	Acetaminophen 160 mg	Ask a doctor	1 tablets**	1½ tablets**	2 tablets	2½ tablets	3 tablets	4 tablets	5 times in 24 hrs

* Ask a doctor for children under 2 years or under 24 lb.
** Ask a doctor for children under 6 years or under 48 lb.

Tylenol Conc./Children's/Jr.—Cont.

How Supplied
Concentrated TYLENOL® Infants' Drops: (purple-colored grape): bottles of ½ oz (15 mL) and 1 oz (30 mL); (red-colored cherry): bottles of ½ oz and 1 oz, and dye-free cherry each with calibrated plastic dropper.
Children's TYLENOL® Suspension Liquid: (red-colored cherry blast): bottles of 2 and 4 fl oz. (pink-colored bubblegum yum, purple-colored grape splash, red-colored very berry strawberry and dye-free cherry): bottles of 4 fl. oz.
Children's TYLENOL® Meltaways: (purple-colored grape punch, pink-colored bubblegum burst, scored, imprinted "TY80"). Bottles of 30 and also blister packaged 48's and 64's.
Jr. TYLENOL® Meltaways: (pink-colored bubblegum burst, imprinted "TY 160"). Blister packaged 24's and 48's. All packages listed above are safety sealed and use child-resistant safety caps or blisters.

CHILDREN'S TYLENOL®   OTC
Dosing Chart

[See table on pages 650 and 651]

REGULAR STRENGTH TYLENOL®   OTC
acetaminophen Tablets
EXTRA STRENGTH TYLENOL®
acetaminophen Caplets, Cool Caplets, and EZ Tabs
EXTRA STRENGTH TYLENOL®
acetaminophen Rapid Release Gels
EXTRA STRENGTH TYLENOL®
acetaminophen Adult Rapid Blast Liquid
TYLENOL® Arthritis Pain Acetaminophen Extended Release Geltabs/Caplets
TYLENOL® 8 Hour Acetaminophen Extended Release Caplets

Product information for all dosage forms of Adult TYLENOL acetaminophen have been combined under this heading.

Description
Each Regular Strength TYLENOL® Tablet contains acetaminophen 325 mg. Each Extra Strength TYLENOL® Caplet, Cool Caplet, EZ Tab, or Rapid Release Gel contains acetaminophen 500 mg. Extra Strength TYLENOL® Adult Liquid is alcohol-free and each 15 mL (1 tablespoonful) contains 500 mg acetaminophen. Each TYLENOL® Arthritis Pain Extended Relief Geltab/Caplet and each TYLENOL® 8 Hour Extended Release Caplet contains acetaminophen 650 mg.

Actions
Acetaminophen is a clinically proven analgesic/antipyretic. Acetaminophen is thought to produce analgesia by elevation of the pain threshold and antipyresis through action on the hypothalamic heat-regulating center. Acetaminophen is equal to aspirin in analgesic and antipyretic effectiveness and it is unlikely to produce many of the side effects associated with aspirin and aspirin-containing products. *Tylenol Arthritis Pain Extended Release* and *TYLENOL 8 Hour Extended Release* use a bilayer geltab/caplet. The first layer dissolves quickly to provide prompt relief while the second layer is time released to provide up to 8 hours of relief.

Uses
Regular Strength Tylenol Tablets; Extra Strength Tylenol Caplets, Rapid Release Gels, Cool Caplets, EZ tabs; Tylenol Adult Liquid; Tylenol 8 Hour Extended Release Caplets: temporarily relieves minor aches and pains due to:
- the common cold • headache • backache
- minor pain of arthritis • toothache
- muscular aches • premenstrual and menstrual cramps
- temporarily reduces fever

TYLENOL® Arthritis Pain Extended Release Caplets: temporarily relieves minor aches and pains due to:
- arthritis • the common cold • headache • toothache
- muscular aches • backache • menstrual cramps
- temporarily reduces fever

TYLENOL® Arthritis Pain Extended Release Geltabs: temporarily relieves minor aches and pains due to:
- minor pain of arthritis • muscular aches • backache
- premenstrual and menstrual cramps • the common cold • headache • toothache
- temporarily reduces fever

Directions
Regular Strength TYLENOL® Tablets:
- **do not take more than directed (see overdose warning)**

adults and children 12 years and over	• take 2 tablets every 4 to 6 hours while symptoms last • do not take more than 12 tablets in 24 hours • do not use for more than 10 days unless directed by a doctor
children 6–11 years	• take 1 tablet every 4 to 6 hours as needed • do not take more than 5 tablets in 24 hours • do not use for more than 5 days unless directed by a doctor
children under 6 years	• do not use this adult product in children under 6 years of age; this will provide more than the recommended dose (overdose) and may cause liver damage

Extra Strength TYLENOL® Caplets, EZ Tabs, or Rapid Release Gels:
- **do not take more than directed (see overdose warning)**

adults and children 12 years and over	• take 2 tablets, gelcaps, or caplets every 4 to 6 hours while symptoms last • do not take more than 8 tablets, gelcaps, or caplets in 24 hours • do not use for more than 10 days unless directed by a doctor
children under 12 years	do not use this adult product in children under 12 years of age; this will provide more than the recommended dose (overdose) and may cause liver damage

Extra Strength TYLENOL® Adult Liquid:
- **do not take more than directed (see overdose warning)**
- use only enclosed dosing cup designed for use with this product. Do not use any other dosing device.

adults and children 12 years and over	• take 2 tablespoons (tbsp.) or 1 oz in dose cup provided every 4 to 6 hours while symptoms last • do not take more than 8 tablespoons (tbsp) or 4 oz in 24 hours • do not take for more than 10 days unless directed by a doctor
children under 12 years	do not use this adult product in children under 12 years of age; this will provide more than the recommended dose (overdose) and may cause liver damage

Extra Strength TYLENOL® Cool Caplets:
- **do not take more than directed (see overdose warning)**

adults and children 12 years and over	• take 2 caplets every 4 to 6 hours while symptoms last • swallow whole - do not crush, chew or dissolve • do not take more than 8 caplets in 24 hours • do not take for more than 10 days unless directed by a doctor
children under 12 years	do not use this adult product in children under 12 years of age; this will provide more than the recommended dose (overdose) and may cause liver damage

TYLENOL® 8 Hour Extended Release Caplets
• do not take more than directed (see overdose warning)

adults and children 12 years and over	• take 2 caplets every 8 hours with water • swallow whole – do not crush, chew or dissolve • do not take more than 6 caplets in 24 hours • do not use for more than 10 days unless directed by a doctor
children under 12 years	• do not use

TYLENOL® Arthritis Pain Extended Release Geltabs/Caplets
• do not take more than directed (see overdose warning)

adults	• take 2 geltabs or caplets every 8 hours with water. Swallow only one geltab at a time. (Geltabs only) • take a sip of water before swallowing each geltab and wash each geltab down with water (up to a full 8 oz glass) (geltabs only) • swallow whole – do not crush, chew or dissolve • do not take more than 6 geltabs or caplets in 24 hours • do not use for more than 10 days unless directed by a doctor
under 18 years of age	• ask a doctor

Warnings
Regular Strength Tylenol
Liver warning: This product contains acetaminophen. Severe liver damage may occur if
• adult takes more than 12 tablets in 24 hours, which is the maximum daily amount
• child takes more than 5 doses in 24 hours
• taken with other drugs containing acetaminophen
• adult has 3 or more alcoholic drinks every day while using this product
Do not use
• with any other drug containing acetaminophen (prescription or nonprescription). If you are not sure whether a drug contains acetaminophen, ask a doctor or pharmacist.
• if you are allergic to acetaminophen or any of the inactive ingredients in this product.
Ask a doctor before use if the user has liver disease
Ask a doctor or pharmacist before use if the user is taking the blood thinning drug warfarin
Extra Strength Tylenol
Liver warning: This product contains acetaminophen. Severe liver damage may occur if you take
• more than 8 tablets, caplets, gelcaps or tablespoons in 24 hours, which is the maximum daily amount
• with other drugs containing acetaminophen
• 3 or more alcoholic drinks every day while using this product

Do not use
• with any other drug containing acetaminophen (prescription or nonprescription). If you are not sure whether a drug contains acetaminophen, ask a doctor or pharmacist.
• if you are allergic to acetaminophen or any of the inactive ingredients in this product.
Ask a doctor before use if you have liver disease
Ask a doctor or pharmacist before use if you are taking the blood thinning drug warfarin
Tylenol Arthritis Pain and Tylenol 8 Hour
Liver warning: This product contains acetaminophen. Severe liver damage may occur if you take
• more than 6 caplets or geltabs in 24 hours, which is the maximum daily amount
• with other drugs containing acetaminophen
• 3 or more alcoholic drinks every day while using this product
Do not use
• with any other drug containing acetaminophen (prescription or nonprescription). If you are not sure whether a drug contains acetaminophen, ask a doctor or pharmacist.
• if you have difficulty swallowing large tablets or capsules. People over 65 may have difficulty swallowing these tablets.
• if you are allergic to acetaminophen or any of the inactive ingredients in this product.
Ask a doctor before use if you have liver disease
Ask a doctor or pharmacist before use if you are taking the blood thinning drug warfarin
Stop use and ask a doctor if:
• the tablet got stuck in your throat (Geltabs only)
• pain gets worse or lasts more than 10 days
• fever gets worse or lasts more than 3 days
• new symptoms occur
• redness or swelling is present
These could be signs of a serious condition.
If pregnant or breast-feeding, ask a health professional before use.
Keep out of reach of children.
Overdose warning: Taking more than the recommended dose (overdose) may cause liver damage. In case of overdose, get medical help or contact a Poison Control Center right away. (1-800-222-1222) Quick medical attention is critical for adults as well as for children even if you do not notice any signs or symptoms.
Other information:
Regular Strength TYLENOL® Tablets
• store between 20–25°C (68–77°F)
Extra Strength TYLENOL® Caplets, Cool Caplets, EZ Tabs, or Rapid Release Gels:
• store between 20–25°C (68–77°F) (*Caplet, Cool Caplets and EZ Tabs*)
• store between 20–25°C (68–77°F). Avoid high humidity. (*Rapid Release Gel*)
Extra Strength TYLENOL® Adult Liquid
• each tablespoon contains: **sodium 9 mg**
• store between 20–25°C (68–77°F)
TYLENOL® Arthritis Pain Extended Release Geltabs/Caplets and *TYLENOL® 8 Hour Extended Release Caplets*
• store at 20–25°C (68–77°F)
• avoid excessive heat 40°C (104°F)

Professional Information:
Overdosage information for all adult TYLENOL products
Acetaminophen: Acetaminophen in massive overdosage may cause hepatic toxicity in some patients. In adults and adolescents ($\geq$ 12 years of age), hepatic toxicity may occur following ingestion of greater than 7.5 to 10 grams over a period of 8 hours or less. Fatalities are infrequent (less than 3–4% of untreated cases) and have rarely been reported with overdoses of less than 15 grams. In children (<12 years of age), an acute overdosage of less than 150 mg/kg has not been associated with hepatic toxicity. Early symptoms following a potentially hepatotoxic overdose may include: nausea, vomiting, diaphoresis and general malaise. Clinical and laboratory evidence of hepatic toxicity may not be apparent until 48 to 72 hours postingestion. In adults and adolescents, any individual presenting with an unknown amount of acetaminophen ingested or with a questionable or unreliable history about the time of ingestion should have a

Continued on next page

Tylenol—Cont.

plasma acetaminophen level drawn and be treated with N-acetylcysteine. For full prescribing information, refer to the N-acetylcysteine package insert. Do not await results of assays for plasma acetaminophen levels before initiating treatment with N-acetylcysteine. The following additional procedures are recommended: Promptly initiate gastric decontamination of the stomach. A plasma acetaminophen assay should be obtained as early as possible, but no sooner than four hours following ingestion. If an acetaminophen *extended release* product is involved, it may be appropriate to obtain an additional plasma acetaminophen level 4–6 hours following the initial acetaminophen level. If either acetaminophen level plots above the treatment line on the acetaminophen overdose nomogram, N-acetylcysteine treatment should be continued for a full course of therapy. Liver function studies should be obtained initially and repeated at 24-hour intervals. Serious toxicity or fatalities have been extremely infrequent following an acute acetaminophen overdose in young children, possibly because of differences in the way they metabolize acetaminophen. In children, the maximum potential amount ingested can be more easily estimated. If more than 150 mg/kg or an unknown amount was ingested, obtain a plasma acetaminophen level as soon as possible, but no sooner than 4 hours following ingestion. If an acetaminophen *extended release* product is involved, it may be appropriate to obtain an additional plasma acetaminophen level 4–6 hours following the initial acetaminophen level. If either acetaminophen level plots above the treatment line on the acetaminophen overdose nomogram, N-acetylcysteine treatment should be initiated and continued for a full course of therapy. If an assay cannot be obtained and the estimated acetaminophen ingestion exceeds 150 mg/kg, dosing with N-acetylcysteine should be initiated and continued for a full course of therapy. For additional emergency information, call your regional poison center or call the Rocky Mountain Poison Center toll-free, (1-800-525-6115).

Our adult Tylenol® combination products contain active ingredients in addition to acetaminophen. The following is basic overdose information regarding those ingredients.
Chlorpheniramine: Chlorpheniramine toxicity should be treated as you would an anthihistamine/anticholinergic overdose and is likely to be present within a few hours after acute ingestion.
Dextromethorhphan: Acute dextromethorphan overdose usually does not result in serious signs and symptoms unless massive amounts have been ingested. Signs and symptoms of a substantial overdose may include nausea and vomiting, visual disturbances, CNS disturbances and urinary retention.
Diphenhydramine: Diphenhydramine toxicity should be treated as you would an antihistamine/anticholinergic overdose and is likely to be present within a few hours after acute ingestion.
Doxylamine: Doxylamine toxicity should be treated as you would an antihistamine/anticholinergic overdose and is likely to be present within a few hours after acute ingestion.
Guaifenesin: Guaifenesin should be treated as a nontoxic ingestion.
Phenylephrine: Symptoms from phenylephrine overdose most often consist of hypertension, anxiety, nervousness, restlessness, tachycardia, bradycardia, headache, dizziness, and/or palpitations. Symptoms usually are transient and typically require no treatment.
Pseudoephedrine: Symptoms from pseudoephedrine overdose consist most often of mild anxiety, tachycardia and/or mild hypertension. Symptoms usually appear within 4 to 8 hours of ingestion and are transient, usually requiring no treatment.
For additional emergency information, please contact your local poison control center.
Alcohol Information: Chronic heavy alcohol abusers may be at increased risk of liver toxicity from excessive acetaminophen use, although reports of this event are rare. Reports usually involve cases of severe chronic alcoholics and the dosages of acetaminophen most often exceed recommended doses and often involve substantial overdose. Healthcare professionals should alert their patients who regularly consume large amounts of alcohol not to exceed recommended doses of acetaminophen.

Inactive ingredients:
Regular Strength TYLENOL® Tablets: cellulose, corn starch, magnesium stearate, sodium starch glycolate.
Extra Strength TYLENOL® Caplets: carnauba wax*, castor oil*, corn starch, FD&C red #40 aluminum lake, hypromellose, magnesium stearate, polyethylene glycol*, powdered cellulose, pregelatinized starch, propylene glycol, shellac, sodium starch glycolate, titanium dioxide. *contains one or more of these ingredients. **Cool Caplets:** castor oil, cellulose, corn starch, FD&C red #40, flavors, hypromellose, magnesium stearate, sodium starch glycolate, sucralose, titanium dioxide. **EZ Tabs:** anhydrous citric acid, carnauba wax, corn starch, D&C yellow #10 aluminum lake, FD&C red #40 aluminium lake, FD&C yellow #6 aluminum lake, iron oxide, magnesium stearate polyethylene glycol, polyvinyl alcohol, potassium sorbate, powdered cellulose, pregelatinized starch, propylene glycol, shellac, sodium benzoate, sodium citrate, sodium starch glycolate, sucralose, talc, titanium dioxide. **Rapid Release Gels:** benzyl alcohol, butylparaben, carboxymethylcellulose sodium, corn starch, D&C yellow #10, edetate calcium disodium, FD&C blue #1, FD&C red #40, gelatin, hypromellose, iron oxide, magnesium stearate, methylparaben, polyethylene glycol, polysorbate 80, powdered cellulose, pregelatinized starch, propylene glycol propylparaben, red iron oxide, sodium lauryl sulfate, sodium propionate, sodium starch glycolate, titanium dioxide, yellow iron oxide.
Extra Strength TYLENOL® Adult Liquid: citric acid, corn syrup, D&C red #33, FD&C red #40, flavor, polyethylene glycol, propylene glycol, purified water, saccharin sodium, sodium benzoate, sorbitol
TYLENOL® Arthritis Pain Extended Release **Caplets:** carnauba wax, corn starch, hydroxyethyl cellulose, hypromellose, magnesium stearate, microcrystalline cellulose, povidone, powdered cellulose, pregelatinized starch, sodium starch glycolate, titanium dioxide, triacetin. **Geltabs:** butylparaben, castor oil, corn starch, edetate calcium disodium, FD&C blue #1 aluminum lake, FD&C blue #2 aluminum lake, gelatin, hydroxyethyl cellulose, hypromellose, magnesium stearate, microcrystalline cellulose, povidone, powdered cellulose, pregelatinized starch, shellac, sodium lauryl sulfate, sodium propionate, sodium starch glycolate, titanium dioxide.
Tylenol 8 Hour Extended Release **Caplets:** corn starch, D&C yellow #10 aluminum lake, FD&C red #40 aluminum lake, FD&C yellow #6 aluminum lake, hydroxyethyl cellulose, magnesium stearate, microcrystalline cellulose, polyethylene glycol, polyvinyl alcohol, povidone, powdered cellulose, pregelantinized starch, sodium starch glycolate, sucralose, talc, titanium dioxide.

How Supplied
Regular Strength TYLENOL® Tablets: (colored white, scored, imprinted "TYLENOL" and "325")—tamper-evident bottles of 100.
Extra Strength TYLENOL® Caplets: (colored white, imprinted "TYLENOL 500 mg")—vials of 10, and tamper-evident bottles of 24, 50, 100, 150, 225, and 325. *Cool Caplets* 8, 24, 50, 100, 150. *Rapid Release Gels* (colored red and light blue with an exposed grey band; gelcaps are imprinted with "TY 500") tamper-evident bottles of 8, 24, 50, 100, 150, 225, and 290. *EZ Tabs* (colored red, imprinted "tylenol EZ Tabs") tamper-evident bottles of 24, 50, 100, and 225.
Extra Strength TYLENOL® Adult Rapid Blast Liquid: Cherry-flavored liquid (colored red) 8 fl. oz. tamper-evident bottle with child resistant safety cap and special dosage cup.
TYLENOL® Arthritis Pain Extended Release Caplets: (colored white, engraved "TYLENOL ER") tamper-evident bottles of 24, 50, 100, 150, 225 and 290
Geltabs: available in bottles of 20, 40 and 80
TYLENOL® 8 Hour Extended Release Caplets: (colored red, imprinted "8 HOUR") available in 24's, 50's, 100's, and 150's.

ZYRTEC® ALLERGY Tablets   OTC

Active ingredient (in each tablet)   *Purpose*
Cetirizine HCl 10 mg .... Antihistamine

Uses
temporarily relieves these symptoms due to hay fever or other upper respiratory allergies:
• runny nose • sneezing • itchy, watery eyes • itching of the nose or throat

Warnings
Do not use if you have ever had an allergic reaction to this product or any of its ingredients or to an antihistamine containing hydroxyzine.
Ask a doctor before use if you have liver or kidney disease. Your doctor should determine if you need a different dose.
Ask a doctor or pharmacist before use if you are taking tranquilizers or sedatives.
When using this product
• drowsiness may occur
• avoid alcoholic drinks
• alcohol, sedatives, and tranquilizers may increase drowsiness
• be careful when driving a motor vehicle or operating machinery
Stop use and ask a doctor if an allergic reaction to this product occurs. Seek medical help right away.
If pregnant or breast-feeding:
• if breast-feeding: not recommended
• if pregnant: ask a health professional before use.
Keep out of reach of children. In case of overdose, get medical help or contact a Poison Control Center right away. (1-800-222-1222)

Directions

adults and children 6 years and over	one 10 mg tablet once daily; do not take more than one 10 mg tablet in 24 hours. A 5 mg product may be appropriate for less severe symptoms.
adults 65 years and over	ask a doctor
children under 6 years of age	ask a doctor
consumers with liver or kidney disease	ask a doctor

Other information
• store between 20° to 25°C (68° to 77°F)
Inactive Ingredients colloidal silicon dioxide, croscarmellose sodium, hypromellose, lactose monohydrate, magnesium stearate, microcrystalline cellulose, polyethylene glycol, titanium dioxide or
carnauba wax, corn starch, hypromellose, lactose monohydrate, magnesium stearate, polyethylene glycol, povidone, titanium dioxide.

How Supplied
Zyrtec® Allergy Tablets are white, film-coated, rounded off rectangular shaped tablets—bottles of 5, 14, 30, 45, 75.

CHILDREN'S ZYRTEC® ALLERGY SYRUP   OTC
1 mg/mL oral solution

Active ingredient (in each 5 mL teaspoonful)   *Purpose*
Cetirizine HCl 5 mg .... Antihistamine

Uses
temporarily relieves these symptoms due to hay fever or other upper respiratory allergies:
■ runny nose ■ sneezing ■ itchy, watery eyes ■ itching of the nose or throat

Warnings
Do not use if you have ever had an allergic reaction to this product or any of its ingredients or to an antihistamine containing hydroxyzine.
Ask a doctor before use if you have liver or kidney disease. Your doctor should determine if you need a different dose.

Ask a doctor or pharmacist before use if you are taking tranquilizers or sedatives.
When using this product
■ drowsiness may occur
■ avoid alcoholic drinks
■ alcohol, sedatives, and tranquilizers may increase drowsiness
■ be careful when driving a motor vehicle or operating machinery
Stop use and ask a doctor if an allergic reaction to this product occurs. Seek medical help right away.
If pregnant or breast-feeding:
■ if breast-feeding: not recommended
■ if pregnant: ask a health professional before use.
Keep out of reach of children. In case of overdose, get medical help or contact a Poison Control Center right away. (1-800-222-1222)

Directions
■ use only with enclosed dosing cup

adults and children 6 years and over	1 teaspoonful (5 mL) or 2 teaspoonfuls (10 mL) once daily depending upon severity of symptoms; do not take more than 2 teaspoonfuls (10 mL) in 24 hours.
adults 65 years and over	1 teaspoonful (5 mL) once daily; do not take more than 1 teaspoonful (5 mL) in 24 hours.
children 2 to under 6 years of age	1/2 teaspoonful (2.5 mL) once daily. If needed, dose can be increased to a maximum of 1 teaspoonful (5 mL) once daily or 1/2 teaspoonful (2.5 mL) every 12 hours. Do not give more than 1 teaspoonful (5 mL) in 24 hours.
children under 2 years of age	ask a doctor
consumers with liver or kidney disease	ask a doctor

Other information
■ store between 20° to 25°C (68° to 77°F)
Inactive ingredients flavors, glacial acetic acid, glycerin, methylparaben, propylene glycol, propylparaben, purified water, sodium acetate, sodium hydroxide, sugar
Professional Information:
For Rx information, please refer to pg. 1920

HOW SUPPLIED
Children's Zyrtec Allergy Syrup: grape flavored bottles of 4 Fl oz (118 mL)

CHILDREN'S ZYRTEC® HIVES RELIEF   OTC
SYRUP

Active ingredient (in each 5 mL*)   *Purpose*
Cetirizine HCl 5 mg .... Antihistamine
*5 mL = one teaspoon

Use
relieves itching due to hives (urticaria). This product will not prevent hives or an allergic skin reaction from occurring.

Warnings
Severe Allergy Warning: Get emergency help **immediately** if you have hives along with any of the following symptoms:
■ trouble swallowing
■ dizziness or loss of consciousness
■ swelling of tongue
■ swelling in or around mouth
■ trouble speaking
■ drooling
■ wheezing or problems breathing

Continued on next page

Children's Zyrtec Hives—Cont.

These symptoms may be signs of anaphylactic shock. This condition can be life threatening if not treated by a health professional **immediately**. Symptoms of anaphylactic shock may occur when hives first appear or up to a few hours later. **Not a Substitute for Epinephrine.** If your doctor has prescribed an epinephrine injector for "anaphylaxis" or severe allergy symptoms that could occur with your hives, never use this product as a substitute for the epinephrine injector. If you have been prescribed an epinephrine injector, you should carry it with you at all times.

Do not use
■ to **prevent** hives from any known cause such as:
   ■ foods ■ insect stings ■ medicines ■ latex or rubber gloves

because this product will not stop hives from occurring. Avoiding the cause of your hives is the only way to prevent them. Hives can sometimes be serious. If you do not know the cause of your hives, see your doctor for a medical exam. Your doctor may be able to help you find a cause.
■ if you have ever had an allergic reaction to this product or any of its ingredients or to an antihistamine containing hydroxyzine.

Ask a doctor before use if you have
■ liver or kidney disease. Your doctor should determine if you need a different dose.
■ hives that are an unusual color, look bruised or blistered
■ hives that do not itch

Ask a doctor or pharmacist before use if you are taking tranquilizers or sedatives.

When using this product
■ drowsiness may occur
■ avoid alcoholic drinks
■ alcohol, sedatives, and tranquilizers may increase drowsiness
■ be careful when driving a motor vehicle or operating machinery

Stop use and ask a doctor if
■ an allergic reaction to this product occurs. Seek medical help right away.
■ symptoms do not improve after 3 days of treatment
■ the hives have lasted more than 6 weeks

If pregnant or breast-feeding:
■ if breast-feeding: not recommended
■ if pregnant: ask a health professional before use.

Keep out of reach of children. In case of overdose, get medical help or contact a Poison Control Center right away. (1-800-222-1222)

Directions
■ use only with enclosed dosing cup

adults and children 6 years and over	1 teaspoonful (5 mL) or 2 teaspoonfuls (10 mL) once daily depending upon severity of symptoms; do not take more than 2 teaspoonfuls (10 mL) in 24 hours.
adults 65 years and over	1 teaspoonful (5 mL) once daily; do not take more than 1 teaspoonful (5 mL) in 24 hours
children under 6 years of age	ask a doctor
consumers with liver or kidney disease	ask a doctor

Other information
■ store between 20° to 25°C (68° to 77°F)
Inactive ingredients flavors, glacial acetic acid, glycerin, methylparaben, propylene glycol, propylparaben, purified water, sodium acetate, sodium hydroxide, sugar

HOW SUPPLIED
Children's Zyrtec Hives Relief comes in 4 FL OZ (118 mL)

CHILDREN'S ZYRTEC® ALLERGY   OTC
cetirizine HCl/antihistamine

Active ingredient (in each 5 mg chewable tablet)   *Purpose*
Cetirizine HCl 5 mg .... Antihistamine
Active ingredient (in each 10 mg chewable tablet)
Cetirizine HCl 10 mg .... Antihistamine

Uses
temporarily relieves these symptoms due to hay fever or other upper respiratory allergies:
■ runny nose ■ sneezing ■ itchy, watery eyes ■ itching of the nose or throat

Warnings
Do not use if you have ever had an allergic reaction to this product or any of its ingredients or to an antihistamine containing hydroxyzine.
Ask a doctor before use if you have liver or kidney disease. Your doctor should determine if you need a different dose.
Ask a doctor or pharmacist before use if you are taking tranquilizers or sedatives.
When using this product
■ drowsiness may occur
■ avoid alcoholic drinks
■ alcohol, sedatives, and tranquilizers may increase drowsiness
■ be careful when driving a motor vehicle or operating machinery
Stop use and ask a doctor if an allergic reaction to this product occurs. Seek medical help right away.
If pregnant or breast-feeding:
■ if breast-feeding: not recommended
■ if pregnant: ask a health professional before use.
Keep out of reach of children. In case of overdose, get medical help or contact a Poison Control Center right away. (1-800-222-1222)

Directions
Children's Zyrtec Allergy 5 mg Chewable Tablets
■ may be taken with or without water

adults and children 6 years and over	1 to 2 tablets once daily depending upon severity of symptoms; do not take more than 2 tablets in 24 hours.
adults 65 years and over	1 tablet once a day; do not take more than 1 tablet in 24 hours
children under 6 years of age	ask a doctor
consumers with liver or kidney disease	ask a doctor

Children's Zyrtec Allergy 10 mg Chewable Tablets
■ may be taken with or without water

adults and children 6 years and over	one 10 mg tablet once daily; do not take more than one 10 mg tablet in 24 hours. A 5 mg product may be appropriate for less severe symptoms.
adults 65 years and over	ask a doctor
children under 6 years of age	ask a doctor
consumers with liver or kidney disease	ask a doctor

Other Information
■ store between 20° to 25°C (68° to 77°F)
Inactive Ingredients 5 mg: acesulfame potassium, beta-cyclodextrin, calcium silicate, carmine, colloidal silicon diox-

ide, disodium inosinate/guanylate, ethyl acetate, FD&C blue no. 2 aluminum lake, flavors, lactose monohydrate, magnesium stearate, maltodextrin, mannitol, microcrystalline cellulose, modified cornstarch, sorbitol
10 mg tablets: acesulfame potassium, betacyclodextrin, carmine, colloidal silicon dioxide, ethyl acetate, FD&C blue no. 2 aluminum lake, flavors, lactose monohydrate, magnesium stearate, maltodextrin, mannitol, microcrystalline cellulose, modified cornstarch

HOW SUPPLIED

5mg Chewable tablets comes in blister packs of 5.
10mg Chewable tablets comes in blister packs of 12 and 24.

ZYRTEC-D® Allergy & Congestion   OTC
Extended Release Tablets

Active ingredients	Purpose
(in each extended release tablet)	

Cetirizine HCl 5 mg .... Antihistamine
Pseudoephedrine HCl 120 mg .... Nasal decongestant

Uses

- temporarily relieves these symptoms due to hay fever or other upper respiratory allergies: ■ runny nose ■ sneezing ■ itchy, watery eyes ■ itching of the nose or throat ■ nasal congestion
- reduces swelling of nasal passages
- temporarily relieves sinus congestion and pressure
- temporarily restores freer breathing through the nose

Warnings

Do not use
- if you have ever had an allergic reaction to this product or any of its ingredients or to an antihistamine containing hydroxyzine.
- if you are now taking a prescription monoamine oxidase inhibitor (MAOI) (certain drugs for depression, psychiatric or emotional conditions, or Parkinson's disease), or for 2 weeks after stopping the MAOI drug. If you do not know if your prescription drug contains an MAOI, ask a doctor or pharmacist before taking this product.

Ask a doctor before use if you have
- heart disease
- thyroid disease
- diabetes
- glaucoma
- high blood pressure
- trouble urinating due to an enlarged prostate gland
- liver or kidney disease. Your doctor should determine if you need a different dose.

Ask a doctor or pharmacist before use if you are taking tranquilizers or sedatives.

When using this product
- **do not use more than directed**
- drowsiness may occur
- avoid alcoholic drinks
- alcohol, sedatives, and tranquilizers may increase drowsiness
- be careful when driving a motor vehicle or operating machinery

Stop use and ask a doctor if
- an allergic reaction to this product occurs. Seek medical help right away.
- you get nervous, dizzy, or sleepless
- symptoms do not improve within 7 days or are accompanied by fever

If pregnant or breast-feeding:
- if breast-feeding: not recommended
- if pregnant: ask a health professional before use.

Keep out of reach of children. In case of overdose, get medical help or contact a Poison Control Center right away. (1-800-222-1222)

Directions

- do not break or chew tablet; swallow tablet whole

adults and children 12 years and over	take 1 tablet every 12 hours; do not take more than 2 tablets in 24 hours

adults 65 years and over	ask a doctor
children under 12 years of age	ask a doctor
consumers with liver or kidney disease	ask a doctor

Other information
- store between 20° to 25°C (68° to 77°F)

Inactive ingredients
colloidal silicon dioxide, croscarmellose sodium, hypromellose, lactose monohydrate, magnesium stearate, microcrystalline cellulose, polyethylene glycol, titanium dioxide

How Supplied
Zyrtec D® Allergy & Congestion Tablets are white, round, bilayer tablets - in blister packs of 12 and 24

Merz Pharmaceuticals
Division of Merz, Inc.
4215 TUDOR LANE (27410)
P.O. BOX 18806
GREENSBORO, NC 27419

Direct Inquiries to:
Medical/Regulatory Affairs
(336) 856-2003
FAX: (336) 217-2439
For Medical Information Contact:
In Emergencies:
Medical/Regulatory Affairs
(336) 856-2003
FAX: (336) 217-2439

MEDERMA®   OTC
[mə-der-mă]
Skin Care for Scars™
Cosmetic

DESCRIPTION

Reduces the appearance of old and new scars resulting from: Surgery, Burns, Injury, Acne, Stretch Marks
Mederma® Skin Care for Scars™ helps make old and new scars appear softer, smoother and less noticeable. Mederma® is a greaseless, topical gel that contains Cepalin®, a proprietary botanical extract. Mederma® is easy to use, safe for sensitive skin, and now, has a fresh new scent.

INGREDIENTS

Water (Purified), PEG-4, Aloe Barbadensis Leaf Juice, Allium Cepa (Onion) Bulb Extract, Xanthan Gum, Allantoin, Methylparaben, Sorbic Acid, Fragrance.

DOSAGE AND ADMINISTRATION

Gently massage Mederma® into your scar 3 to 4 times daily. Mederma should be used for 8 weeks on new scars and 3-6 months on existing scars.

STORAGE

Store at room temperature

HOW SUPPLIED

MEDERMA® is available in:
- 20g tube (a three-month supply for scars up to three inches long)
- 50g tube (a three-month supply for scars up to ten inches long)

Manufactured for:
Merz Pharmaceuticals, Greensboro, NC 27410
5011179   Rev. 08/06

MEDERMA® CREAM PLUS SPF 30   OTC
[ma-der-mă]

DESCRIPTION

Mederma® Cream helps old and new scars appear softer, smoother and less noticeable. Mederma® Cream offers the added protection of SPF 30 in a cream formulation to help protect scars from the sun's UV rays. Mederma® Cream is a greaseless, topical cream that is safe for use on all skin types.

ACTIVE INGREDIENTS

Avobenzone 3%, Octocrylene 10%, Oxybenzone 6%

INACTIVE INGREDIENTS

Water, Allium Cepa (Onion) Bulb Extract, C12-15 Alkyl Benzoate, Dicaprylyl Carbonate, Hydrogenated Lecithin, Caprylic/Capric Triglyceride, Panthenol, Pentylene Glycol, Phenoxyethanol, Butyrospermum Parkii (Shea Butter), Glycerin, Ammonium Acryloyl – Dimethyltaurate/VP Copolymer, Fragrance, Squalane, Methylparaben, Xanthan Gum, Disodium EDTA, Ceramide 3, Sodium Hyaluronate, Butylparaben, Ethylparaben, Propylparaben, Isobutylparaben.

DOSAGE AND ADMINISTRATION

Evenly apply a small amount of Mederma® Cream and gently massage into the scar 3 times daily and as needed before sun exposure. Mederma® Cream should be used for 8 weeks on new scars and 3-6 months on existing scars. Children under 6 months of age: ask a doctor.

WARNINGS

For external use only. When using this product keep out of eyes. Rinse with water to remove. Stop use and ask doctor if rash or irritation develops and lasts. Do not use on open wounds. Keep out of reach of children. If swallowed, get medical help or contact a Poison Control Center right away.

STORAGE

Store at room temperature

HOW SUPPLIED

Mederma® Cream is available in:
• 20g tube (a three-month supply for scars up to three inches long)
• 50g tube (a three-month supply for scars eight to ten inches long)
Manufactured for:
Merz Pharmaceuticals, Greensboro, NC 27410
5011234   Rev. 09/07

MEDERMA® for Kids™   OTC
[ma-der-mă]
Cosmetic

DESCRIPTION

Helps soften and smooth old and new scars resulting from: cuts and scrapes, stitches, burns, bug bites, and surgery. Mederma® for Kids™ is a greaseless, pleasant-smelling purple topical gel that turns clear as it is massaged into the scar. Mederma® for Kids™ is the first and only scar product formulated especially for children ages 2 to 12.

INGREDIENTS

Water (Purified), PEG-4, Allium Cepa (Onion) Bulb Extract, Xanthan Gum, Allantoin, Fragrance, Methylparaben, Sorbic Acid, D&C Violet No. 2, FD&C Red No. 4.

DOSAGE AND ADMINISTRATION

Apply a thin coat of Mederma® for Kids™ to the scar and gently massage in 3 times per day for 8 weeks on new scars and 3 times a day for 3 to 6 months on existing scars.
NOT INTENDED FOR USE ON OPEN WOUNDS
FOR TOPICAL USE ONLY
THIS PRODUCT SHOULD BE USED UNDER ADULT SUPERVISION

STORAGE

Store at room temperature

HOW SUPPLIED

Mederma® for Kids™ is supplied in 20 g tubes. The 20g tube will last approximately 3 months when treating a scar up to 3 inches in length.
Manufactured for Merz Pharmaceuticals, Greensboro, NC 27410
34554   Rev 07/04

Paddock Laboratories, Inc.
**3940 QUEBEC AVENUE NORTH
MINNEAPOLIS, MN 55427-1244**

Direct Inquiries to:
Professional Affairs
(800) 328-5113

ACTIDOSE® with SORBITOL   OTC
[act 'ĭ –dose]
(Activated Charcoal with Sorbitol Suspension)

DESCRIPTION

Actidose with Sorbitol is supplied in bottles and tubes. Each 120 mL package contains 25 grams of activated charcoal in suspension and 48 grams of sorbitol. Each 240 mL package contains 50 grams of activated charcoal in suspension and 96 grams of sorbitol. Each milliliter contains 208 mg (0.208 gram) activated in charcoal and 400 mg (0.4 gram) sorbitol.

HOW SUPPLIED

25 g unit-of-use bottle NDC 0574-0120-04
50 g unit-of-use bottle NDC 0574-0120-08
25 g unit-of-use tube NDC 0574-0120-74
50 g unit-of-use tube NDC 0574-0120-76
Shown in Product Identification Guide, page 403

ACTIDOSE®–AQUA   OTC
[act 'ĭ 'dose a–qua]
(Activated Charcoal Suspension)

DESCRIPTION

Actidose-Aqua is supplied in bottles and tubes. Each 72 mL package contains 15 grams of activated charcoal in suspension, each 120 mL package contains 25 grams of activated charcoal in suspension and each 240 mL package contains 50 grams of activated charcoal in suspension. Each milliliter contains 208 mg (0.208 gram) activated charcoal.

HOW SUPPLIED

25 g unit-of-use bottle NDC 0574-0121-04
50 g unit-of-use bottle NDC 0574-0121-08
15 g unit-of-use tube NDC 0574-0121-25
25 g unit-of-use tube NDC 0574-0121-74
50 g unit-of-use tube NDC 0574-0121-76
Shown in Product Identification Guide, page 403

EZ-CHAR® Pellets   OTC
Activated Charcoal Pellets

DESCRIPTION

EZ-Char is a pelletized form of activated charcoal designed to be mixed with water and used as a poison adsorbent in poisoning emergencies.

HOW SUPPLIED

25 gram bottle NDC 0574-0122-25
Shown in Product Identification Guide, page 404

GLUTOSE 15™   OTC
GLUTOSE 45™
(Oral Glucose Gel)

DESCRIPTION
Glutose gel is a dye-free oral glucose gel for treatment of insulin reaction or hypoglycemia. Glutose gel contains Dextrose (d-glucose) USP 40%. Available in lemon and grape.

HOW SUPPLIED
Glutose 15 Lemon: 3 x 15g unit-of-use tubes per package NDC 0574-0069-30
Glutose 15 Grape: 3 x 15g unit-of-use tubes per package NDC 0574-0070-30
Glutose 45 Lemon: 1 x 45g multi-use tube per package NDC 0574-0069-45
Shown in Product Identification Guide, page 404

Schering-Plough HealthCare Products, Inc.
ROSELAND, NJ 07068 USA

Direct Product Requests to:
Schering-Plough HealthCare Products, Inc.
Roseland, NJ 07068 USA
For Medical Emergencies Contact:
Consumer Relations Department
P.O. Box 377
Memphis, TN 38151
(901) 320-2998 (Business Hours)

CORRECTOL®   ℞
(bisacodyl)
Stimulant Laxative, Delayed-Release Tablets, USP

Professional Labeling
Active ingredient: Each enteric coated tablet contains 5 mg bisacodyl, stimulant laxative.

INDICATIONS
For use as part of a bowel cleansing regimen in preparing the patient for surgery or for preparing the colon for x-ray endoscopic examination. This product generally produces a bowel movement in 6 to 12 hours.

WARNINGS
Patients should not use laxative products when abdominal pain, nausea or vomiting is present unless directed by a doctor. Patients should consult a doctor before use if they notice a sudden change in bowel habits that persists over a period of two weeks. Laxative products should not be used for a period longer than 1 week unless directed by a doctor. Rectal bleeding or failure to have a bowel movement after use of a laxative may indicate a serious condition. In these circumstances, patients should discontinue use and consult their doctor.
Because these bisacodyl tablets are enteric coated, patients should not chew or crush tablets. This product should not be used by persons who cannot swallow without chewing.
Patients should not take this product within 1 hour after taking an antacid or milk.
This product may cause abdominal pain, discomfort, faintness or cramps.
Pregnant or breast-feeding patients should ask a health professional before use. **Keep out of reach of children.** In case of overdose, patients should get medical help or contact a Poison Control Center right away.

DIRECTIONS
Adults and children 12 years of age and over: oral dosage is 5 mg to 15 mg (1 to 3 tablets) in a single daily dose. **Children 6 to under 12 years of age:** oral dosage is 5 mg (1 tab-

let) in a single daily dose. **Children under 6 years of age:** safety and effectiveness of bisacodyl have not been established.
Other information
Each tablet contains: calcium 20 mg. Do not expose to temperatures above 30°C (86°F), store between 20° to 25°C (68° to 77°F).
Inactive ingredients: calcium sulfate, carnauba wax, confectioner's sugar, croscarmellose sodium, D&C red No. 27 aluminum lake, FD&C blue No. 1 aluminum lake, FD&C yellow No. 6 aluminum lake, gelatin, kaolin, lactose anhydrous, magnesium stearate, methacrylic acid copolymer, microcrystalline cellulose, pharmaceutical ink, polyethylene glycol, polysorbate 80, povidone, sodium lauryl sulfate, sucrose, talc, titanium dioxide, white wax.
Questions or comments? If you have questions or need more information on this product, call toll free 1-800-317-2165 between 8:00 AM and 5:00 PM Central Standard Time, Monday through Friday.

HOW SUPPLIED
Boxes of 10, 30 and 90 comfort-coated tablets
© Copyright and Distributed by Schering-Plough Health-Care Products, Inc. Memphis, TN 38151. Product of Italy. All rights reserved.

Hyland's, A Division of Standard Homeopathic Company
210 WEST 131ST STREET
BOX 61067
LOS ANGELES, CA 90061

Direct Inquiries to:
Jay Borneman
(800) 624-9659 Ext. 20

HYLAND'S CALMS FORTÉ™   OTC

ACTIVE INGREDIENTS
Passiflora (Passion Flower) 1X triple strength HPUS, *Avena Sativa* (Oat) 1X double strength HPUS, *Humulus Lupulus* (Hops) 1X double strength HPUS, *Chamomilla* (Chamomile) 2X HPUS, *Calcarea Phosphorica* (Calcium Phosphate) 3X HPUS, *Ferrum Phosphorica* (Iron Phosphate) 3X HPUS, *Kali Phosphoricum* (Potassium Phosphate) 3X HPUS, *Natrum Phosphoricum* (Sodium Phosphate) 3X HPUS, *Magnesia Phosphoricum* (Magnesium Phosphate) 3X HPUS.

INACTIVE INGREDIENTS
Lactose, N.F., Calcium Sulfate, Starch (Corn and Tapioca), Magnesium Stearate.

INDICATIONS
Temporary symptomatic relief of simple nervous tension and sleeplessness.

DIRECTIONS
Adults: As a relaxant: Swallow 1–2 tablets with water as needed, three times daily, preferably before meals. For insomnia: 1 to 3 tablets 1/2 to 1 hour before retiring. Repeat as needed without danger of side effects. Children: As a relaxant: Swallow 1 tablet with water as needed, three times daily, preferably before meals. For insomnia: 1 to 2 tablets ½ to 1 hour before retiring. Repeat as needed without danger of side effects.

WARNING
Do not use if imprinted cap band is broken or missing. If symptoms persist for more than seven days or worsen, consult a licensed health care professional. As with any drug, if

Continued on next page

Hyland's Calms Forte—Cont.

you are pregnant or nursing a baby, seek the advice of a licensed health care professional before using this product. Keep this and all medications out of the reach of children. In case of accidental overdose, contact a Poison Control Center immediately. In case of emergency, the manufacturer may be reached 24 hours a day, 7 days a week by calling 800/624-9659.

HOW SUPPLIED

Bottles of 100 4-grain tablets (NDC 54973-1121-02), 50 4-grain tablets (NDC 54973-1121-01) and 32 5.5-grain caplets (NDC 54973-1121-68). Store at room temperature.

HYLAND'S CALMS FORTÉ 4 KIDS™   OTC

ACTIVE INGREDIENTS

ACONITUM NAP. 6X HPUS, CALC. PHOS. 12X HPUS, CHAMOMILLA 6X HPUS, CINA 6X HPUS, LYCOPODIUM 6X HPUS, NAT. MUR. 6X HPUS, PULSATILLA 6X HPUS, SULPHUR 6X HPUS

INACTIVE INGREDIENTS

Lactose, N.F.

INDICATIONS

Temporarily relieves the symptoms restlessness, sleeplessness, night terrors, growing pains, causeless crying, occasional sleeplessness due to travel and lack of focus in children.

DIRECTIONS

Children ages 2–5: dissolve 2 tablets under tongue every 15 minutes for up to 8 doses until relieved; Then every 4 hours as required.
Children ages 6–11: Dissolve 3 tablets under tongue every 15 minutes for up to 8 doses until relieved; Then every 4 hours as required.
Children 12 years and over: Dissolve 4 tablets under tongue every 15 minutes for up to 8 doses until relieved; then every 4 hours as are required or as recommended by a health care professional

WARNINGS

Ask a doctor before use if: pregnant or nursing, child is taking any prescription medications. If symptoms don't improve within 7 days, discontinue use and seek the advice of a licensed medical practitioner.
Keep this and all medications out of reach of children. Do not use if imprinted tamper band is broken or missing. In case of accidental overdose, contact a poison control center immediately. In case of emergency, the manufacturer may be contacted 24 hours a day, 7 days a week at 800/624-9659.

HOW SUPPLIED

Bottles of 125 1-grain tablets (NDC 54973-7518-03). Store at room temperature.

HYLAND'S COLD 'N COUGH 4 KIDS   OTC

Active Ingredient: *Allium Cepa* 6X HPUS, *Hepar Sulph Calc* 12X HPUS, *Nat Mur* 6X HPUS, *Phosphorus* 12X HPUS, *Pulsatilla* 6X HPUS, *Sulphur* 12X HPUS, *Hydrastis* 6X HPUS
Inactive Ingredients: Purified Water USP, Vegetable Glycerine USP, Citric Acid USP, Sodium Benzoate NF, Glycyrrhiza Extract

INDICATIONS

Temporarily relieves multi-symptom of the common cold.

DIRECTIONS

Children 2 to under 6 years: 1 teaspoon up to 6 times per day (every 4 hours) or as directed by a licensed health care professional.
Children 6 to under 12 years: 2 teaspoons up to 6 times per day (every 4 hours) or as directed by a licensed health care professional.

Adults and children 12 years and over: 3 teaspoons up to 6 times per day (every 4 hours) or as directed by a licensed health care professional.

WARNINGS

Ask your doctor before use if pregnant or nursing. Consult a physician if: Symptoms persist for more than 7 days or worsen; inflammation, fever or infection develops; symptoms are accompanied by a high fever (over 101° F); cough tends to recur or is accompanied by a high fever, rash or persistent headache. Keep this and all medications out of the reach of children. Do not use this product for persistent or chronic cough such as occurs with asthma, smoking or emphysema; or if cough is accompanied with excessive mucus, unless directed by a licensed health care professional. A persistent cough may be the sign of a serious condition. Do not use if imprinted tamper band is broken or missing. In case of accidental overdose, contact a poison control center immediately. In case of emergency, the manufacturer may be contacted 24 hours a day, 7 days a week at 800-624-9659.

HOW SUPPLIED

Bottles of 4 fluid oz (NDC 54973-3075-1). Store at room temperature.
Shown in Product Identification Guide, page 404

HYLAND'S COLIC TABLETS   OTC

ACTIVE INGREDIENT

Dioscorea 3X HPUS, *Chamomilla* 3X HPUS, *Colocynthis* 3X HPUS

INACTIVE INGREDIENTS

Lactose N.F.

INDICATIONS

Temporarily relieves the symptoms of colic and gas pains caused by irritating food, feeding too quickly, swallowing air and similar conditions during teething, colds and other minor upset periods in children.

DIRECTIONS

For Children up to 2 years: Dissolve 2 tablets on tongue every 15 minutes for up to 8 doses until relieved; then every 2 hours as required. For Children over 2 years: Dissolve 3 tablets as above or as recommended by a licensed health care professional. If you prefer, tablets may be dissolved in a teaspoon of water and then given to the child. Colic Tablets are very soft and dissolve almost instantly under the tongue. Please note: if your baby has been crying or is very upset, your baby may fall asleep after using this product because the pain has been relieved and your child can rest.

WARNINGS

Ask a doctor before use if pregnant or nursing. Consult a physician if symptoms persist for more than 7 days or worsen. Keep out of the reach of children. Do not use if imprinted tamper band is broken or missing. In case of accidental overdose, contact a Poison Control Center immediately. In case of emergency, the manufacturer may be contacted 24 hours a day, 7 days a week at 800/624-9659.

HOW SUPPLIED

Bottle of 125 1-grain, sublingual tablets (NDC 54973-7502-1)

HYLAND'S COUGH SYRUP WITH 100% NATURAL HONEY 4 KIDS   OTC

Active Ingredient: *Ipecacuanha* 6X HPUS, *Acontinum Napellus* 6X HPUS, *Spongia Tosta* 6X HPUS, *Antimonium Tartaricum* 6X HPUS
Inactive Ingredients: Orange Honey, Purified Water USP, Cane Sugar, Vegetable Glycerine USP, Sodium Benzoate NF

INDICATIONS

Temporarily relieves symptoms of simple, dry, tight or tickling coughs due to colds in children.

DIRECTIONS

Children 2 to under 6 years: 1 teaspoon up to 6 times per day (every 4 hours) or as directed by a licensed health care professional.
Children 6 to under 12 years: 2 teaspoons up to 6 times per day (every 4 hours) or as directed by a licensed health care professional.
Adults and children 12 years and over: 3 teaspoons up to 6 times per day (every 4 hours) or as directed by a licensed health care professional.

WARNINGS

Ask a doctor before use if pregnant or nursing. Consult a physician if: Symptoms persist for more than 7 days; cough tends to recur or is accompanied by a high fever, rash or persistent headache. Keep this and all medications out of the reach of children. Do not use this product for persistent or chronic cough such as occurs with asthma, smoking or emphysema; or if cough is accompanied with excessive mucus, unless directed by a licensed health care professional. A persistent cough may be the sign of a serious condition. Do not use if imprinted tamper band is broken or missing. In case of accidental overdose, contact a poison control center immediately. In case of emergency, the manufacturer may be contacted 24 hours a day, 7 days a week at 800/624-9659.

HOW SUPPLIED

Bottles of 4 fluid oz (NDC 54973-7520-1). Store at room temperature.

HYLAND'S EARACHE DROPS   OTC

ACTIVE INGREDIENTS

Pulsatilla 30C HPUS, Chamomilla 30C HPUS, Sulphur 30C HPUS, Calc Carb 30C HPUS, Belladonna 30C HPUS, Lycopodium 30C HPUS.

INACTIVE INGREDIENTS

Citric Acid USP, Purified Water, Sodium Benzoate USP, Vegetable Glycerin USP.

INDICATIONS

Temporarily relieves the symptoms of fever, pain, irritability and sleeplessness associated with earaches after diagnosis by a physician. Relieves common pain and itching of "swimmer's ear." If symptoms persist for more than 48 hours, or if there is a discharge from the ear, discontinue use and contact your physician.

DIRECTIONS

Adults and children of all ages: Tilt head sideways and apply 3–4 drops into involved ear 4 times daily or as needed. Tilt ear upward for at least 2 minutes after application or gently place cotton in ear to keep drops in.

WARNINGS

Keep away from eyes. Do not take by mouth. Earache drops are only to be used in the ears. Tip of applicator should not enter ear canal. Ask a doctor before use if pregnant or nursing. Consult a physician if symptoms persist for more than 48 hours or if there is discharge from the ear. Keep this and all medications out of reach of children. Do not use if imprinted tamper band is broken or missing. In case of accidental overdose, contact a poison control center immediately. In case of emergency, the manufacturer may be contacted 24 hours a day, 7 days a week at 800/624-9659.

HOW SUPPLIED

Bottle of .33 ounce (NDC 54973-7516-1)

HYLAND'S LEG CRAMPS WITH QUININE   OTC

ACTIVE INGREDIENTS

Cinchona Officinalis 3X, HPUS (Quinine), Viscum Album 3X, HPUS; Gnaphalium Polycephalum 3X, HPUS; Rhus Toxicodendron 6X, HPUS; Aconitum Napellus 6X, HPUS; Ledum Palustre 6X, HPUS; Magnesia Phosphorica 6X, HPUS.

INACTIVE INGREDIENTS

Lactose, N.F.

INDICATIONS

Hyland's Leg Cramps is a traditional homeopathic formula for the relief of symptoms of cramps and pains in lower back and legs often made worse by damp weather. Working without contraindications or side effects, Hyland's Leg Cramps stimulates your body's natural healing response to relieve symptoms. Hyland's Leg Cramps is safe for adults and can be used in conjuction with other medications.

DIRECTIONS

Adults: Dissolve 2–3 tablets under tongue every 4 hours as needed.

WARNINGS

Do not use if imprinted cap band is missing or broken. If symptoms persist for more than seven days or worsen, contact a licensed health care professional. As with any drug, if you are pregnant or nursing a baby, seek the advice of a licensed health care professional before using this product. Do not use if pregnant, sensitive to quinine or under 12 years of age. Keep this and all medications out of the reach of children. In case of accidental overdose, contact a poison control center immediately. In case of emergency, the manufacturer may be reached 24 hours a day, 7 days a week at 800-624-9659.

HOW SUPPLIED

Bottles of 100 3-grain sublingual tablets (NDC 54973- 2956-02), Bottles of 50 3-grain sublingual tablets (NDC 54973-2956-01), Bottles of 40 5.5 grain caplets (NDC 54973-2956-68). Store at room temperature.

HYLAND'S LEG CRAMPS PM WITH QUININE   OTC

Active Ingredients: *Calcarea Carbonica* 12X HPUS, *Causticum* 12X HPUS, *Chamomilla* 6X HPUS, *Cinchona Officinalis* 3X HPUS (Quinine), *Cuprum Metallicum* 12X HPUS, *Lycopodium* 12X HPUS, *Magnesia Phosphorica* 6X HPUS, *Rhus Toxicodendron* 6X HPUS, *Silicea* 12X HPUS, *Sulphur* 6X HPUS
INACTIVE INGREDIENTS: Lactose, N.F.

INDICATIONS

Temporarily relieves the symptoms of pain and cramps in lower body, legs, feet and toes with accompanying sleeplessness and disrupted sleep.

DIRECTIONS

Adults and children 12 years and over: Take 1-3 tablets before bed to help you fall asleep, stay asleep and relieve leg cramps. **After being woken by cramps:** Take 1-2 tablets to relieve pain and help you get back to sleep.

WARNINGS

As with any drug, ask a doctor before use if: You are pregnant or nursing a baby; sensitive to quinine; under 12 years of age. Keep this and all medications out of the reach of children. Do not use if imprinted tamper band is broken or missing. In case of accidental overdose, contact a poison control center immediately. In case of emergency, Hyland's may be contacted 24 hours a day, 7 days a week at 800-624-9659.

HOW SUPPLIED

Bottles of 50 3-grain tablets (NDC 54973-3093-01). Store at room temperature.
Shown in Product Identification Guide, page 404

HYLAND'S NERVE TONIC   OTC

ACTIVE INGREDIENTS

Calcarea Phosphorica (Calcium Phosphate) 3X HPUS; Ferrum Phosphorica (Iron Phosphate) 3X HPUS; Kali Phosphoricum (Potassium Phosphate) 3X HPUS; Natrum Phosphoricum (Sodium Phosphate) 3X HPUS; Magnesia Phosphoricum (Magnesium Phosphate) 3X HPUS.

Continued on next page

Hyland's Nerve Tonic—Cont.

INACTIVE INGREDIENTS

Lactose, N.F.

INDICATIONS

Temporary symptomatic relief of simple nervous tension and stress.

DIRECTIONS

Adults take 2–6 tablets before each meal and at bedtime. Children: 2 tablets. In severe cases take 3 tablets every 2 hours.

WARNINGS

Do not use if imprinted cap band is broken or missing. If symptoms persist for more than seven days or worsen, contact a licensed health care professional. As with any drug, if you are pregnant or nursing a baby, seek the advice of a licensed health care professional before using this product. Keep this and all medications out of the reach of children. In case of accidental overdose, contact a poison control center immediately. In cases of emergency, the manufacturer may be contacted 24 hours a day, 7 days a week at 800/624-9659.

HOW SUPPLIED

Bottles of 32 5.5-grain caplets (NDC 54973-1129-68), Bottles of 500 1-grain tablets (NDC 54973-1129-1), Bottles of 100 3-grain tablets (NDC 54973-3014-02)

HYLAND'S RESTFUL LEGS   OTC

ACTIVE INGREDIENTS

ARSENICUM ALBUM 12X HPUS, LYCOPODIUM 6X HPUS, PULSATILLA 6X HPUS, RHUS TOXICODENDRON 6X HPUS, SULPHUR 6X HPUS, ZINC METALLICUM 12X HPUS.

INACTIVE INGREDIENTS

Lactose, N.F.

INDICATIONS

Temporarily relieves the symptoms of the compelling urge to move legs to relieve sensations of itching, tingling, crawling, and restlessness of legs. Symptoms may occur while sitting or lying down, and improve with activity.

DIRECTIONS

Adults dissolve 2–3 quick dissolving tablets under tongue every 4 hours or as needed. Children ages 6–12 ½ adult dose.

WARNINGS

Ask a doctor before use if pregnant or nursing a baby. Consult a physician if symptoms persist for more than 7 days. Keep this and all medications out of reach of children. Do not use if imprinted tamper band is broken or missing. In case of accidental overdose, contact a poison control center immediately. In case of emergency, the manufacturer may be contacted 24 hours a day, 7 days a week at 800/624-9659.

HOW SUPPLIED

Bottles of 50 3-grain tablets (NDC 54973-2966-1). Store at room temperature.

HYLAND'S SNIFFLES 'N SNEEZES 4 KIDS OTC

ACTIVE INGREDIENTS

ACONITUM NAPELLUS 6X HPUS, ALLIUM CEPA 6X HPUS, ZINCUM GLUCONICUM 2X HPUS, GELSENIUM SEMPERVIRENS 6X HPUS.

INACTIVE INGREDIENTS

Lactose, N.F.

INDICATIONS

Temporarily relieves the symptoms of the common cold.

DIRECTIONS

Children ages 2–5: dissolve 2 tablets under tongue every 15 minutes for up to 8 doses until relieved; then every 4 hours as required. Children ages 6–11: dissolve 3 tablets under tongue every 15 minutes for up to 8 doses until relieved; then every 4 hours as required. Children 12 years and older: dissolve 4 tablets under tongue every 15 minutes for up to 8 doses until relieved; then every 4 hours as required or as recommended by a health care professional.

WARNINGS

Ask a doctor before use if pregnant or nursing. Consult a physician if: symptoms persist for more than 7 days or worsen. Inflammation, fever or infection develops. Symptoms are accompanied by high fever. (over 101° F) Keep this and all medications out of the reach of children. Do not use if imprinted tamper band is broken or missing. In case of accidental overdose, contact a poison control center immediately. In case of emergency, the manufacturer may be contacted 24 hours a day, 7 days a week at 800/624-9659.

HOW SUPPLIED

Bottles of 125 1-grain tablets (NDC 54973-7519-1). Store at room temperature.

HYLAND'S TEETHING GEL   OTC

ACTIVE INGREDIENTS

Calcarea Phosphorica (Calcium Phosphate) 12X, HPUS; Chamomilla (Chamomile) 6X, HPUS; Coffea Cruda (Coffee) 6X, HPUS; and Belladonna 6X, HPUS (Alkaloids 0.0000003%)

INACTIVE INGREDIENTS

Deionized water, Vegetable Glycerin, Hydroxyethyl Cellulose, Methyl Paraben and Propyl Paraben.

INDICATIONS

A homeopathic combination for the temporary relief of symptoms of simple restlessness and wakeful irritability due to cutting teeth.

DIRECTIONS

Apply to gums as necessary. If symptoms persist for more than seven days or worsen, discontinue use and contact your health care professional. Please note, if your baby has been crying or has been very upset, your baby may fall asleep after using this product because the pain has been relieved and your child can rest.

WARNINGS

Do not use if tube tip is broken or missing. If symptoms persist for more than seven days or if irritation persists, inflammation develops or fever or infection develop, discontinue use and consult a licensed health care professional. As with any drug, if you are pregnant or nursing a baby, seek the advice of a licensed health care professional before using this product. Keep this and all medications out of the reach of children. In case of accidental overdose, contact a poison control center immediately. In case of emergency, the manufacturer may be contacted 24 hours a day, 7 days a week at 800/624-9659.

HOW SUPPLIED

Tubes of 0.5 OZ. (NDC 54973-7521-1). Store at room temperature.

HYLAND'S TEETHING TABLETS   OTC

ACTIVE INGREDIENTS

Calcarea Phosphorica (Calcium Phosphate) 3X HPUS, *Chamomilla* (Chamomile) 3X HPUS, *Coffea Cruda* (Coffee) 3X HPUS, *Belladonna* 3X HPUS (Alkaloids 0.0003%).

INACTIVE INGREDIENTS

Lactose N.F.

INDICATIONS

A homeopathic combination for the temporary relief of symptoms of simple restlessness and wakeful irritability due to cutting teeth.

DIRECTIONS

Dissolve 2 to 3 tablets under the tongue 4 times per day. If you prefer, tablets may first be dissolved in a teaspoon of water and then given to the child. If the child is restless or wakeful, 2 tablets every hour for 6 doses or as recommended by a licensed health care professional. Teething Tablets are very soft and dissolve almost instantly under the tongue. Please note, if your baby has been crying or has been very upset, your baby may fall asleep after using this product because the pain has been relieved and your child can rest.

WARNINGS

Do Not use if imprinted cap band is broken or missing. If symptoms persist for more than seven days, or if irritation persist, inflammation develops or fever or infection develop, discontinue use and consult a licensed health care professional. As with any drug, if you are pregnant or nursing a baby, seek the advice of a health care professional before using this product. Keep this and all medications out of the reach of children. In case of accidental overdose, contact a poison control center immediately. In case of emergency, the manufacturer may be contacted 24 hours a day, 7 days a week at 800/624-9659.

HOW SUPPLIED

Bottles of 125 1-grain tablets (NDC 45973-7504-1), Bottles of 145 1-grain tablets (NDC 45973-7512-1), Bottles of 250 1-grain tablets (NDC 45973-7504-2). Store at room temperature.

IVYBLOCK®   OTC

ACTIVE INGREDIENT

Bentoquatam 5% (skin protectant)

INACTIVE INGREDIENTS

Bentonite, Benzyl Alcohol, Diisopropyl Adipate, Methylparaben, Purified Water, SDA 40 Denatured Alcohol (25% By Weight)

INDICATIONS

Helps prevent poison ivy, oak and sumac rash when applied before exposure.

DIRECTIONS

Shake well before use. Apply 15 minutes before risk of exposure. Avoid intentional contact with poison ivy, oak, and sumac. For adults and children 6 and older: apply every 4 hours for continued protection or sooner if needed. For children under 6 years: ask a doctor before use. Remove with soap and water after risk of exposure.

WARNINGS

For external use only. Keep away from fire or flame. Do not use if you are allergic to any ingredients, or have an open rash. When using this product, do not get into eyes. If contact occurs, rinse eyes thoroughly with water. Keep out of reach of children. If swallowed, get medical help or contact a Poison Control Center right away.

HOW SUPPLIED

Bottle of 4 ounces (NDC 62333-111-40)

SMILE'S PRID®   OTC

INGREDIENTS

Acidum Carbolicum 2X HPUS, Ichthammol 2X HPUS, Arnica Montana 2X HPUS, Calendula Off 3X HPUS, Echinacea Ang 3X HPUS, Sulphur 12X HPUS, Hepar Sulph 12X HPUS, Silicea 12X HPUS, Rosin, Beeswax, Petrolatum, Stearyl Alcohol, Methyl & Propyl Paraben.

INDICATIONS

Temporary topical relief of pain symptoms associated with boils, minor skin eruptions, redness and irritation. Also aids in relieving the discomfort of superficial cuts, scratches and wounds.

DIRECTIONS

Wash affected parts with hot water, dry and apply PRID® twice daily on clean bandage or gauze. Do not squeeze or pressure irritated skin area. After irritation subsides, repeat application once a day for several days. Children under two years: consult a physician.

CAUTION: If symptoms persist for more than seven days or worsen, or if fever occurs, contact a licensed health care professional. Do not use on broken skin. Keep out of reach of children. In case of accidental ingestion, seek professional assistance or contact a poison control center. For external use only. Avoid contact with eyes.

HOW SUPPLIED

18GM tin (NDC 0619- 4202-54). Keep in a cool dry place.

Topical BioMedics, Inc.

PO BOX 494
RHINEBECK, NY 12572-0494

Direct Inquiries to:
Professional Services at Topricin
Phone: (845) 871-4900 ext. 1115
Fax: (845) 876-0818
E-mail: info@topicalbiomedics.com for Free samples and prescription pads

TOPRICIN®   OTC

KEY FACTS

Topricin® is an odorless non-irritating anti-inflammatory pain relief cream that provides excellent adjunctive support in medical treatments such as post surgical, physical and occupational therapy, chiropractic. Greaseless and contains no lanolin, menthol, capsaicin, or fragrances.

ACTIVE INGREDIENTS

(HPUS) Arnica Montana 6X, Echinacea 6X, Aesculus 6X, Ruta Graveolens 6X, Lachesis 8X, Rhus Tox 6X Belladonna 6X, Crotalus 8X, Heloderma 8X, Naja 8X, Graphites 6X. Fomitopsis officinalis IX.

MAJOR USES

Topical relief of inflammation & pain, and a healing treatment for soft tissue & trauma/sports injuries.

BENEFITS

relieves swelling, stiffness, numbness, tingling and burning pain associated with these soft tissue ailments: carpal tunnel syndrome, other neuropathic pain, arthritis, lower back pain, muscle spasm of the back, neck, legs, and feet, muscle soreness, crushing injury, and sprains. First aid: bruises, minor burns. Use before and after exercise

DIRECTIONS

Apply generously 3–4 times a day or more often if needed making sure to cover the entire joint or area of pain. Massage in until absorbed. Reapply before bed and at the start of the day for best results.
For further information go to www.topicalbiomedics.com

SAFETY INFORMATION

For external use only, use only as directed, if pain persists for more that 7 days or worsens, Consult a doctor. This homeopathic medicine has no known side effects or contraindications. Complies with FDA standards as an OTC medicine. Safe to use for children, adults, pregnant women and the elderly. Paraben free.

Continued on next page

Topricin—Cont.

INACTIVE INGREDIENTS
purified water, highly refined vegetable oils, glycerin, medium-chain-triglyceride.

HOW SUPPLIED
Consumer size 4 oz jar or 2 oz tube or 8 oz pump
For professional use only: 16 oz or 32 oz pump bottle
Topricin Junior 1.5oz tube
Topricin Foot Therapy Cream 8 oz bottle
Topricin Consumer size....
Shown in Product Identification Guide, page 404

Unicity International
THE MAKE LIFE BETTER COMPANY
1201 NORTH 800 EAST
OREM, UT 84097

Direct Inquiries to:
(801) 226 2600
www.unicity.net
science@unicity.net
Products of Unicity International are distributed through independent distributors.

CM PLEX™ AND CM PLEX™ CREAM   OTC
[*CM plĕks*]
Proprietary fatty acid blend to help alleviate symptoms of osteoarthritis*

DESCRIPTION
CM Plex and CM Plex Cream are a softgel and topical cream, respectively, that contain a proprietary blend of cetylated fatty acids, soy and fish oil.
CM Plex is an opaque powder that is insoluble in water. One softgel capsule of CM Plex contains 350 mg of cetylated fatty acids, 160 mg of soy oil and 25 mg of salmon oil. In addition to these active ingredients, each softgel capsule contains glycerin and St. John's Bread.
CM Plex Cream is an off-white powder that is insoluble in water. One gram of CM Plex Cream contains 7.7 mg of cetylated fatty acids and olive oil. In addition to these active ingredients CM Plex Cream also contains glyceryl stearate, glycerin, lecithin, tocopheryl acetate, benzyl alcohol, phenoxyethanol, carbomer, PEG-100 stearate, sodium hydroxide, methylparaben, propylparaben, butylparaben, ethylparaben, isobutylparaben and citrus aurantium bergamia (Bergamot) fruit oil.

BENEFITS AND RESEARCH
Cetyl myristoleate and related fatty acids have been proven to improve joint health through their anti-inflammatory effects. A clinical study indicated that subjects exhibited improvements in knee flexion compared to placebo. A second study indicated the cream is effective for improving knee range of motion, ability to climb stairs, rise from a chair and walk, balance, strength, and endurance.*

SUGGESTED USE
Softgels: Take one to two softgels three times daily with meals.
Cream: Apply generously onto clean skin and gently massage until the cream disappears. Repeat 3 to 4 times daily as necessary. For maximum results combine both products.

SAFETY AND WARNINGS
CM Plex Softgels and Cream are well tolerated. Some gastrointestinal discomfort may be experienced with CM Plex Softgels as with any dietary supplement.

HOW SUPPLIED
CM Plex is available in soft gels and as a topical cream.

REFERENCES
Hesslink, R et al (2002), Journal of Rheumatology 29, 1708–1712.
Kraemer, WJ et al (2004), Journal of Rheumatology 31, 767–774.
* THESE STATEMENTS HAVE NOT BEEN EVALUATED BY THE FOOD AND DRUG ADMINISTRATION. THIS PRODUCT IS NOT INTENDED TO DIAGNOSE, TREAT CURE, OR PREVENT ANY DISEASE.
Shown in Product Identification Guide, page 404

IMMUNIZEN®   OTC
[*ĭm mōō nĭ zĕn*]

DESCRIPTION
Immunizen® is a nutritional supplement for boosting the immune system.
Immunizen® is a modestly water soluble, white crystalline powder. Immunizen® consists of a proprietary ingredient blend of colostrum, arabinogalactan, 1,3, 1,6 yeast beta-glucans and lactoferrin. In addition to the active ingredients, each 835 mg capsule of Immunizen® contains natural gelatin, stearic acid and silicon dioxide.

BENEFITS AND RESEARCH
Immunizen® combines the positive immune modulating effects of colostrum, arabinogalactans, yeast beta-glucans and lactoferrin to boost your body's natural defenses to foreign antigens. Colostrum is composed of immunoglobulins that bolster the body's immune system by providing immunity against various pathogens.
Beta-glucans are generally derived from the cell walls of the yeast species *Saccharomyces cerevisiae*. Beta-glucans are potent immuno-modulating agents that prime both the innate and adaptive immune systems.

USAGE
Take six capsules with water one to two hours before a meal for 10 days as needed.

SAFETY AND WARNINGS
Immunizen® is well tolerated. Some gastrointestinal discomfort may be experienced as with any dietary supplement.

HOW SUPPLIED
Available in capsules.

REFERENCES
Lilius EM, Marnila P. (2001), Current Opinion in Infectious Diseases 14:295-300.
Hammarström L, Weiner CK. (2008), Advances in Experimental Medicine and Biology 606: 321-343.
Chan GC, Chan WK, Sze DM. (2009), The Journal of Hematology and Oncology, 2: 25-
* THESE STATEMENTS HAVE NOT BEEN EVALUATED BY THE FOOD AND DRUG ADMINISTRATION. THIS PRODUCT IS NOT INTENDED TO DIAGNOSE, TREAT, CURE, OR PREVENT ANY DISEASE.

VISUTEIN®   OTC
[*vĭ s-u-tēn*]
Clinically proven to support healthy eyes and vision.*

DESCRIPTION
VISUtein® is a nutritional supplement for maintaining healthy eyes. VISUtein® contains lutein, anthocyanidins from bilberry, N-acetyl cysteine, zinc, mixed carotenoids (β−carotene, α−carotene and zeaxanthin) and riboflavin.
VISUtein® is a purple crystalline powder that is water soluble. In addition to the active ingredients lutein, anthocyanidins, N-acetyl cysteine, zinc, mixed carotenoids and riboflavin, each 600 mg capsule contains magnesium stearate.

BENEFITS AND RESEARCH
Antioxidants from the carotenoid chemical family, such as lutein and zeaxanthin, play an important role in eye health. Low concentrations of these compounds in the retina are associated with age-related macular degeneration (AMD).

Supplementation with high levels of lutein can restore the lutein concentration in the retina. Further supplementation of vitamins C and E along with zinc, copper and β-carotene delayed the onset of AMD. Low glutathione levels have been shown to reduce protection of the eye against oxidative stress. N-acetyl cysteine has been shown to elevate glutathione levels in the retina. A recent clinical study with VISUtein® has shown that AMD patients experience clear improvements in visual acuity, contrast sensitivity, and recovery from a flash.*

USAGE

Take two capsules per day with a meal.

SAFETY AND WARNINGS

VISUtein® is well tolerated. Some gastrointestinal discomfort may be experienced as with any dietary supplement.

HOW SUPPLIED

Available in capsules.

REFERENCES

Newsome, DA and Meyers, L (2004), "A Randomized Prospective Clinical Trial of Two Commercially Available Ocular Diet Supplements", In press.
* THESE STATEMENTS HAVE NOT BEEN EVALUATED BY THE FOOD AND DRUG ADMINISTRATION. THIS PRODUCT IS NOT INTENDED TO DIAGNOSE, TREAT, CURE, OR PREVENT ANY DISEASE.

Shown in Product Identification Guide, page 404

Upsher-Smith Laboratories, Inc.
6701 EVENSTAD DRIVE
MINNEAPOLIS, MN 55369

For Medical Information Contact:
Write: Medical Information Department
or call: (800) 654-2299
(during business hours-8:00 am to 5:00 pm CST)

AMLACTIN®   OTC
Moisturizing Body Lotion and Cream
[ăm-lăk-tĭn]
Cosmetic Lotion and Cream

DESCRIPTION

AMLACTIN® Moisturizing Body Lotion and Cream are special formulations of 12% lactic acid neutralized with ammonium hydroxide to provide a lotion or cream pH of 4.5–5.5. Lactic acid, an alpha-hydroxy acid, is a naturally occurring humectant for the skin. AMLACTIN® moisturizes and softens rough, dry skin.

HOW SUPPLIED:

225g (8oz) plastic bottle: List No. 0245-0023-22
400g (14oz) plastic bottle: List No. 0245-0023-40
140g (4.9oz) tube: List No. 0245-0024-14

AMLACTIN XL®   OTC
[ăm-lăk-tĭn X-L]
Moisturizing Lotion, ULTRAPLEX® Formulation

PRODUCT DESCRIPTION

AmLactin XL® Moisturizing Lotion is a clinically proven moisturizer, which provides powerful moisturizing for rough, dry skin. AmLactin XL® Moisturizing Lotion contains ULTRAPLEX® formulation, a proprietary blend of alpha-hydroxy moisturizing compounds. Alpha-hydroxy acids are naturally occurring humectants, which moisturize and soften rough, dry skin.

HOW SUPPLIED

AmLactin XL® Moisturizing Lotion is available in single 160g tubes packed in an outer carton (List 0245-0022-16).

U.S. Pharmaceutical Corporation
2401 MELLON COURT, SUITE C
DECATUR, GA 30035

Direct Inquiries to:
Allison Krebs-Bensch
Vice President
(770) 987-4745
a.bensch@uspco.com

HEMOCYTE® TABLETS   OTC
[hē-mō-sīt]
(ferrous fumarate 324 mg.)

HOW SUPPLIED

Boxes of 100 child-proof tablets NDC 52747-307-70
Boxes of 30 child-proof tablets NDC 52747-307-30

TANDEM®   OTC
[tan' dem]
Ferrous Fumarate/Polysaccharide Iron Complex Capsules

NDC 52747-900-90

HOW SUPPLIED

Tandem® are light brown opaque capsules imprinted radially "Tandem" "US, US, US, US/US, US, US, US": 9 units of 10 capsules, each blister pack in containers of 90 capsules (NDC 52747-900-90).

Westlake Laboratories, Inc.
24700 CENTER RIDGE ROAD
CLEVELAND, OH 44145

Direct Inquiries to:
Customer Service
(888) WSTLAKE (978–5253)
Fax (440) 835–2177
Internet: www.westlake-labs.com

AUTHIA® CREAM   OTC
TTFD & Methyl B$_{12}$ Supplement

DESCRIPTION

Thiamine (Vitamin B$_1$) disulfide and methyl Vitamin B$_{12}$ is a pink liposomal cream for topical application designed for transdermal delivery (TD) of the two vitamins. It has a mild odor due to its sulfur content.

CLINICAL OBSERVATIONS

TD application is a more efficient way of administering these vitamins and they are solely responsible for any therapeutic benefit from the cream. Use of TTFD has been shown to result in clinical improvement in 8 of 10 autistic children in a pilot study.

CONTRAINDICATIONS

None known other than a rare sensitivity to excipients in the cream. (Paraben Free)

ADVERSE REACTIONS

Occasional localized rash may result at the site of application. An abnormal metabolism of the patient may create a skunk-like odor. This gradually disappears as clinical improvement occurs and can often be modified by taking 10 mg of Biotin daily.

Continued on next page

Authia—Cont.

DOSAGE

¼ tsp. (approximately 1 ml) of AUTHIA® CREAM topically will provide a pharmacological dose of 1000 mcg methyl cobalamin and 50 mg TTFD. Usual dose is once to twice daily.

HOW SUPPLIED

AUTHIA® CREAM is supplied in a 2 oz. plastic tube that does not require refrigeration.
Also available in enteric coated tablets.
Covered by U.S. Patent Number 6,585,996

Shown in Product Identification Guide, page 404

BEVITAMEL®   OTC
[bē-vīt 'ə-měl]
Melatonin-B-Vitamin Supplement

DESCRIPTION

Each tablet contains:

	Amount	% U.S. RDA*
Melatonin	3 mg	***
Methylcobalamin (Vitamin B12)	1000 µg	16667
Folic Acid	400 µg	100

*   U.S. Recommended Daily Amount (RDA) established by the U.S. Food and Drug Administration (FDA).
*** The U.S.RDA has not been established by the U.S. FDA.

INDICATIONS

Bevitamel can be used to enhance the natural sleep process. Vitamin B12 and Folic Acid can be used to assist the metabolism of blood homocysteine.

CONTRAINDICATIONS

Product NOT intended for the treatment of Pernicious anemia

WARNINGS

Keep out of reach of children and store in a cool dry place. Tamper-resistant package, do not use if outer seal is missing or broken.

PRECAUTIONS

The dose size and timing may need to be adjusted by the physician to provide maximum effect for individual patients.
Individuals taking other medications, or with autoimmune, seizure or endocrine disorders and pregnant or lactating women, should consult a physician prior to use.

ADVERSE REACTIONS

None known.

DOSAGE AND ADMINISTRATION

One tablet sub-lingual approximately 30 minutes before bedtime as directed by a physician. Fractional tablets may be taken when indicated.

OVERDOSAGE

None known.

HOW SUPPLIED

BEVITAMEL is supplied as a pink bisected sub-lingual tablet (60 per bottle).

Shown in Product Identification Guide, page 404

DIETARY SUPPLEMENT INFORMATION

This section presents information on natural remedies and nutritional supplements marketed under the Dietary Supplement Health and Education Act of 1994. The information on each product described has been provided by the manufacturer for publication in the 2010 *PDR* or 2010 *PDR for Ophthalmic Medicines*.

Products found in this section include vitamins, minerals, and other substances intended to supplement the diet. The descriptions of these products are designed to provide all information necessary for informed use, including, when applicable, active ingredients, inactive ingredients, actions, warnings, cautions, interactions, symptoms and treatment of oral overdosage, dosage and directions for use, and how supplied. Descriptions in this section must be in full compliance with the Dietary Supplement Health and Education Act, which permits claims regarding a product's effect on the structure or functioning of the body, but forbids claims regarding a product's ability to treat, diagnose, cure, or prevent any specific disease. **Note:** Descriptions of products marketed under the Dietary Supplement Health and Education Act do not receive formal evaluation or approval from the Food and Drug Administration.

The publisher does not warrant or guarantee any product described here, and does not perform any independent analysis of the information provided. Inclusion of a product in this book does not represent an endorsement, and the publisher does not advocate the use of any product listed.

America Pharma Co.
750 STIMSON AVENUE
CITY OF INDUSTRY, CA 91745

Direct Inquiries to:
Phone: (626) 336-8889
Fax: (626) 336-1299
Email: ac.usa.inc@gmail.com
http://www.acusainc.net

HEPLIVE   DS

INGREDIENTS
Each Softgel Capsule Contains:
Vitamin A (Palmitate) 1200iu
Vitamin E (d-Alpha Tocopherol) 10iu
Vitamin C (Ascorbic Acid) 10mg
Folic Acid 0.06mg
Vitamin B1 (Thiamine Mononitrate) 1mg
Vitamin B2 (Riboflavin) 1mg
Niacinamide 10mg
Vitamin B6 (Pyridoxine HCl) 0.5mg
Vitamin B12 (Cobalamin) 1mg
Biotin 3.3mg
Pantothenia Acid 2mg
Choline Bitartrate 21mg
Zinc (Zinc Sulfate) 2mg
Desiccated Liver 194.4mg
Liver Concentrate 64.8mg
Liver Fraction Number#2 64.8mg
Yeast (Dried) 64.8mg
dl-Methionine 10mg
Inositol 10mg

INTRODUCTION
HEPLIVE is a balanced formulation of vitamins, minerals, lipotropic factors, and vitamin-protein supplements. It's of value as a nutritional supplement for persons who are receiving professional treatment for alcoholism, hepatic dysfunction due to hepatotoxic drugs and liver poisons, male and female infertility due to hormonal imbalance caused by hepatic dyfunction, and for nutritional supplementation after treatment.

DOSAGE
Three to Six Capsules Daily.

HOW SUPPLIED
30/60/90/100/120/300/1000 Softgel Capsules Per Bottle.
Shown in Product Identification Guide, page 402

MEILI   DS

Each Soft Capsule Contains:
Placenta extract Powder 300mg
Elastin 120mg
Collagen 100mg
Spiralina 100mg
Desiccated Liver 100mg
Avocado Oil 50mg
Blackcurrant Berry 50mg
Kelp 50mg
Bee Pollen 50mg
Royal Jelly 40mg

INTRODUCTION
With advances in medicine, people nowadays live in longer life. People are not satisfied with just living longer. They also want to be healthy, to look young at any age. They try many ways to minimize appearances of aging. Besides using skin care and cosmetic products to preserve physical appearance, people should also look into oral supplements, which will enhance beauty from within. Oral intake of MeiLi can work wonder in the body, increase hormone functions, make skin to glow from within, for younger and firmer skin texture.

DOSAGE
Twice daily, 1-2 capsules/time, increase as necessary

HOW SUPPLIED
30-1000 soft capsules/1box
Shown in Product Identification Guide, page 402

MEILI CLEAR SOFT CAPSULES   DS

Each Soft Capsule Contains:
Bilberry extract 20mg
Eyebright extract 50mg
Marigold (Lutein 2mg) 10mg
Marine Algae (Zeaxanthin 800mcg) 4mg
Folic Acid 0.4mg
Ascorbic Acid 60mg
Lycii Powder 20mg
Beta Carotene 30% 30mg

INTRODUCTION
It is very common for people to have some minor problems with their eyes such as red eyes, dry eyes, itchiness, sensitivity to light, constant tearing, etc. By lacking just one type of vitamin, it can lead to various eye problems. For example: cataract, glaucoma, eye pressure or inflammation, blurry eyesight, dried eyes, itchiness, etc. In order to avoid these kinds of health issues, it is necessary to include all sorts of vitamins and minerals in the diet. Meili Clear is one of these supplements that can help provide nutrients that cannot be formed naturally. Meili Clear can help protect eyes from harm.

DOSAGE
Twice daily, 1-2 capsules/time, increase as necessary

HOW SUPPLIED
30-1000 soft capsules/1box
Shown in Product Identification Guide, page 402

SPRINGCODE SPRAY   DS

Without containing macromolecule protein and hormones, this product is deemed the most upscale preparation of sheep placenta, which only retains more than 8,000 primitive life elements such as the micro molecules, polysaccharide factor, and nucleotides. Springcode Spray has the advantages of injection-free, allergy-free, effective and low-price properties.

INDICATION
1. Adjustment of endocrine secretion and metabolism, enhancement of liver function, and anti-inflammation.
2. Boost of regeneration ability of tissue, improvement of blood circulation.
3. Increase of body immunity and adjustment of autonomic nervous system.
4. Neurasthenia, insomnia, malnutrition, in appetence, climacteric disorder.
5. Delay of aging, anti-fatigue, beauty and skin care.
Applicable to:
1. Youth in the development period
2. Women in the climacteric period
3. Daily health care for the general public
4. Anti-aging and health protection for middle and old persons
Application:
Each bottle contains 10 ml. Use two to three times daily, apply two sprays each time to sublingual mucosa and swallow it after two minutes.
For the amount taken for different physical constitution and illness, please follow the directions of doctors or professionals.

DOSAGE
10ml/bottle, 1ml/40mg
Shown in Product Identification Guide, page 402

Bausch & Lomb Incorporated
ONE BAUSCH & LOMB PLACE
ROCHESTER NY 14604

7 GIRALDA FARMS
MADISON, NJ 07940

Direct Inquiries to:
Main Office
(585) 338-6000
Consumer Affairs
1-800-553-5340

BAUSCH & LOMB
PRESERVISION® AREDS   DS
Eye Vitamin and Mineral Supplement
AREDS: Soft Gels Formula.
Convenient to take 2 per day Soft Gels Formula
(AREDS daily dose)

DESCRIPTION
see Supplement Facts (table A)
[See table A below]

Other Ingredients: Gelatin, Glycerin, Soybean Oil, Soy
Lecithin, Yellow Beeswax, Silicon Dioxide, Titanium
Dioxide, FD&C Yellow 6, FD&C Red #40, FD&C Blue #1,
Contains Soy.
- Age-related macular degeneration (AMD) is the leading
  cause of vision loss and blindness in people over 55. The
  landmark National Institutes of Health AREDS trial
  proved that a high potency antioxidant vitamin and mineral supplement was effective in helping to preserve the
  sight of certain people most at risk.*
- The patented Bausch & Lomb PreserVision® Soft Gels
  are based on the AREDS Formula that is the ONLY eye
  vitamin and mineral supplement clinically proven effective in the 10 year National Institutes of Health (NIH)
  Age Related Eye Disease Study (AREDS). US Patent
  6,660,297.
- Bausch & Lomb PreserVision® Soft Gels are a high potency antioxidant and mineral supplement with the antioxidant vitamins A, C, E, and selected minerals in
  amounts above those in ordinary multivitamins and generally cannot be obtained through diet alone.
- **Recommended Intake:** Instead of taking 4 tablets per day
  to get the high levels proven effective in the National Institutes of Health (NIH) Age Related Eye Disease Study
  (AREDS), you only need to take: 2 softgels per day – 1 in
  the morning. 1 in the evening with a full glass of water
  and during meals.
Bausch & Lomb PreserVision® is the #1 recommended eye
vitamin and mineral supplement among vitreoretinal eye
doctors for AMD.**
CURRENT AND FORMER SMOKERS:
Consult your eye doctor or eye care professional about the
risks associated with smoking and Beta-Carotene.

* This statement has not been evaluated by the Food
and Drug Administration. This product is not intended
to diagnose, treat, cure or prevent any disease.

** Data on file, Bausch & Lomb Incorporated.

HOW SUPPLIED
NDC 24208-532-10 60 ct. NDC 24208-532-30 120 ct. NDC
24208-532-40 150 ct. Available in bottles of 60 count, 120
and 150 count soft gels.
Oval shaped soft gelatin capsule.
DO NOT USE IF SEAL UNDER CLOSURE IS BROKEN
Keep this product out of the reach of children.
STORE AT ROOM TEMPERATURE
For more information or to report a serious side effect, call
1-800-553-5340
Made in the USA
Marketed by:
Bausch & Lomb Incorporated, Rochester NY 14609
Bausch & Lomb and Preservision are registered trademarks
of Bausch & Lomb Incorporated.
© Bausch & Lomb Incorporated. All rights reserved.
Shown in Product Identification Guide, page 402

BAUSCH & LOMB
PRESERVISION® LUTEIN   DS
Eye Vitamin and Mineral Supplement Beta-carotene
free formulation.
Convenient to take 2 per day Soft Gels

DESCRIPTION
see Supplement Facts (table A)
[See first table at top of next page]

Other Ingredients: Gelatin, Glycerin, Soybean Oil, Soy
Lecithin, Yellow Beeswax, Silicon Dioxide, Titanium
Dioxide, FD&C Red #40, FD&C Blue #1. Contains Soy.
This product is Vitamin A (beta-carotene) Free.
- The Bausch & Lomb PreserVision® Lutein patented formula is based on the Bausch & Lomb PreserVision®
  AREDS formula*, with the beta-carotene substituted with
  5 mg of FloraGlo® Lutein.
- Lutein is a carotenoid found in dark leafy green vegetables such as spinach. Carotenoids are concentrated in
  the macula, the part of the eye responsible for central vision. Studies suggest that lutein plays an essential role in
  maintaining healthy central vision by protecting against
  free radical damage and filtering blue light.**
- Lutein levels in your eye are related to the amount in
  your diet. Bausch & Lomb PreserVision® Lutein contains
  5 mg of lutein per soft gel, which gives you 10 mg of
  lutein per day. The leading multivitamin contains only a
  fraction of the amount of lutein used in clinical studies.
*Bausch & Lomb Ocuvite® PreserVision® AREDS formula
was the only antioxidant vitamin and mineral supplement
proven effective in the 10-year National Institutes of Health
(NIH) Age-Related Eye Disease Study (AREDS). AREDS
was a 10-year, independent study conducted by the National
Eye Institute (NEI) of the National Institutes of Health
(NIH).

RECOMMENDED INTAKE
2 soft gels per day – 1 in the morning, 1 in the evening
taken with a full glass of water and during meals.

**This statement has not been evaluated by the Food
and Drug Administration. This product is not intended
to diagnose, treat, cure or prevent any disease.

HOW SUPPLIED
NDC 24208-632-10. Available in bottles of 50 count soft gels.
Oval shaped soft gelatin capsule.
DO NOT USE IF SEAL UNDER CLOSURE IS BROKEN.

Continued on next page

Table A

Supplement Facts
Serving Size: 1 soft gel

Amount per serving	1 soft gel	% DV
Vitamin A (beta-carotene)	14,320 IU	286%
Vitamin C (ascorbic acid)	226 mg	377%
Vitamin E (dl-alpha tocopheryl acetate)	200 IU	667%
Zinc (zinc oxide)	34.8 mg	232%
Copper (cupric oxide)	0.8 mg	40%

Supplement Facts
Serving Size: 1 soft gel

Amount per serving	1 Soft Gel	% Daily Value
Vitamin C (ascorbic acid)	226 mg	377%
Vitamin E (dl-alpha tocopheryl acetate)	200 IU	667%
Zinc (zinc oxide)	34.8 mg	232%
Copper (cupric oxide)	0.8 mg	40%
Lutein	5 mg	†

† Daily value not established

Table A

Supplement Facts
Serving Size: 4 tablets daily; 2 in the morning, 2 in the evening taken with meals.

Contents	Two tablets		Daily Dosage (4 tablets)	
	Amount	% of Daily Value	Amount	% of Daily Value
Vitamin A (100% as beta-carotene)	14,320 IU	286%	28,640 IU	573%
Vitamin C (ascorbic acid)	226 mg	377%	452 mg	753%
Vitamin E (dl-alpha tocopheryl acetate)	200 IU	667%	400 IU	1333%
Zinc (zinc oxide)	34.8 mg	232%	69.6 mg	464%
Copper (cupric oxide)	0.8 mg	40%	1.6 mg	80%

B&L Preservision Lutein—Cont.

Keep out of reach of children.
STORE AT ROOM TEMPERATURE
For more information or to report a serious side effect, call 1-800-553-5340
®FloraGLO is a registered trademark of Kemin Industries, Inc.
Made in the USA
Marketed by:
Bausch & Lomb Incorporated, Rochester NY 14609
© Bausch & Lomb Incorporated. All rights reserved.
Bausch & Lomb, Preservision and Ocuvite are registered trademarks of Bausch & Lomb Incorporated.
Shown in Product Identification Guide, page 402

BAUSCH & LOMB PRESERVISION® DS AREDS
High Potency Eye Vitamin and Mineral Supplement Original, 4 per day tablets

DESCRIPTION
see Supplement Facts (table A)
[See table A above]

Other Ingredients: Lactose Monohydrate, Microcrystalline Cellulose, Crospovidone, Stearic Acid, Magnesium Stearate, Silicon Dioxide, Polysorbate 80, Triethyl Citrate, Titanium Dioxide Yellow #6, Yellow 6 Lake, Red #40, Red 40 Lake. Contains Soy.
• Age-related macular degeneration is the leading cause of vision loss and blindness in people over 55. The National Institutes of Health (NIH) Age Related Eye Disease Study (AREDS) proved that a unique high- potency vitamin and mineral supplement was effective in helping to preserve the sight of certain people most at risk.*
• Bausch & Lomb **PreserVision®** was the only eye vitamin and mineral supplement clinically proven effective in the NIH AREDS Study.
• Bausch & Lomb **PreserVision®** is a high-potency antioxidant supplement with the antioxidant vitamins A, C, E and select minerals at levels that are well above those in ordinary multivitamins and generally cannot be attained through diet alone.
For a FREE 16-page brochure on Age-Related Macular Degeneration call toll-free 1-866-467-3263 (1-866-HOPE-AMD)

RECOMMENDED INTAKE
To get the same levels proven in the NIH AREDS Study it is important to take 4 tablets per day – 2 in the morning, 2 in the evening taken with meals.
Current and Former Smokers: Consult your eye care professional about the risks associated with smoking and using Beta-Carotene.
Bausch & Lomb PreserVision is the #1 recommended eye vitamin and mineral supplement brand among Retinal Specialists.[1]

*This statement has not been evaluated by the Food and Drug Administration. This product is not intended to diagnose, treat, cure or prevent any disease.

HOW SUPPLIED
NDC 24208-432-62 (120 ct) NDC 24208-432-72 (240 ct) Eye shaped film coated tablet, engraved BL 01 on one side, scored on the other side. Available in bottles of 120 or 240 count tablets
DO NOT USE IF SEAL UNDER CLOSURE IS BROKEN.
Keep this product out of the reach of children.
STORE AT ROOM TEMPERATURE.
For more information or to report a serious side effect, call 1-800-553-5340
Made in USA
Marketed by
Bausch & Lomb Incorporated
Rochester, NY 14609

REFERENCES
1. Data on file, Bausch & Lomb, Incorporated
© Bausch & Lomb Incorporated. All Rights Reserved.
Bausch & Lomb, and PreserVision are registered trademarks of Bausch & Lomb Incorporated or its affiliates. Other brand names are trademarks of their respective owners.
Shown in Product Identification Guide, page 402

BAUSCH & LOMB OCUVITE® DS
Adult 50+ Formula
Eye Vitamin and Mineral Supplement
Lutein & Omega 3 Formula

Nutritional support for those at risk for AMD
Convenient to take soft gels.
• Advanced Eye Nutrition
• Contains 6 mg Lutein and 150 mg of Omega-3

Table A

Supplement Facts
Serving Size: 1 Soft Gel

Amount per Serving	1 Soft Gel	% of Daily Value
Vitamin C (ascorbic acid)	150 mg	250%
Vitamin E (d-alpha tocopherol)	30 IU	100%
Zinc (as zinc oxide)	9 mg	60%
Copper (as cupric oxide)	1 mg	50%
Lutein	6 mg	+
Omega-3	150mg	+

+ Daily Value not established

Table A

Supplement Facts
Serving Size: 1 capsule

	Amount	% Daily Value
Vitamin C (ascorbic acid)	60 mg	100%
Vitamin E (dl-alpha tocopheryl acetate)	30 IU	100%
Zinc (zinc oxide)	15 mg	100%
Copper (cupric oxide)	2 mg	100%
Crystalline Lutein Lutein, Zeaxanthin	6 mg	†

† Daily value not established

DESCRIPTION

see Supplement Facts (table A)
[See first table A above]
Other Ingredients: Gelatin, Fish Oil (anchovy, sardine), Glycerin, Yellow Beeswax, Silicon Dioxide, Soy Lecithin (Contains peanut oil), Caramel color, Titanium Dioxide, Blue 2 Lake, Yellow #6, Yellow 6 Lake, Red #40, Red 40 Lake.

- Ocuvite® Adult 50+ formula is an antioxidant supplement with 6 mg of Lutein and 150 mg of Omega-3
- As we age, free radicals pose a greater threat to eye health. Our bodies don't neutralize them as effectively as before. The right amount of natural antioxidants, such as 6 mg of Lutein found in Ocuvite® Adult 50+ can help maintain eye health as you age.*
- Omega-3 essential fatty acids are structural components of retinal tissues. The retina is particularly rich in long-chain polyunsaturated fatty acids (PUFA) like Omega-3.[1] DHA is a major component of Omega-3. The brain and retina show the highest content of DHA in any tissues. DHA is used continuously for the biogenesis and maintenance of photoreceptor membranes.[2]

---

*This statement has not been evaluated by the Food and Drug Administration. This product is not intended to diagnose, treat, cure or prevent any disease.

REFERENCES
1. Uauy R, Lipids, 2001; Vertuani S, Current Pharmac Des, 2004.
2. San Giovanni JP, Progr Ret Eye Res, 2005.

DIRECTIONS FOR USE
Take 1 Soft Gel daily, in the morning with a full glass of water and during meals. Do not exceed the dose indicated without seeking medical advice.

HOW SUPPLIED
NDC 24208-465-30. – Available in bottles of 50 count soft gels
DO NOT USE IF SEAL UNDER CLOSURE IS BROKEN
Keep out of reach of children
STORE AT ROOM TEMPERATURE
For more information or to report a serious side effect, call 1-800-553-5340

Bausch & Lomb – Committed to research and leadership in ocular nutritionals
Bausch & Lomb and Ocuvite are registered trademarks of Bausch & Lomb Incorporated.
©Bausch & Lomb Incorporated.
All Rights Reserved
Marketed by:
Bausch & Lomb Incorporated, Rochester, NY 14609
Shown in Product Identification Guide, page 402

BAUSCH & LOMB OCUVITE®   DS
LUTEIN
[lu 'teen]
Vitamin and Mineral Supplement

DESCRIPTION

see Supplement Facts (table A)
[See second table A above]

Other Ingredients: Lactose monohydrate, Gelatin, Crospovidone, Magnesium Stearate, Titanium dioxide, Silicon dioxide Yellow #6, Blue #2.

- Lutein is a carotenoid. Carotenoids are the yellow pigments found in fruits and vegetables, particularly dark, leafy green vegetables such as spinach. Carotenoids are concentrated in the macula, the part of the eye responsible for central vision. Clinical studies suggest that Lutein plays an essential role in maintaining healthy central vision by protecting against free radical damage and filtering blue light.*
- Lutein levels in your eye are related to the amount in your diet. Ocuvite® Lutein contains 6 mg of Lutein per capsule. The leading multi-vitamin contains only a fraction of the amount of lutein used in clinical studies.
- Ocuvite® Lutein helps supplement your diet with 100% of the US Daily Values for the antioxidant vitamins C, E, and essential minerals, zinc and copper that can play an important role in your ocular health.*

Continued on next page

Ocuvite Lutein—Cont.

• Ocuvite® Lutein is an advanced antioxidant supplement formulated to provide nutritional support for the eye.* The Ocuvite® Lutein formulation contains essential antioxidant vitamins, minerals and 6 mg of Lutein.

RECOMMENDED INTAKE

Adults: One capsule, one or two times daily or as directed by their physician.

---

*These statements have not been evaluated by the Food and Drug Administration. This product is not intended to diagnose, treat, cure or prevent any disease.

HOW SUPPLIED

Yellow capsule with Ocuvite Lutein printed in black.
NDC 24208-403-19—Bottle of 36
NDC 24208-403-73—Bottle of 72
DO NOT USE IF SEAL UNDER CLOSURE IS BROKEN.
Keep this product out of the reach of children.
STORE AT ROOM TEMPERATURE
For more information or to report a serious side effect, call 1-800-323-0000
Made in U.S.A.
Marketed by
Bausch & Lomb Incorporated
Rochester, NY 14609
© Bausch & Lomb Incorporated. All rights reserved.
Bausch & Lomb, Ocuvite are registered trademarks of Bausch & Lomb Incorporated.
Shown in Product Identification Guide, page 402

Beach Pharmaceuticals
Division of Beach Products, Inc.
5220 SOUTH MANHATTAN AVENUE
TAMPA, FL 33611

Direct Inquiries to:
Richard Stephen Jenkins
(813) 839-6565
FAX (813) 837-2511

BEELITH Tablets   DS
MAGNESIUM SUPPLEMENT
with PYRIDOXINE HCl
Each tablet supplies 362 mg (30 mEq) of magnesium and 25 mg of pyridoxine hydrochloride.

DESCRIPTION

Each tablet contains magnesium oxide 600 mg and pyridoxine hydrochloride (Vitamin B_6) 25 mg equivalent to Vitamin B_6 20 mg. Each tablet yields 362 mg of magnesium and supplies 90% of the Adult U.S. Recommended Daily Allowance (RDA) for magnesium and 1000% of the Adult RDA for Vitamin B_6.

INACTIVE INGREDIENTS

FD&C Yellow No. 6, hydroxypropyl methylcellulose, magnesium stearate, microcrystalline cellulose, polyethylene glycol, sodium starch glycolate, titanium dioxide. May also contain D&C Yellow No. 10, FD&C Yellow No. 5 (Tartrazine), hydroxypropyl cellulose, polydextrose, stearic acid and/or triacetin.

INDICATIONS

As a dietary supplement for patients with magnesium and/or Vitamin B_6 deficiencies resulting from malnutrition, alcoholism, magnesium depleting drugs, chemotherapy, and inadequate nutritional intake or absorption. Also, increases urinary magnesium levels.

DOSAGE

One tablet daily or as directed by a physician.

DRUG INTERACTION PRECAUTION

Do not take this product if you are presently taking a prescription drug without consulting your physician or other health professional.

WARNINGS

Do not take this product if you are presently taking a prescription drug without consulting your physician or other health professional. Ask a physician before use if you have kidney disease or if you are on a magnesium-restricted diet. Excessive dosage may cause laxation. If pregnant or breast-feeding, ask a health professional before use. Keep out of the reach of children.

HOW SUPPLIED

Golden yellow, film-coated tablet with the letters **BP** and the number **132** imprinted on each tablet. Packaged in bottles of 100 (Item No. 0486-1132-01) tablets.
Shown in Product Identification Guide, page 403

J.R. Carlson Laboratories, Inc.
15 COLLEGE DRIVE
ARLINGTON HEIGHTS, IL 60004-1985

Direct Inquiries to:
Customer Service
(888) 234-5656
FAX: (847) 255-1605
www.carlsonlabs.com
For Medical Information Contact:
In Emergencies:
Customer Service
(888) 234-5656
FAX: (847) 255-1605

DDROPS   DS
Dietary Supplement

DESCRIPTION

Pure, natural liquid vitamin D3 simply drops onto your food or tongue. Carlson Ddrops is highly concentrated: receive 400 IU, 1000 IU, or 2000 IU in only 1 drop. Vitamin D supports healthy immune system function, supports a healthy mood and promotes muscle strength.*
Ingredient: Vitamin D3
Other Ingredient: Fractionated Coconut Oil

DIRECTIONS

Take 1 drop (0.027 ml) once or twice daily or as directed. May be put on food or mixed in other liquids such as water or juice.

WARNINGS

KEEP OUT OF REACH OF CHILDREN. BOTTLE SHOULD BE STORED UPRIGHT BETWEEN 60°F AND 85°F.

HOW SUPPLIED

Supplied in 11 ml bottles 400 IU, 1000 IU and 2000 IU
*These statements have not been evaluated by the FDA. These products are not intended to diagnose, treat, cure or present diseases.
Shown in Product Identification Guide, page 403

MED OMEGA™ FISH OIL 2800   DS
[*měd ōměga*]
Balanced Concentrate
DHA 1200 mg & EPA 1200 mg
Professional Strength Dietary Supplement

DESCRIPTION

From Norway: The finest fish oil from deep, cold ocean-water fish. Concentrated to supply 2800 mg (2.8 grams) of total omega 3's per teaspoonful. Bottled in Norway to ensure maximum freshness. Refreshing natural orange taste.

Supplement Facts

Serving Size 1 Teaspoonful (5 ml)	Servings Per Container 20

Each Teaspoonful Contains		% D.V.
Omega-3 Fatty Acids	2.8 g (2800 mg)	*
EPA (eicosapentaenoic acid)	1.2 g (1200 mg)	*
DHA (docosahexaenoic acid)	1.2 g (1200 mg)	*
Other Omega-3 Fatty acids	.4 g (400 mg)	*
Vitamin E (d-Alpha Tocopherol)	10 IU	33%

This product is regularly tested (using AOAC international protocols) for freshness, potency and purity by an independent, FDA-registered laboratory and has been determined to be fresh, fully-potent and free of detectable levels of mercury, cadmium, lead, PCB's and 28 other contaminants.
Other Ingredients: Natural orange flavor, rosemary extract, ascorbyl palmitate, natural tocopherols.

HOW SUPPLIED
Supplied in 100 mL (3.35 Fl. oz.) bottles. Orange Flavor.

CARLSON NORWEGIAN COD LIVER OIL   DS

Each Teaspoonful of Carlson Norwegian Cod Liver Oil provides:

		% DV
Total Omega 3 Fatty Acids	1100 mg to 1250 mg**	*
DHA (Docosahexaenoic Acid)	500 mg to 590 mg**	*
EPA (Eicosapentaenoic Acid)	360 mg to 500 mg**	*
ALA (Alpha-linolenic Acid)	40 mg to 60 mg**	*
Vitamin A	700 IU to 1,200 IU**	14% to 24%
Vitamin D	400 IU	100%
Vitamin E	10 IU	33%
Norwegian Cod Liver Oil	4.6 g	*

**Naturally Occurring Variations.

DESCRIPTION
Carlson Norwegian Cod Liver oil comes from the livers of fresh cod fish found in the arctic coastal waters of Norway.
Suggested Use: Take one teaspoonful daily at mealtime. This product is regularly tested (using AOAC international protocols) for freshness, potency, and purity by an independent, FDA-registered laboratory and has been determined to be fresh, fully-potent and free of detectable levels of mercury, cadmium, lead, PCB's and 28 other contaminants.

HOW SUPPLIED
Supplied in bottles of 250ml and 500ml. Lemon or regular flavor.

SUPER OMEGA-3   DS

DESCRIPTION
Carlson Super Omega-3 soft gels contain a special concentrate of fish body oils from deep cold-water fish, which are rich in EPA & DHA.
Each soft gelatin capsule provides 1000 mg of omega-3 fish oils consisting of:

		% U.S. RDA
EPA (eicosapentaenoic acid)	300 mg	*
DHA (docosahexaenoic acid)	200 mg	*
Other Omega-3's	100 mg	*
Vitamin E (d-alpha tocopherol)	10 IU	33%

This product is regularly tested (using AOAC international protocols) for freshness, potency and purity by an independent, FDA-registered laboratory and has been determined to be fresh, fully-potent and free of detectable levels of mercury, cadmium, lead, PCB's and 28 other contaminants.

HOW SUPPLIED
In bottles of 50, 100, 250.

Immunotec Inc.
300 JOSEPH CARRIER
VAUDREUIL, DORION, QC
CANADA J7V 5V5

For Direct Inquiries Contact:
450-424-9992 Ext 4449

IMMUNOCAL®   DS
NUTRACEUTICAL
(Bonded cysteine supplement) glutathione precursor Powder Sachets

DESCRIPTION and CLINICAL PHARMACOLOGY
IMMUNOCAL® is a U.S. patented natural food protein concentrate in the FDA category of GRAS (generally recognized as safe) which assists the body in maintaining optimal concentrations of glutathione (GSH) by supplying the precursors required for intracellular glutathione synthesis. It is clinically proven to raise glutathione values.
Glutathione is a tripeptide made intracellularly from its constituent amino acids L-glutamate, L-cysteine and glycine. The sulfhydryl (thiol) group (SH) of cysteine is responsible for the biological activity of glutathione. Provision of this amino acid is the rate-limiting factor in glutathione synthesis by the cells since bioavailable cysteine is relatively rare in foodstuffs
Immunocal® is a bovine whey protein isolate specially prepared so as to provide a rich source of bioavailable cysteine. Immunocal® can thus be viewed as a cysteine delivery system.
The disulphide bond in cystine is pepsin and trypsin resistant but may be split by heat, low pH or mechanical stress releasing free cysteine. When subject to heat or shearing forces (inherent in most extraction processes), the fragile disulfide bonds within the peptides are broken and the bioavailablility of cysteine is greatly diminished.
Glutathione is a tightly regulated intracellular constituent and is limited in its production by negative feedback inhibition of its own synthesis through the enzyme gamma-glutamylcysteine synthetase, thus greatly minimizing any possibility of overdosage.
Glutathione has multiple functions:
1. It is the major endogenous antioxidant produced by the cells, participating directly in the neutralization of free radicals and reactive oxygen compounds, as well as maintaining exogenous antioxidants such as vitamins C and E in their reduced (active) forms.
2. Through direct conjugation, it detoxifies many xenobiotics (foreign compounds) and carcinogens, both organic and inorganic.
3. It is essential for the immune system to exert its full potential, e.g. (1) modulating antigen presentation to lymphocytes, thereby influencing cytokine production and type of response (cellular or humoral) that develops, (2) enhancing proliferation of lymphocytes thereby increasing magnitude of response, (3) enhancing killing ac-

Continued on next page

Immunocal—Cont.

tivity of cytotoxic T cells and NK cells, and (4) regulating apoptosis, thereby maintaining control of the immune response.

4. It plays a fundamental role in numerous metabolic and biochemical reactions such as DNA synthesis and repair, protein synthesis, prostaglandin synthesis, amino acid transport and enzyme activation. Thus, most systems in the body can be affected by the state of the glutathione system, especially the immune system, the nervous system, the gastrointestinal system and the lungs.

INDICATIONS AND USAGE

IMMUNOCAL® is a natural food supplement and as such is limited from stating medical claims per se. Statements have not been evaluated by the FDA. As such, this product is thus not intended to diagnose, cure, prevent or treat any disease. Glutathione augmentation is a strategy developed to address states of glutathione deficiency, high oxidative stress, immune deficiency, and xenobiotic overload in which glutathione plays a part in the detoxification of the xenobiotic in question. Glutathione deficiency states include, but are not limited to: HIV/AIDS, infectious hepatitis, certain types of cancers, cataracts, Alzheimer's Disease, Parkinsons, chronic obstructive pulmonary disease, asthma, radiation, poisoning by acetominophen and related agents, malnutritive states, arduous physical stress, aging, and has been associated with sub-optimal immune response. Many clinical pathologies are associated with oxidative stress and are elaborated upon in numerous medical references.

Low glutathione is also strongly implicated in wasting and negative nitrogen balance, notably as seen in cancer, AIDS, sepsis, trauma, burns and even athletic overtraining. Cysteine supplementation can oppose this process and in AIDS, for example, result in improved survival rates.

CONTRAINDICATIONS

IMMUNOCAL® is contraindicated in individuals who develop or have known hypersensitivity to specific milk proteins.

PRECAUTIONS

Each sachet of IMMUNOCAL® contains nine grams of protein. Patients on a protein-restricted diet need to take this into account when calculating their daily protein load. Although a bovine milk derivative, IMMUNOCAL® contains less than 1% lactose and therefore is generally well tolerated by lactose-intolerant individuals.

WARNINGS

Patients undergoing immunosuppressive therapy should discuss the use of this product with their health professional. Individuals with the autosomal-recessive metabolic disorder cystinuria, are at higher risk of developing cysteine nephrolithiasis (1–2% of renal calculi).

ADVERSE REACTIONS

Gastrointestinal bloating and cramps if not sufficiently rehydrated. Transient urticarial-like rash in rare individuals undergoing severe detoxification reaction. Rash abates when product intake stopped or reduced.

OVERDOSAGE

Overdosing on IMMUNOCAL® has not been reported.

DOSAGE AND ADMINISTRATION

For mild to moderate health challenges, 20 grams per day is recommended. Clinical trials in patients with AIDS, COPD, cancer and chronic fatigue syndrome have used 30–40 grams per day without ill effect. IMMUNOCAL® is best administered on an empty stomach or with a light meal. Concomitant intake of another high protein load may adversely affect absorption.

RECONSTITUTION

IMMUNOCAL® is a dehydrated powdered protein isolate. It must be appropriately rehydrated before use. Remains bioactive up to 12 hours after mixing. DO NOT heat or use a hot liquid to rehydrate the product. DO NOT use a high-speed blender for reconstitution. These methods will decrease the activity of the product.

Proper mixing is imperative. Consult instructions included in packaging.

HOW SUPPLIED

10 grams of bovine milk protein isolate powder per sachet. 30 sachets per box.

STORAGE

Store in a cool dry environment. Refrigeration is not necessary.

Patent no.'s: 5,230,902 - 5,290,571 - 5,456,924 - 5,451,412 - 5,888,552

REFERENCES

1. Baruchel S, Viau G, Olivier R. et al. Nutraceutical modulation of glutathione with a humanized native milk serum protein isolate, Immunocal®: application in AIDS and cancer. *In*: Oxidative Stress in Cancer, AIDS and Neurodegenerative Diseases. Ed.; Montagnier L, Olivier R, Pasquier C. Marcel Dekker Inc. New York, 447–461, 1998

2. Bounous G, Kongshavn P. Influence of protein type in nutritionally adequate diets on the development of immunity. *In* Absorption and Utilization of Amino Acids Vol.II. Ed. M. Friedman. CRC Press, Inc., Fla. 2:219–32, 1989

3. Bounous G, Gold P. The biological activity of undenatured whey proteins: role of glutathione. Clin Invest Med 14:296–309, 1991

4. Bounous G, Baruchel S, Falutz J. Gold P. Whey proteins as a food supplement in HIV-seropositive individuals. Clin Invest Med. 16:3; 204–209, 1992

5. Bounous G. Whey protein concentrate (WPC) and glutathione modulation in cancer treatment. Anticancer Res. 20:4785–4792, 2000

6. Bounous G. Immunoenhancing properties of undenatured milk serum protein isolate in HIV patients. Int. Dairy Fed: Whey: 293–305, 1998

7. Bray T, Taylor C. Enhancement of tissue glutathione for antioxidant and immune functions in malnutrition. Biochem. Pharmacol. 47:2113–2123, 1994.

8. Droge W, Holm E. Role of cysteine and glutathione in HIV infection and other diseases associated with muscle wasting and immunological dysfunction. FASEB J: 11(13):1077–1089, 1997

9. Herzenberg LA, De Rosa SC, Dubs JG et al. Glutathione deficiency is associated with impaired survival in HIV disease. Proc Natl Acad Sci 94:1967–72, 1997

10. Kennedy R, Konok G, Bounous G et al.. The use of a whey protein concentrate in the treatment of patients with metastatic carcinoma: A phase 1-II clinical study. Anticancer Res. 15:2643–50, 1995

11. Lands LC, Grey VL, Smountas AA. Effect of supplementation with a cysteine donor on muscular performance. J. Appl. Physiol. 87:1381–1385, 1999

12. Locigno R, Castronovo V. Reduced glutathione System: Role in cancer development, prevention and treatment. International Journal of Oncology 19:221–236, 2001

13. Lomaestro B, Malone M. Glutathione in health and disease: pharmacotherapeutic issues. Ann Pharmacother 29: 1263–73, 1995

14. Lothian B, Grey V, Kimoff RJ, Lands. Treatment of obstructive airway disease with a cysteine donor protein supplement: a case report. Chest 117:914–916, 2000

15. Meister A. Glutathione. Ann Rev Biochem 52:711–60, 1983

16. Peterson JD, Herzenberg LA, Vasquez KK, Waltenbaugh C. Glutathione levels in antigen-presenting cells modulate Th1 versus Th2 response patterns. Proc. Natl. Acad. Sci. 95:3071–3076, 1998

17. Tozer RG, Tai P, Falconer W, Ducruet T, Karabadjian A, Bounous G, Molson J, Dröge W. Cysteine-rich protein reverses weight loss in lung cancer patients receiving chemotherapy or radiotherapy. Antioxidants & redox signalling. 10: 395–402, 2008.

18. Watanabe A, Higachi K, Yasumura S. et al. Nutritional modulation of glutathione level and cellular immunity in chronic hepatitis B and C. Hepatology. 24:597A, 1996

19. Witschi A, Reddy S, Stofer B, Lauterberg B. The systemic availability of oral glutathione. Eur. J. Clin. Pharmacol. 43:667–669, 1992.

Manufactured by Immunotec Inc.

Tel: 450-424-9992 Ext. 4449

www.immunocal.com

Kyowa Wellness Co., Ltd.
S-S-I CO., Ltd.

Ishikura Bldg. 3F3
5-2 Oodenma-Cho, Nihonbashi,
Chuo-Ku, Tokyo 103-001, Japan

Direct Inquiries to:
Consumer Relations
Tel: +81-3-3660-1235
Fax: +81-3-3660-1236
URL: http://www.s-s-i.jp

SEN-SEI-RO LIQUID GOLD™   DS
Kyowa's Agaricus blazei Murill Mushroom Extract
100ml liquid
Dietary Supplement

SEN-SEI-RO LIQUID ROYAL™
Kyowa's Agaricus blazei Murill Mushroom Extract
50ml liquid (2 x concentrate of Liquid Gold, v/v)
Dietary Supplement

DESCRIPTION

Sen-Sei-Ro Liquid Gold™, a dietary supplement containing exclusively all-natural, standardized extract of the Kyowa's cultured *Agaricus blazei* Murill mushroom is primarily used to reduce symptoms of fatigue, to promote vitality, overall well-being, and to support immune functions.[†] Normal immune function can decline with age, and are necessary for maintenance of vitality, energy, good health, and quality of life. A few major biomarkers for decreased immune functions are decreased natural killer cell (NK) activity, and the number of lymphocytes and macrophage cells. These cells, primarily attack diseased cells and thereby, maintain body homeostasis, promote health and quality of life. For the past half a century in Brazil and other countries, *Agaricus blazei* Murill mushroom has been used to restore vitality, and energy, and to serve as a potent tonic conducive to general health and aging concerns.[†]

CLINICAL TRIALS

Preclinical genetic toxicity studies in Ames' test, chromosome aberration, and micronuclei tests were negative. In addition, subchronic toxicity studies in F344 male and female rats, and SPF-bred beagle dogs showed no toxicities based on a comprehensive microscopic pathology of all organs in both species. All GLP toxicity studies were in compliance to US, FDA guidelines.

The effectiveness of ABMK22 in Sen-Sei-Ro Gold™ and Sen-Sei-Ro Royal™ for health benefits were tested in several controlled pre- and clinical trials in animals and in humans.[†] Recent studies in Japan led researchers to report that in humans, ABMK22 in Sen-Sei-Ro Gold™ and Sen-Sei-Ro Royal™ enhanced NK cell activity, promoted maturation and activation of dendritic cells indicated by increased cell kill, elevated expression of CD80 and CD83 expressions (Biotherapy 15(4): 503–507, 2001), increased the number of macrophage (Anticancer Research 17(1A): 274–284, 1997; Japanese Association of Cancer Research, no. 2268, 1999) and tumor necrosis factor α (TNF-α)(Japanese Association of Cancer Research, no. 1406, 1999; Japanese J. Veterinary Clin. Medicine 17(2):31–42, 1998).[†] Recently, the molecular basis of its potential mechanism(s) of action and the current safety status of the product was published (Jap. J. Complimentary Altern. Med. 6(2):75–87, 2009). Further clinical studies with Sen-Sei-Ro Gold™ and Sen-Sei-Ro Royal™ among 100 cancer patients undergoing chemotherapy in Korea have shown that NK cell activity were significantly enhanced, while NK cell activity in the placebo group was markedly diminished (Int. J. Gynecol. Cancer 14: 589–594, 2004).[†] This finding is further supported by a retrospective study of 782 cancer patients, who consumed Sen-Sei-Ro products demonstrated consumer's perception of relief of symptoms and functional well being (Cronbach's alpha: Relief of symptoms, α = .74; Functional well being, α = .91) (BMC Complimentary and Alternative Medicine, 7:32, 2008) Earlier and recent both pre- and clinical studies in Japan, and Korea, led researchers to report that Kyowa's *Agaricus blazei* Murill mushroom extract can be part of an effective treatment for supporting the immune systems of cancer patients by stimulating host defense system (Biotherapy 15(4): 503–507, 2001; Carbohydrate Res. 186(2): 267–273, 1989; Japanese J. Pharmacology 662: 265–271, 1994; Agricultural and Biological Chemistry 54: 2889–2905, 1990).[†]

INGREDIENTS

Each 100ml heat-treated high pressure pack of all natural Kyowa's *Agaricus blazei* Murill water extract is scientifically standardized to contain 300mg% carbohydrate, 700mg% protein, 0mg% fat,; 1.4mg% sodium, 0% food quality cellulose, and 4 Kcal energy.

Molecular weights of polysaccharopeptides ranges between 600~8,000. Water: 99.2g%,; includes a variety of amino acids and vitamins (arginine 12mg%, lysine 6mg%, histidine 2mg%, phenylalanine 4mg%, tyrosine 4mg%, leucine 5mg%, isoleucine 3mg%, methionine 1mg%, valine 5mg%, alanine 13mg%, glycine 7mg%, proline 13mg%, glutamic acid 53mg%, serine 6mg%, threonine 5mg%, and asparagine 10mg%.

RECOMMENDED USE

As a dietary supplement, take 1~3 packs per day. Pour the liquid content into a cup or drink directly from the pack. Do not heat the pack either in a microwave oven or heating range or leave the pack open since the product does not contain any preservatives. If warming is necessary, place the pack in warm to mildly hot water for desired length of time. Once the pack is open, drink immediately.

ADVERSE REACTIONS

No subjects have reported any side effects since the dietary supplement was placed for consumers in Japan, and Korea for the past 17, and 9 years, respectively. The use of this dietary supplements (Sen-Sei-Ro Gold™, Royal™, and ABMK22) is generally safe based on FDA's INDA required tripartite genotoxicities, and 28-day subacute toxicity involving a comprehensive microscopic pathology of rats and dogs. In addition, two-year chronic toxicity studies of the products were carried out by Toxicology Research Center, which is both GLP (Good Laboratory Practice) and AAALAC (American Association of Accreditation of Laboratory Animal Certification) certified. Toxicity evaluation of general, CNS, reproductive and developmental, cardiovascular, immunology, and the two-year bioassay for carcinogenicity was negative. Recent clinical studies with 100 cancer patients undergoing chemotherapy in Korea have shown no known side effects or contraindications (Int. J. Gynecol. Cancer 14: 589–594, 2004).[†]

WARNINGS

Sen-Sei-Ro Liquid Gold™ and Sen-Sei-Ro Liquid Royal™ have not been evaluated in pregnant and breast feeding mothers or children and should consult a physician prior to use. Also consult a physician prior to use if taking a prescription medication. **Keep this product out of the reach of children. Do not use if you are pregnant, can become pregnant or breast feeding.**

HOW SUPPLIED

Sen-Sei-Ro Liquid Gold™ 100ml, and Sen-Sei-Ro Liquid Royal™ 50ml in water extract are high pressure heat sealed. A box contains 30, 100ml packs, and can be purchased directly from company representatives, health food stores, and independent pharmacies. Storage condition keep at room temperature and avoid any direct heat or sun light.

[†] **These statements have not been evaluated by the Food and Drug Administration. These products are not intended to diagnose, treat, cure or prevent any disease.**

Shown in Product Identification Guide, page 403

SEN-SEI-RO POWDER GOLD™   DS
KYOWA'S Agaricus blazei Murill Mushroom
1800mg standard granulated powder
Dietary Supplement

DESCRIPTION

Sen-Sei-Ro Powder Gold™ slim pack, a dietary supplement containing an exclusively all natural and prepared from

Sen-Sei-Ro Powder—Cont.

Kyowa's *Agaricus blazei* Murill mushroom is primarily used to reduce symptoms of fatigue, to promote vitality, overall well-being, and to support immune functions.[†] Normal immune function can decline with age, and are necessary for maintenance of vitality, energy, good health, and quality of life. A few major biomarkers for decreased immune functions are decreased natural killer cell (NK) activity, and the number of lymphocytes and macrophage cells. These cells, primarily attack diseased cells and thereby, maintain body homeostasis, promote health and quality of life. For the past half a century in Brazil and other countries, *Agaricus blazei* Murill mushroom has been used to restore vitality, and energy, and to serve as a potent tonic conducive to general health and aging concerns.[†]

CLINICAL TRIALS

Preclinical 2-year chronic cancer bioassay in compliance to FDA GLP Guideline demonstrated no increase in carcinogenicity in all treatment groups as compared to controls with Sen-Sei-Ro product. Furthermore, survival of Sen-Sei-Ro consumed groups were increased by 20–34% over that of controls at the end of life-time feeding studies (2-years) and incidence of cataract in males at the end of 2-year study showed only 20–30% of control and demonstrating highly significant survival and prevention of cataracts (*SAS version* 9; p<0.006).[†]

The effectiveness of Sen-Sei-Ro Powder Gold™ for health benefits were tested in several controlled pre- and clinical trials in animals and in humans.[†] Recent studies in Japan, and Korea led researcher to report that in humans, Sen-Sei-Ro Powder Gold™ enhanced NK cell activity, increased the number of macrophage cells (Anticancer Research 17 (1A): 274–284, 1997; Japanese Association of Cancer Research, no. 2268, 1999) and tumor necrosis factor α (TNF-α) (Japanese Association of Cancer Research, no. 1406, 1999).[†] Antitumor effects of Sen-Sei-Ro against various murine and dog tumors were thought to be mediated by stimulation of NK cell activity, increased number of macrophage cells, and increased activity of tumor necrosis factor α (TNF-α)(Japanese J. Veterinary Clin. Medicine 17(2): 31–42, 1998).[†] Recent clinical studies in Japan, and Korea, led researchers to report that *Agaricus blazei* Murill mushroom extract can be part of an effective treatment for supporting the immune systems of cancer patients by stimulating host defense system (Biotherapy 15(4): 503–507, 2001; Carbohydrate Res. 186(2): 267–273, 1989; Japanese J. Pharmacology 662: 265–271, 1994; Agricultural and Biological Chemistry 54: 2889–2905, 1990).[†]

INGREDIENTS

Each 1800mg granulated powder in a slim pack contains 488 mg protein, 820 mg carbohydrate, 47 mg fat, 0.19 mg Sodium; 284 mg food grade cellulose; 5.7 kcal energy. Water: 68mg, includes 0.1 mg Fe, 0.24 mg Ca, 37 mg K, 0.01mg thiamine, 0.04mg ergosterol, 0.59mg niacin.

RECOMMENDED USE

As a dietary supplement, take 1~3 packs per day. Pour the content into a cup containing warm water or other desirable beverage and mix and drink. Do not heat the pack either in a microwave oven or heating range or leave the pack open since the product does not contain any preservatives. Once the pack is open, drink immediately.

ADVERSE REACTIONS

No subjects have reported any side effects since the dietary supplement was placed for consumers in Japan and Korea for the past 17, and 9 years, respectively. The use of this dietary supplement is generally safe based on two-year chronic toxicity studies of the products by Toxicology Research Center, which is both GLP (Good Laboratory Practice) and AAALAC (American Association of Accreditation of Laboratory Animal Certification) certified. Toxicity evaluation of general, CNS, reproductive and developmental, cardiovascular, immunology, and the two-year bioassay for carcinogenicity was negative.[†]

WARNINGS

Sen-Sei-Ro Powder Gold™ has not been evaluated in pregnant and breast feeding mothers or children and should consult a physician prior to use. Also consult a physician prior to use if taking a prescription medications.. **Keep this product out of the reach of children. Do not use if you are pregnant, can become pregnant or breast feeding.** Quality of the dietary supplement is guaranteed for 2 years from the manufactured date, but for more information, please write or call 81-72-257-8568 or 81-3-3512-5032.

HOW SUPPLIED

Sen-Sei-Ro Powder Gold™ is high pressure heat sealed. A box contains 30 slim packs of each with 1800mg per pack, and can be purchased directly from company representatives, health food stores, and independent pharmacies. Storage condition keep at room temperature and avoid any direct heat or sun light.

[†]**These statements have not been evaluated by the Food and Drug Administration. These products are not intended to diagnose, treat, cure or prevent any disease.**

Shown in Product Identification Guide, page 403

Marlyn Nutraceuticals, Inc.
4404 E. ELWOOD STREET
PHOENIX, AZ 85040

Direct Inquiries to:
4404 E. Elwood St.
Phoenix, AZ 85040
(800) 899-4499
480 991-0200
EMAIL info@naturallyvitamins.com
WEBSITE www.naturally.com

HEP-FORTE®   DS
[*hep-for'tay*]

DESCRIPTION

Hep-Forte is a comprehensive formulation of protein, B factors and other nutritional factors which can be important as a dietary supplement for maintenance and support of normal hepatic function.

COMPOSITION

Each capsule contains:

Vitamin A (Palmitate)	1,200I.U.
Vitamin E (d-Alpha Tocopherol)	10I.U.
Vitamin C (Ascorbic Acid)	10mg.
Folic Acid	0.06mg.
Vitamin B1 (Thiamine)	1mg.
Vitamin B2 (Riboflavin)	1mg.
Niacinamide	10mg.
Vitamin B6 (Pyridoxine HCl)	0.5mg.
Vitamin B12 (Cobalamin)	1mcg.
Biotin	3.3mg.
Pantothenic Acid (Calcium Pantothenate)	2mg.
Choline Bitartrate	21mg.
Zinc (Zinc Sulfate)	2mg.
Desiccated Liver	194.4mg.
Liver Concentrate	64.8mg.
Liver Fraction Number 2	64.8mg.
Yeast (Dried)	64.8mg.
dl-Methionine	10mg.
Inositol	10mg.

INDICATIONS

Hep-Forte is a balanced formulation of vitamins, minerals, lipotropic factors, and vitamin-protein supplements. It is of value as a nutritional supplement for persons who are receiving professional treatment for alcoholism, hepatic dysfunction due to hepatotoxic drugs and liver poisons, male and female infertility due to hormonal imbalance caused by hepatic dysfunction, and for nutritional supplementation after treatment.

CONTRAINDICATIONS

There are no known contraindications to Hep-Forte.

DOSAGE

Three to six capsules daily.

HOW SUPPLIED

Bottles of 100, 200 or 500 capsules.
Literature Available.

MEDIZYM®   DS

[mĕd-ĭ-zīm]

DESCRIPTION

Medizym is a combination of proteolytic enzymes and the antioxidant Rutin that work systemically by targeting various tissues and organs in the body. Proteolytic enzymes, such as those found in Medizym, modulate the immune response by activating alpha-2-macroglobulin and supporting a healthy balance between anti-inflammatory and pro-inflammatory cytokines.*

COMPOSITION

- Each serving contains
- Pancreatin***78,000 USP-units • protease (pancreas) Sus scrofa 300 mg
- Papain***2.9 million USP-units • Carica papaya 180 mg
- Bromelain***324 GDU Ananas comosus 135 mg
- Trypsin 180,000 USP-units (pancreas) Sus scrofa 72 mg
- Chymotrypsin 22,500 USP-units (pancreas) Sus scrofa 3 mg
- Rutosid Sophora japonica 150 mg

MAJOR USES

Orally administered enzymes work as biocatalysts, which accelerate and control the bodily metabolism without themselves being altered. They support enzymatic catabolism. They have great significance for optimal functioning of the immune system and the body's own defense forces. Enzymes are responsible for the physiological discharge of inflammation and reestablishment of the affected tissue's function.*

SAFTEY INFORMATION

Daily dosage of Medizym should be calibrated when dispensed simultaneously with blood thinners by measuring relevant laboratory parameters in peripheral blood on a regular basis.

DOSAGE AND ADMINISTRATION

As a dietary supplement, three tablets on a relatively empty stomach two times a day.

HOW SUPPLIED

Bottles of 100, 200, 400 and 800 tablets. Vegetarian and topical also available. Literature available upon request.

---

*This statement has not been evaluated by the Food and Drug Administration. This product is not intended to diagnose, treat, cure or prevent any disease.

Mericon Industries, Inc.

8819 N. PIONEER ROAD
PEORIA, IL 61615

Direct Inquiries to:
William R. Connelly
(309) 693-2150
FAX: (309) 693-2158

FLORICAL®   DS

[flor ĭ cal]
(fluoride and calcium supplement)

ACTIVE INGREDIENTS

Florical contains 3.75mg fluoride (as sodium fluoride) and 145mg calcium (as calcium carbonate)

DESCRIPTION

Otosclerosis is an inherited disease of the small bones of the middle ear. Florical supports the stimulation of bone mineral density and supports the repair of small cracks (microfractures) in the small bones in the otic capsule. The leakage of enzymes that occurs at this time is also neutralized by Florical halting the progression of hearing loss in a large percentage of patients.[1]

SIDE EFFECTS

Gastrointestinal upset, joint pain. Most side effects can be alleviated by staying below 15mg elemental fluoride (4 capsules of Florical).

PRECAUTIONS

Florical should not be used in patients with a known allergy or hypersensitivity to any of its ingredients.

INDICATIONS

Florical may be used in otosclerosis.

DOSAGE

1–4 capsules daily as recommended by your physician. Use only one capsule daily during pregnancy.
These statements have not been evaluated by the FDA. This product is not intended to diagnose, treat, cure, or prevent any disease.

HOW SUPPLIED

Florical® is supplied as tablets or capsules in bottles of 100 or 500
NDC 00394-0102-02 (Capsules 100's)
NDC 00394-0102-05 (Capsules 500's)
NDC 00394-0100-02 (Tablets 100's)
NDC 00394-0100-05 (Tablets 500's)

---

[1]Causse, JR et aI, Sodium Fluoride Therapy, The American Journal of Otology (14) Sep 1993, p. 482.

Shown in Product Identification Guide, page 403

MERIBIN®   DS

(biotin 5mg)

DESCRIPTION

Biotinidase deficiency is an autosomal inherited disorder that is the cause of most cases of late-onset multiple carboxylase deficiency. Affected children usually exhibit seizures, hypotonia, developmental delay, ataxia, hyperventilation and/or coma between one week and two years of age. Visual and hearing abnormalities as well as alopecia, skin rash, conjunctivitis and recurrent infections often occur later.[1]
All symptomatic children have responded to pharmacologic doses of Meribin (biotin 5mg) with resolution of symptoms, with the exception of visual and hearing impairments and severe developmental delay.

ADVERSE REACTIONS

Urticaria and gastrointestinal upset have been reported.

PRECAUTIONS

Meribin should not be used in patients with known allergy or hypersensitivity to any of its ingredients.

INDICATIONS

Meribin is recommended as the product of choice for biotinidase deficiency.

DOSAGE

1 capsule daily. Capsule may be emptied into babies' bottles. Contents of capsule will pass through nipple of baby bottle.

HOW SUPPLIED

MERIBIN (biotin 5mg) is uspplied in bottles of 120 capsules (120-day supply)

Continued on next page

Meribin—Cont.

These statements have not been evaluated by the Food and Drug Administration. This product is not intended to diagnose, treat, cure, or prevent any disease.

---

[1]Bousounis, D.P., Canfield, P.R., Wolf, B. Reversal of Brain Atrophy with Biotin Treatment in Biotinidase Deficiency. Neuropediatrics 24 (1993) 214-217.

Merz Pharmaceuticals
Division of Merz, Inc.
4215 TUDOR LANE (27410)
P.O. BOX 18806
GREENSBORO, NC 27419

Direct Inquiries to:
Medical/Regulatory Affairs
(336) 856-2003
FAX: (336) 217-2439
For Medical Information Contact:
In Emergencies:
Medical/Regulatory Affairs
(336) 856-2003
FAX: (336) 217-2439

APPEAREX®   DS
(biotin 2.5 mg)
Dietary Supplement

DESCRIPTION
Appearex® is a small, easy-to-swallow tablet that contains 2.5mg of biotin, the dose clinically proven to strengthen nails and improve nail quality. When taken as directed each day, Appearex® stimulates healthy nail growth and smoothes brittle ridges, increases nail strength, and produces firmer, healthier nails in approximately 3 to 6 months.

INGREDIENTS
Each tablet contains 2.5mg pharmaceutical-grade biotin, a nutritional supplement for nail health, lactose monohydrate, cornstarch, povidone (K25), and magnesium stearate.

INDICATIONS
For the treatment of weak, brittle, splitting, or soft nails.

WARNINGS
As with any drug or supplement, consult your physician before taking this product if you are pregnant or nursing. Do not use this product if you have any known allergies or hypersensitivities to any of the ingredients.

CAUTION
Do not use tablets if protective blister pack has been broken. Keep this product out of the reach of small children.

SIDE EFFECTS
Although very rare, allergic skin reactions (urticaria) and gastrointestinal upset have occurred in some cases. If you experience any side effects not described here, inform your physician or pharmacist immediately and discontinue use.

DOSAGE
Take one tablet daily with water. Consult a physician for use in children under 12.

HOW SUPPLIED
Cartons of either 28 tablets (4-week supply) or 84 tablets (12-week supply).

STORAGE
Store in a dry place at room temperature (15°C-25°C or 59°F-77°F). Avoid excessive heat.

NU-IRON® 150 CAPSULES   DS
(polysaccharide-iron complex)
Dietary Supplement

Each NU-IRON® 150 Capsule contains:
Iron (elemental) .... 150 mg
   (as a Polysaccharide Iron Complex)

INACTIVE INGREDIENTS
Sucrose, Gelatin, Starch, Pharmaceutical Glaze, Titanium Dioxide, FD&C Red #40, Carnauba Wax, and FD&C Blue #1.

> **WARNING**
> Accidental overdose of iron-containing products is a leading cause of fatal poisoning in children under 6. Keep this product out of reach of children. In case of accidental overdose, call a doctor or poison control center immediately.

The treatment of any anemic condition should be under the advice and supervision of a doctor.

DOSAGE
Adults: One or two capsules daily or as recommended by a physician.
Children: Consult a physician.
If pregnant or breastfeeding, ask a health care professional before use.

HOW SUPPLIED
NU-IRON® 150 CAPSULES in bottles of 100.
Non-USP
Distributed by Merz Pharmaceuticals, Greensboro, NC 27410
Store at controlled room temperature, 15°–30°C (59°–86°F)

Pharmanex, LLC
75 WEST CENTER STREET
PROVO, UT 84601

For Information and Product Support:
Phone: 1-800-487-1000
Website: www.pharmanex.com

CORDYMAX® Cs-4®   DS
[kōr-dē-măks CS-4]
Dietary Supplement

DESCRIPTION
CordyMax® Cs-4® (Patent Pending) is a dietary supplement used to reduce symptoms of fatigue, and to promote vitality and overall well-being.* It is an exclusive fermentation product derived from the renowned *Cordyceps sinensis* mushroom.

INGREDIENTS
Each capsule contains 525 mg *Cordyceps sinensis* (Berk.) Sacc. mycelia (*Paecilomyces hepiali* Chen, Cs-4), standardized 0.14% adenosine and 5% mannitol.

RECOMMENDED USE
Take 2 capsules bid or tid with water and food.

WARNINGS
Keep out of reach of children. Consult a physician prior to use if pregnant or breastfeeding, or using anticoagulants, MAO inhibitors, or any other prescription medication. Discontinue use of this product 2 weeks prior to and after surgery.

HOW SUPPLIED
20–30 day supply, 120 count bottle.

LIFEPAK® ANTI-AGING FORMULA DS
[līf-păk]
Dietary Supplement

DESCRIPTION
LifePak® is a comprehensive nutritional wellness program, delivering the optimum types and amounts of vitamins, minerals, trace elements, antioxidants, and phytonutrients for general health and well-being. LifePak addresses all common nutrient deficiencies, provides key anti-aging nutrients that promote cellular protection, and supports cardiovascular health, bone metabolism, nutrient metabolism, and normal immune function.*

INGREDIENTS
LifePak provides an optimal blend of vitamins, minerals, trace elements, antioxidants, and phytonutrients. Contact Pharmanex for a detailed ingredient list.

RECOMMENDED USE
Take 1 packet bid with water and food.

WARNINGS
Keep this product out of reach of children. Consult a physician prior to use if pregnant or lactating, or taking a prescription medication. Discontinue use of this product 2 weeks prior to and after surgery.

HOW SUPPLIED
60 individual packets, 30 day supply. Additional LifePak® products include: LifePak® nano, Prime, Women, Prenatal, Teen, and Jungamals.

MARINEOMEGA™ DS
[mă-rēn-ō-mĕ-gă]
Dietary Supplement

DESCRIPTION
MarineOmega™ is a dietary supplement of ultra-pure omega-3 (n-3) fatty acids formulated to promote normal immune function, cardiovascular health, joint mobility, brain function, and skin health*.

INGREDIENTS
Each softgel capsule contains 1,100 mg of Marine Lipid Concentrate (150 mg of EPA, 100 mg of DHA, and 50 mg of other Omega 3 Fatty Acids), 50 mg of krill oil, and 5 IU of Vitamin E (as Natural Mixed Tocopherols).

RECOMMENDED USE
Take 2 softgel capsules bid with water and food.

WARNINGS
Keep this product out of reach of children. Consult a physician if pregnant or lactating, taking anticoagulants, or any other prescription medication. Discontinue use of this product 2 weeks prior to and after surgery.

HOW SUPPLIED
30 day supply, 120 count bottle.

REISHIMAX GLp® DS
[rīsh-ĭ-măks GL-p]
Dietary Supplement

DESCRIPTION
ReishiMax® GLp is a proprietary, standardized extract of Reishi (Ganoderma lucidum) mushroom. ReishiMax supports healthy immune system function by stimulating cell-mediated immunity.*

INGREDIENTS
Each capsule contains 495 mg of standardized Reishi mushroom extract and 5 mg of Reishi cracked spores, standardized to 6% triterpenes and 13.5% polysaccharides.

WARNINGS
Keep out of reach of children. If you are pregnant or nursing, or taking a prescription medication, including immuno-suppressive therapies, consult a physician before using this product. Discontinue use of this product 2 weeks prior to and after surgery.

RECOMMENDED USE
Take 1-2 capsules bid with water and food.

HOW SUPPLIED
15-30 day supply, 60 count bottle.

TēGREEN 97® DS
[tē-grēn 97]
Dietary Supplement

DESCRIPTION
Tēgreen® is a standardized, decaffeinated polyphenol extract of fresh green tea leaves, with proven free radical scavenging and antioxidant properties.*

INGREDIENTS
Each 250 mg capsule contains a 20:1 extract of green tea leaves (Camellia sinensis) standardized to a minimum 97% pure polyphenols including 162 mg catechins, of which 95 mg is EGCg.

RECOMMENDED USE
Take 1–2 capsules bid with water and food. Maximum recommended dose of 4 capsules daily (1,000 mg). Do not exceed 1,200 mg green tea extract in combination with other green tea-containing supplements.

WARNINGS
Keep out of reach of children. Consult a physician prior to use if pregnant or lactating, taking anticoagulants, or other prescription medications. Discontinue use of this product 2 weeks prior to and after surgery.

HOW SUPPLIED
30-day supply, 30 and 120 count bottles.

---

*These statements have not been evaluated by the Food and Drug Administration. This product is not intended to diagnose, treat, cure or prevent any disease.

Unicity International
THE MAKE LIFE BETTER COMPANY
1201 NORTH 800 EAST
OREM, UT 84097

Direct Inquiries to:
(801) 226 2600
www.unicity.net
science@unicity.net
Products of Unicity International are distributed through independent distributors.

BIO-C™ DS
[bīō sē]

DESCRIPTION
Bio-C™ is a vitamin C nutritional supplement. Bio-C™ is a yellow, water-soluble, crystalline powder pressed into a tablet. Each Bio-C™ tablet consists of a proprietary blend of ascorbyl palmitate, calcium ascorbate, ascorbic acid, magnesium ascorbate and 75 mg of citrus bioflavonoids. In addition to the active ingredients, each 803 mg tablets contains dextrose, microcrystalline cellulose, silicon dioxide, magnesium stearate, and stearic acid.

BENEFITS AND RESEARCH
Vitamin C (ascorbic acid) is a water-soluble vitamin that is used in the body to form cartilage, collagen, muscles and

Continued on next page

Bio-C—Cont.

blood vessels. Vitamin C is a potent antioxidant that can protect small molecules such as proteins, carbohydrates, nucleic acids and lipids from damage caused by free radicals that are generated through the course of normal metabolism or through exposure to external toxins and pollutants (e.g. ultraviolet radiation from the sun or smoking). Vitamin C can also regenerate other antioxidants like vitamin E. Additionally, vitamin C is required for the synthesis of carnitine, a molecule involved in the transport of fats across the mitochondrial membrane, as well as the synthesis of norepinephrine, a neurotransmitter.*

USAGE
Take one tablet morning and night with a meal.

SAFETY AND WARNINGS
Bio-C™ is well tolerated. Some gastrointestinal discomfort may be experienced as with any dietary supplement.

HOW SUPPLIED
Available in tablets.

REFERENCES
Carr, AC and Frei B. (1999), American Journal of Clinical Nutrition 96: 1086-1107.
Jacob, RA and Sotoudeh G. (2002), Nutrition in Clinical Care 5: 66-74.
Deruelle F, Baron B. (2008), Journal of Alternative and Complementary Medicine 14:1291-1298.
Levine M, Rumsey SC, Daruwala R, Park JB, Wang Y. (1999), The Journal of the American Medical Association 281: 1415-1423.
* THESE STATEMENTS HAVE NOT BEEN EVALUATED BY THE FOOD AND DRUG ADMINISTRATION. THIS PRODUCT IS NOT INTENDED TO DIAGNOSE, TREAT, CURE, OR PREVENT ANY DISEASE.

BIOS LIFE® C   DS
[bī-ōs līf sē]
Advanced Fiber and Nutrient Drink

DESCRIPTION
Bios Life® C is a fiber-based, vitamin-rich nutritional supplement. Bios Life® C contains a blend of soluble and insoluble fibers, phytosterols, policosanol, an extract of *Chrysanthemum morifolium*, vitamins, and minerals that when combined with a healthy diet and exercise may lower total serum cholesterol, lower triglyceride levels and reduce the risk of heart disease.
Bios Life® C is light orange in color. It is a hygroscopic crystalline powder that is generally soluble in water. Each serving of Bios Life® C contains 3 g of fiber, 1 g of phytosterols, 6 mg of policosanol, and 12.5 mg of an extract of *Chrysanthemum morifolium*. In addition to these active ingredients, each serving of Bios Life® C contains maltodextrin, citric acid, orange juice powder, sucralose and orange flavor.

BENEFITS AND RESEARCH
It's estimated that Americans consume 10-12 g of total fiber per day, less than half the amount of the recommended daily intake. Epidemiological and clinical studies have correlated low daily fiber intake with higher incidences of hyperinsulinemia, hypercholesterolemia, and elevated risks of cardiovascular disease.
Bios Life® C is a nutritional supplement designed to increase daily fiber intake. Each serving of Bios Life® C contains three grams of dietary fiber. When taken three times a day, this achieves nearly half of the recommended daily value of fiber. Fiber supplementation has been shown to decrease preprandial and postprandial glucose levels and lower LDL cholesterol and apolipoprotein B levels.
In addition to fiber supplementation, Bios Life® C contains a patented blend of phytosterols, policosanol, *Chrysanthemum morifolium*, vitamins and minerals. This blend of ingredients optimizes cholesterol levels through a combination of four mechanisms. First, the soluble fiber matrix prevents cholesterol reabsorption in the gastrointestinal tract through bile-acid sequestration. Second, the phytosterols reduce dietary absorption of cholesterol. Third, policosanol inhibits hepatic synthesis of cholesterol mediated through HMG-CoA reductase. Fourth, *Chrysanthemum morifolium* provides phytonutrients that enhance conversion of cholesterol to 7-α-hydroxycholesterol. The four mechanisms provide a synergistic approach to optimizing cholesterol levels. Research has shown that this product may serve as a first line treatment option for mild hypercholesterolemia, as well as adjunct therapy for lipid lowering pharmaceutical intervention.

SUGGESTED USAGE
Dissolve the contents of one packet or one scoop into 8 to 10 fl. oz. of liquid (water or juice) and stir vigorously. Drink immediately. Use 15-20 minutes prior to meals up to three times daily.

SAFETY AND WARNINGS
Bios Life® C is well tolerated. There may be mild gastrointestinal discomfort, such as increased flatulence or loose stools, during the first month of initial use due to the increased uptake of dietary fiber. This GI disturbance usually disappears within the first thirty days. If the GI discomfort persists, reduce the number of servings of Bios Life® C. If the GI discomfort further persists, stop taking the product and consult your physician. Taking this product without adequate liquid can result in complications. If you are a diabetic, consult a physician for proper use of this product, as the chromium may reduce the need for medication.

HOW SUPPLIED
Bios Life® C is packaged in single-serving foil packets or in bulk canisters.

REFERENCES
Sprecher, DL and Pearce GL (2002), Metabolism 51: 1166-70.
Verdegem, PJE; Freed, S and Joffe D (2005), American Diabetes Assocation 65th Scientific Sessions, San Diego, CA.
Duenas, V; Duenas, J; Burke, E and Verdegem, PJE (2006), 7th International Conference on Arteriosclerosis, Thrombosis, and Vascular Biology, American Heart Association, Denver, CO.
Verdegem, PJE (2007), Current Topics in Nutraceutical Research 5: 1-6
US Patent 6,933,291.
* THESE STATEMENTS HAVE NOT BEEN EVALUATED BY THE FOOD AND DRUG ADMINISTRATION. THIS PRODUCT IS NOT INTENDED TO DIAGNOSE, TREAT, CURE, OR PREVENT ANY DISEASE.
Shown in Product Identification Guide, page 404

BIOS LIFE® SLIM™   DS
[bī-ōs līf slim]
Advanced Fiber and Nutrient Drink

DESCRIPTION
Bios Life® Slim™ is a fiber-based, vitamin-rich nutritional supplement. Bios Life® Slim™ contains a blend of soluble and insoluble fibers, Unicity® 7× technology, phytosterols, policosanol, an extract of *Chrysanthemum morifolium*, vitamins, and minerals that when combined with a healthy diet and exercise may lower total serum cholesterol, reduce the risk of heart disease and help achieve and maintain a healthy body weight.
Bios Life® Slim™ is light orange in color. It is a hygroscopic crystalline powder that is generally soluble in water. Each serving of Bios Life® Slim™ contains 4 g of fiber, 1 g of phytosterols, 750 mg of Unicity 7×, 6 mg of policosanol and 12.5 mg of an extract of *Chrysanthemum morifolium*. In addition to these active ingredients each serving of Bios Life® Slim™ contains maltodextrin, citric acid, orange juice powder, sucralose and orange flavor.

BENEFITS AND RESEARCH
It's estimated that Americans consume 10-12 g of total fiber per day, less than half the amount of the recommended daily intake. Epidemiological and clinical studies have correlated low daily fiber intake with higher incidences of obesity, hyperinsulinemia, hypercholesterolemia, and elevated risks of cardiovascular disease.
Bios Life® Slim™ is a nutritional supplement designed to increase fiber intake. Each serving of Bios Life® Slim™ con-

tains four grams of fiber. When taken three times a day this achieves half of the recommended daily value of fiber. Fiber supplementation has been shown to decrease preprandial and postprandial glucose levels; lower LDL cholesterol and apolipoprotein B levels; increase satiety and facilitate weight loss.

In addition to fiber supplementation, Bios Life® Slim™ contains a patented blend of phytosterols, policosanol, *Chrysanthemum morifolium*, vitamins and minerals. Bios Life® Slim™ facilitates weight loss through five distinct mechanisms. First, the soluble fiber matrix promotes an increase in satiety. Second, Bios Life® Slim™ improves cholesterol levels. Reduction in LDL content removes a potent inhibitor of lipolysis. Third, Bios Life® Slim™ improves blood glucose levels. Maintaining appropriate serum glucose levels reduces hyperinsulinemia and promotes insulin sensitivity. Reducing insulin levels permits fatty acid oxidation to occur. Fourth, Bios Life® Slim™ restores appropriate leptin signaling. Lastly, Bios Life® Slim™, reduces triglyceride levels allowing for leptin to cross the blood-brain barrier and effect its mechanism of action. Research has shown that this product may serve as a first line treatment option for mild hypercholesterolemia, as well as adjunct therapy for lipid lowering pharmaceutical intervention.

SUGGESTED USAGE

Dissolve the contents of one packet or one scoop into 8 to 10 fl. oz. of liquid (water or juice) and stir vigorously. Drink immediately. Use 15-20 minutes before meals up to three times daily.

SAFETY AND WARNINGS

Bios Life® Slim™ is well tolerated. There may be mild gastrointestinal discomfort, such as increased flatulence or loose stools, during the first month of initial use due to the increased uptake of dietary fiber. This GI disturbance usually disappears within the first thirty days. If the GI discomfort persists, reduce the number of servings of Bios Life® Slim™. If the GI discomfort further persists, stop taking the product and consult your physician. Taking this product without adequate liquid can result in complications. If you are a diabetic, consult a physician for proper use of this product, as the chromium may reduce the need for medication.

HOW SUPPLIED

Bios Life® Slim™ is packaged in single-serving foil packets or in bulk canisters.

REFERENCES

Sprecher, DL and Pearce GL (2002), Metabolism 51: 1166-70.
Verdegem, PJE; Freed, S and Joffe D (2005), American Diabetes Assocation 65th Scientific Sessions, San Diego, CA.
Slavin, JL, (2005) Nutrition 21: 411-418.
Delzenne NM, Cani PD, (2005) Current Opinion Clincal Nutrition & Metabolic Care 8: 636-640
Duenas, V; Duenas, J; Burke, E and Verdegem, PJE (2006), 7th International Conference on Arteriosclerosis, Thrombosis, and Vascular Biology, American Heart Association, Denver, CO.
Verdegem, PJE (2007), Current Topics in Nutraceutical Research 5: 1-6
US Patent 6,933,291.
* THESE STATEMENTS HAVE NOT BEEN EVALUATED BY THE FOOD AND DRUG ADMINISTRATION. THIS PRODUCT IS NOT INTENDED TO DIAGNOSE, TREAT, CURE, OR PREVENT ANY DISEASE.

BONEMATE® PLUS   DS
[bōn-māt plŭs]
Advanced Bone Health Formula

DESCRIPTION

BoneMate® Plus is specially formulated to help maintain optimal bone health.* It contains three forms of calcium and vitamin D to maximize absorption and aid in the support of healthy bones, teeth, nerves, heart, and muscle tissue. BoneMate® Plus is a light gray in color and is soluble in water. Each serving of BoneMate® Plus contains the following active ingredients 600mg of calcium, 300mg of magne-

sium, 30 mg of vitamin C, 2000 IU of vitamin D, 0.5mg of boron, 5 mg of zinc, 1mg of manganese, 1mg of copper, and 20mg of vitamin K. In addition, it also contains the inactive ingredients microcrystalline cellulose, croscarmellose sodium, and magnesium stearate.

BENEFITS AND RESEARCH

Calcium is the most common mineral in the body. Almost 99% of the calcium in our body is found in the bones and teeth. Bone is a dynamic tissue that is constantly being remodeled throughout our lives. A chronically low calcium intake in growing individuals may prevent the attainment of optimal peak bone mass. Once peak bone mass has been achieved, inadequate calcium intake may contribute to accelerated bone loss and eventually to osteoporosis.

Vitamin D, a secosteroid that is produced by the body upon exposure to the sun, is required for optimal calcium absorption. To ensure that calcium absorption is not limited by inadequate vitamin D levels, BoneMate® Plus contains 2000 IU of vitamin D per serving. In addition to facilitating calcium absorption, Vitamin D has been shown to target over 2000 different genes in the body. Vitamin D deficiency has been associated with increased risks for heart disease, stroke, diabetes, depression, osteoarthritis, chronic pain, and osteoporosis.

USAGE

Take two tablets twice daily with a meal.

SAFETY AND WARNINGS

BoneMate® Plus is well tolerated. Some gastrointestinal discomfort may be experienced as with any dietary supplement. The Food and Nutrition Board of the Institute of Medicine has set the tolerable upper level (UL) of intake for calcium in adults at 2,500 milligrams (mg) of calcium/day.

HOW SUPPLIED

Available as tablets or as a powder.

REFERENCES

Weaver CM, Heaney RP. Calcium. In: Shils M, Olson JA, Shike M, Ross AC, eds. Modern Nutrition in Health and Disease. 9th ed. Baltimore: Williams & Wilkins; 1999: 141-155.
Heaney RP. Calcium, dairy products and osteoporosis. J Am Coll Nutr. 2000;19(2 Suppl):83S-99S.
Food and Nutrition Board, Institute of Medicine. Calcium. Dietary Reference Intakes: Calcium, Phosphorus, Magnesium, Vitamin D, and Fluoride. Washington, D.C.: National Academy Press; 1997:71-145.
Reid IR. Therapy of osteoporosis: calcium, vitamin D, and exercise. Am J Med Sci 1996;312:278-86. Food and Nutrition Board, Institute of Medicine. Calcium. Dietary Reference Intakes: Calcium, Phosphorus, Magnesium, Vitamin D, and Fluoride. Washington, D.C.: National Academy Press; 1997:71-145.
* THESE STATEMENTS HAVE NOT BEEN EVALUATED BY THE FOOD AND DRUG ADMINISTRATION. THIS PRODUCT IS NOT INTENDED TO DIAGNOSE, TREAT, CURE, OR PREVENT ANY DISEASE.

CARDIO-BASICS™   DS
Caring for your heart*

DESCRIPTION

Cardio-Basics™ is a nutritional supplement that combines multivitamins, minerals and antioxidants to support the cardiovascular system.

Cardio-Basics™ is a light orange, water-soluble powder pressed into tablets. Each tablet of Cardio-Basics™ contains the following vitamins, minerals, amino acids and antioxidants: beta-carotene (vitamin A), thiamine (vitamin B1), riboflavin (vitamin B2), niacin (vitamin B3), calcium d-pantothenate (vitamin B5), pyridoxine hydrochloride (vitamin B6), folate (vitamin B9), cyanocobalamin (vitamin B12), ascorbic acid and ascorbyl palmitate (vitamin C), cholecalciferol (vitamin D), d-alpha-tocopherol (vitamin E), biotin, calcium, chromium, copper, magnesium, manganese, molybdenum, phosphorus, potassium, selenium, sodium, zinc, L-arginine, L-carnitine, L-cysteine, L-lysine, L-proline,

Continued on next page

Cardio-Basics—Cont.

inositol, coenzyme Q10, and maritime pine extract. In addition to those active ingredients each tablet also contains microcrystalline cellulose, sucrose, fatty acid esters, silicon dioxide, magnesium stearate, and maltodextrin.

BENEFITS AND RESEARCH

According to the Center for Disease Control and Prevention, one American will die every minute as a result of heart disease. Narrowing of the arterial walls can lead to blocked blood flow to the brain. A healthy lifestyle including being physically active, not smoking, and making good food choices can lead to a reduction of heart disease. Cardio-Basics™ provides the vitamins, minerals and antioxidants needed for a healthy heart. In clinical studies, participants using Cardio-Basics™ and Bio-C™ saw a significant reduction in arterial wall thickness, removal of calcification deposits and a reduced risk for cardiovascular disease when compared to the placebo group. Cardio-Basics™ provides the body with the necessary vitamins and minerals needed to support a healthy vascular system.*

SUGGESTED USE

Take two tablets daily with food.

SAFETY AND WARNINGS

Cardio-Basics™ is well tolerated. Some gastrointestinal discomfort may be experienced as with any dietary supplement.

HOW SUPPLIED

Available in tablets

REFERENCES

Niedzwiekcki, A, Rath, M. (1996) Journal of Applied Nutrition, 48: 67-78.

Jeejeebhoy, F, Keith, M, Freeman, M, Barr, A, McCall, M, Kurian, R, Mazer, D, Errett, L, (2002), American Heart Journal 143: 1092-1100.

Verdgem, PJE, Lonky, S, Curley, S. (2005) 7th Conference on Arteriosclerosis, Thrombosis and Vascular Biology.

Lloyd-Jones D, Adams R, Carnethon M, DeSimone G, Ferguson TB, Flegal K, Ford E, Furie K, Go A, Greenlund K, Haase N, Hailpern S, Ho M, Howard V, Kissela B, Kittner S, Lackland D, Lisabeth L, Marelli A, McDermott M, Meigs J, Mozaffarian D, Nichol G, O'Donnell C, Roger V, Rosamond W, Sacco R, Sorlie P, Stafford R, Steinberger J, Hong Y; (2009) Circulation, 119: 480-486.

* THESE STATEMENTS HAVE NOT BEEN EVALUATED BY THE FOOD AND DRUG ADMINISTRATION. THIS PRODUCT IS NOT INTENDED TO DIAGNOSE, TREAT, CURE, OR PREVENT ANY DISEASE.

CARDIO-ESSENTIALS   DS
Caring for your heart*

DESCRIPTION

Cardio-Essentials is a nutritional supplement for the heart. Cardio-Essentials contains Coenzyme Q-10, L-carnitine, L-taurine and Hawthorn berry.

Cardio-Essentials is a light tan, water-soluble powder. Each capsule of Cardio-Essentials contains 100 mg of Coenzyme Q-10 and 3.5 g of a blend of L-carnitine, L-taurine, and Hawthorn berry. In addition to those active ingredients, each capsule also contains silicon dioxide, stearic acid and calcium silicate.

BENEFITS AND RESEARCH

One of the leading causes of congestive heart failure (CHF), left ventricular dysfunction, affects approximately 1.5% of the population in the United States. CHF patients with left ventricular dysfunction have reduced levels of Coenzyme Q-10, L-carnitine and L-taurine and have an enlarged left ventricle. In a clinical study, the combination of L-carnitine, L-taurine, and Coenzyme Q10 was shown to benefit congestive heart failure patients by reducing left ventricular size. These ingredients are known to be important in providing adequate energy for heart muscle. Cardio-Essentials provides adequate amounts of these ingredients, i.e. 100 mg of CoQ10, Hawthorn extract is traditionally used in supporting the heart function.

SUGGESTED USE

Take three capsules twice a day with food.

SAFETY AND WARNINGS

Cardio-Essentials is well tolerated. Some gastrointestinal discomfort may be experienced as with any dietary supplement.

HOW SUPPLIED

Available in capsules

REFERENCES

Jeejeebhoy, F et al (2002), American Heart Journal 143 1092–1100.

* THESE STATEMENTS HAVE NOT BEEN EVALUATED BY THE FOOD AND DRUG ADMINISTRATION. THIS PRODUCT IS NOT INTENDED TO DIAGNOSE, TREAT, CURE, OR PREVENT ANY DISEASE.

OMEGALIFE-3™   DS
[ōmĕgā-līf 3]
Omega-3 Fatty Acid Supplementation

DESCRIPTION

OmegaLife-3™ is a blend of omega-3 fatty acids designed to help maintain healthy cardiovascular and cerebral function as well as aiding in the prevention of age-related macular degeneration.

OmegaLife-3™ is an amber-colored, semi-viscous, fat-soluble liquid. Each serving of OmegaLife-3™ contains the following active ingredients 800 mg eicosapentaenoic acid (EPA), 400 mg docosahexaenoic acid (DHA), and vitamin E. In addition, it also contains the inactive ingredients gelatin, glycerin, purified water, and orange oil. OmegaLife-3™ has been molecularly distilled to ensure exceptionally pure oil and includes orange oil to prevent a fishy after taste.

BENEFITS AND RESEARCH

Clinical research suggests that fish oil can help support proper brain and visual function. In 2002 the FDA approved supplementation of DHA in infant formula. DHA is potentially important in fetal and infant neural development, in that DHA and arachidonic acid have been shown to be incorporated into brain and retinal cell membranes—particularly during the third trimester and early infant life.

DHA is the predominant structural fatty acid in the central nervous system and in the retina of the eyes.

EPA supports the synthesis of important compounds in the body. EPA is the precursor of thromboxane and leukotriene, compounds involved in supporting healthy circulation. They also promote healthy blood vessels.*

Evidence is accumulating that increasing intakes of EPA and DHA can decrease the risk of cardiovascular disease by preventing arrhythmias, decreasing the risk of thrombosis, decreasing triglyceride levels, slowing the growth of atherosclerotic plaque, and decreasing inflammation.*

The U.S. Food and Drug Administration (FDA) has stated that, "Supportive but not conclusive research shows that consumption of EPA and DHA omega-3 fatty acids may reduce the risk of coronary heart disease."

USAGE

Take two softgels per day with a meal.

SAFETY AND WARNINGS

OmegaLife-3™ is well tolerated. Some gastrointestinal discomfort may be experienced as with any dietary supplement. Common side effects include a "fishy" taste upon eructation.

HOW SUPPLIED

Available in softgels.

REFERENCES

Barter P, Ginsberg HN. Effectiveness of combined statin plus omega-3 fatty acid therapy for mixed dyslipidemia. Am J Cardiol. 2008 Oct 15;102(8):1040-5

Lee JH, Harris WS, et al. Omega-3 fatty acids for cardioprotection. Mayo Clin Proc. 2008 Mar;83(3):324-32.

SanGiovanni JP, Chew EY, Sperduto RD, et al. The relationship of dietary omega-3 long-chain polyunsaturated fatty

acid intake with incident age-related macular degeneration: AREDS report no. 23. Arch Ophthalmol. 2008 Sep;126(9): 1274-9.

SanGiovanni JP, Parra-Cabrera S, Colditz GA, Berkey CS, Dwyer JT. Meta-analysis of dietary essential fatty acids and long-chain polyunsaturated fatty acids as they relate to visual resolution acuity in healthy preterm infants. Pediatrics 2000;105:1292-8.
Kris-Etherton PM, Harris WS, Appel LJ. Omega-3 fatty acids and cardiovascular disease: new recommendations from the American Heart Association. Arterioscler Thromb Vasc Biol. 2003;23(2):151-152.
* THESE STATEMENTS HAVE NOT BEEN EVALUATED BY THE FOOD AND DRUG ADMINISTRATION. THIS PRODUCT IS NOT INTENDED TO DIAGNOSE, TREAT, CURE, OR PREVENT ANY DISEASE.

Upsher-Smith Laboratories, Inc.
6701 EVENSTAD DRIVE
MINNEAPOLIS, MN 55369

For Medical Information Contact:
Write: Medical Information Department
or call: (800) 654-2299
(during business hours-8:00 am to 5:00 pm CST)

SLO–NIACIN® Tablets   DS
(polygel® controlled-release niacin)
Dietary Supplement

DESCRIPTION

Slo-Niacin® Tablets are manufactured utilizing a unique, patented polygel® controlled-release delivery system. This exclusive technology assures the gradual and measured release of niacin (nicotinic acid) and is designed to reduce the incidence of flushing and itching commonly associated with niacin use. Slo-Niacin® Tablets are available in 250 mg, 500 mg, and 750 mg strengths.

HOW SUPPLIED

250 mg tablets in bottles of 100: List 0245–0062–11
500 mg tablets in bottles of 100: List 0245–0063–11
750 mg tablets in bottles of 100: List 0245–0064–11
U.S. Patent No. 5,126,145 and 5,268,181

USANA Health Sciences, Inc.
3838 WEST PARKWAY BOULEVARD
SALT LAKE CITY, UT 84120-6336

Direct Inquiries to:
Ph: (801) 954 7860
Fax: (801) 954 7658

ACTIVE CALCIUM™   DS

COMPOSITION

Each Active Calcium contains the following minerals:

Vitamin D3 (as Cholecalciferol)	100 IU
Vitamin K (as Phylloquinone)	15 mcg
Calcium (as Calcium Citrate and Carbonate)	200 mg
Magnesium (as Magnesium Citrate, Amino Acid Chelate and Oxide)	100 mg
Boron (as Boron Citrate)	0.33 mg
Silicon (as Silicon Amino Acid Complex)	2.25 mg

ADVANTAGES

Each tablet contains a balanced blend of calcium, magnesium, vitamin D, vitamin K, boron and silicon; six nutrients required for bone development, bone remodeling and skeletal health. This non-prescription product meets USP guidelines for potency (as applicable), uniformity and disintegration, and is manufactured according to pharmaceutical cGMP standards.

RECOMMENDED USE

Take 4 tablets by mouth daily, preferably with meals.

SUPPLIED

Capsule-shaped tablet, mottled greenish-white color, with clear film coating, and with USANA imprint. In bottle of 112 tablets.

CHELATED MINERAL   DS
[*key'-lā-tĕd*]
mineral

COMPOSITION

Each Chelated Mineral contains the following minerals:

Calcium (As Calcium Citrate and Carbonate)	67.5 mg
Iodine (As Potassium Iodide)	75 mcg
Magnesium (As Magnesium Citrate and Amino Acid Chelate)	75 mg
Zinc (As zinc citrate)	5 mg
Selenium (As L-selenomethionine and Amino Acid Complex)	50 mcg
Copper (As Copper Gluconate)	0.5 mg
Manganese (As Manganese Gluconate)	1.25 mg
Chromium (As Chromium Polynicotinate and Picolinate**)	75 mcg
Molybdenum (As Molybdenum Citrate)	1.25 mcg
Boron (As boron citrate)	0.75 mg
Silicon (As Silicon Amino Acid Complex)	1 mg
Vanadium (As Vanadium Citrate)	10 mcg
Ultra trace Minerals	0.75 mg

**Licensed under U.S. Patent 4,315,927.

ADVANTAGES

Each tablet contains a complete and balanced blend of essential minerals in bioavailable forms. The Chelated Mineral is designed to be taken with USANA's Mega Antioxidant to provide a full complement of essential nutrients required for health. This non-prescription product meets USP guidelines for potency (as applicable), uniformity and disintegration, and is manufactured according to pharmaceutical cGMP standards.

RECOMMENDED USE

Take two (2) tablets twice daily, preferably with food.

SUPPLIED

Oblong shaped tablets, off-white color, with clear film coating with USANA imprint. In bottle of 112 tablets

---

COQUINONE® 30   DS
[*cō'-kwi-nōn*]

COMPOSITION

Each CoQuinone 30 capsule contains the following:

Coenzyme Q_{10}	30 mg
Alpha Lipoic Acid	12.5 mg

ADVANTAGES

CoQuinone 30 contains a hydrosoluble form of Coenzyme Q_{10} (CoQ$_{10}$) that is 2.5 times more bioavailable than material supplied in dry tablet/capsule formulas. The higher blood levels of CoQ$_{10}$ supplied enhance mitochondrial production of ATP. CoQ$_{10}$ is a rate-limiting factor in the electron transport chain involved in mitochondrial production of ATP. It is also involved in neutralizing free radicals generated during ATP production. As such, CoQ$_{10}$ helps the body maintain healthy skeletal and cardiac muscle. Alpha lipoic acid is included in the formula as a lipid-soluble antioxidant to recycle CoQ$_{10}$ from the prooxidant form to the antioxidant form. This non-prescription product meets USP guide-

Continued on next page

CoQuinone 30—Cont.

lines for potency (where applicable), uniformity and disintegration, and is manufactured according to cGMP standards.

RECOMMENDED USE

Take 1 or 2 capsules by mouth daily.

SUPPLIED

Oval shaped, soft gelatin capsule, annatto-colored, opaque, imprinted with USANA in white edible ink. Capsules contain an orange colored liquid. In bottle of 56 soft-gel capsules.

MEGA ANTIOXIDANT   DS

[mĕ-gă aenti-ŏx'-si-dĕnt]

COMPOSITION

Each Mega Antioxidant contains the following vitamins and Minerals:

Vitamin A (as beta carotene)	3,750 IU
Vitamin C (as Calcium, Potassium, Magnesium, & Zinc Ascorbates)	325 mg
Vitamin D3 (as Cholecalciferol)	450 IU
Vitamin E (as D-alpha Tocopheryl Succinate)	100 IU
Vitamin K (as Phylloquinone)	15 mcg
Thiamin (as Thiamine HCL)	6.75 mg
Riboflavin	6.75 mg
Niacin and Niacinamide	10 mg
Vitamin B6 (as Pyridoxine HCL)	8 mg
Folate (as Folic Acid)	250 mcg
Vitamin B12 (as Cyanocobalamin)	50 mcg
Biotin	75 mcg
Pantothenic Acid (as D-Calcium Pantothenate)	22.5 mg
Olivol ® (Olive Extract)	7.5 mg
Mixed Natural Tocopherols (D-gamma, D-delta, D-beta Tocopherol)	8.5 mg
Bioflavonoid complex (Rutin, Quercetin, Hesperidin, Green Tea Extract-Decaffeinate, Pomegranate Extract, Cinnamon Extract, Bilberry Extract)	49.5 mg
Inositol	37.5 mg
Choline Bitartrate	25 mg
N-Acetyl L-Cysteine	25 mg
Bromelain	12.5 mg
Alpha-Lipoic Acid	5 mg
Coenzyme Q10	3 mg
Turmeric Extract	3.75 mg
Lutein	150 mcg
Lycopene	250 mcg
Broccoli Concentrate	3.75 mg

ADVANTAGES

A comprehensive and balanced formula containing the essential vitamins and antioxidants at levels substantially higher than RDA amounts. In addition to the traditionally recognized essential nutrients, the formula contains a unique blend of dietary antioxidants including carotenoids, a bioflavonoid complex, a glutathione complex, and USANA's patented Olivol™ to provide full-spectrum antioxidant protection. This formula is designed to be taken with USANA's Chelated Mineral to provide a full compliment of essential nutrients required for health. This non-prescription

product meets USP guidelines for potency (as applicable), uniformity and disintegration, and is manufactured according to pharmaceutical cGMP standards.

RECOMMENDED USE

Take two (2) tablets twice daily, preferably with food.

SUPPLIED

Oblong shaped tablets, mottled orange-brown color, with clear film coating with USANA imprint. In bottle of 112 tablets.

PROCOSA II   DS

COMPOSITION

Each Procosa II tablet contains the following:

Vitamin C (As Calcium Ascorbate)	75 mg
Manganese (As Manganese Gluconate)	1.25 mg
Glucosamine Sulfate 2KCl (From Shrimp & Crab Shells)	500 mg
Turmeric Extract (Curcuma longa L., Root)	125 mg
Silicon (As Silicon Amino Acid Complex)	0.75 mg

ADVANTAGES

A comprehensive joint health formula which combines a widely researched, clinically studied dose of Glucosamine Sulfate with Vitamin C, Manganese, and Silicon; three additional nutrients, necessary for the maintenance of healthy cartilage.

Procosa II also contains Turmeric Extract, a potent antioxidant that supports the body's inflammatory response processes. This non-prescription product meets USP guidelines for potency (as applicable), uniformity and disintegration and is manufactured according to pharmaceutical GMP standards.

RECOMMENDED USE

Take two tablets twice daily, preferably with meals

SUPPLIED

Oblong, orange-colored tablet, scored on one side. In bottle of 120 tablets.

PROFLAVANOL® 90   DS

[prŏ-flă' vi-nol]

COMPOSITION

Each Proflavanol 90 tablet contains the following:

Vitamin C (As Calcium, Potassium, Magnesium, Zinc Ascorbates)	300 mg
Grape Seed Extract (Vitis Vinifera L., Seeds)	90 mg

ADVANTAGES

A potent antioxidant formula combining the proanthocyanidins (bioflavonoids) from standardized grape seed extract with vitamin C in the form of ascorbate salts and ascorbyl palmitate. Proflavanol 90 is designed to be taken as a standalone antioxidant, or preferably in combination with USANA's Mega Antioxidant and Chelated Mineral to provide additional antioxidant protection. This non-prescription product meets USP guidelines for potency (where applicable), uniformity and disintegration, and is-manufactured according to pharmaceutical cGMP standards.

RECOMMENDED USE

Take 1–3 tablets by mouth daily.

SUPPLIED

Oblong, buff-colored tablet, with clear film coating, with USANA imprint. In bottles of 56 tablets.

DIETARY SUPPLEMENT PROFILES

This section provides information on commonly used dietary supplements, which are marketed under the federal Dietary Supplement Health and Education Act of 1994. The profiles are derived from clinical monographs appearing in *PDR® for Nutritional Supplements* and have been updated based on recent scientific findings and reviewed by PDR's clinical staff.

Included here is information on vitamins, minerals, and other substances intended to supplement the diet. **Note:** Dietary supplements are not regulated by the Food and Drug Administration and are not intended to diagnose, treat, cure, or prevent any disease.

Dietary Supplements

Alpha Lipoic Acid

EFFECTS

Alpha lipoic acid (ALA) is an important coenzyme with antioxidant and antidiabetic properties. It is an endogenous substance that acts as a cofactor in the pyruvate-dehydrogenase complex, the alpha-ketoglutarate-dehydrogenase complex, and the amino acid-hydrogenase complex. Reduced levels of ALA have been found in patients with liver cirrhosis, diabetes mellitus, atherosclerosis, and polyneuritis. During metabolism, ALA may be transformed from its oxidized form (with the disulfide bridge in the molecule) to its reduced dihydroform with two free sulfide groups. Both forms have strong antioxidant effects. They protect the cell from free radicals that result from intermediate metabolites, from the degradation of exogenous molecules, and from heavy metals. ALA is available in oral and parenteral formulations. The scope of this monograph is limited to the oral formulations.

COMMON USAGE

Unproven uses: Studies of the efficacy of ALA for treating complications of diabetes mellitus are conflicting. ALA may be beneficial for alleviating pain and paresthesia caused by diabetic neuropathy. It is probably ineffective for the treatment of alcohol-related liver disease, *Amanita* ("death cap" mushroom) poisoning, and HIV-associated cognitive impairment. More placebo-controlled trials are needed.

CONTRAINDICATIONS

There are no known contraindications to the oral formulation of ALA.

WARNINGS/PRECAUTIONS

Insulin autoimmune syndrome and hypoglycemia: As ALA has increased in popularity as a supplement, the number of cases of insulin autoimmune syndrome has risen rapidly. Patients with diabetes may need additional blood-sugar monitoring.

Paresthesia: Symptoms may temporarily worsen at the beginning of therapy; some research shows that antidepressants or neuroleptics may be used concurrently to treat the pain.

Pregnancy and breastfeeding: Scientific evidence for the safe use of ALA during pregnancy is not available; it is not recommended during lactation.

DRUG INTERACTIONS

Antidiabetic agents: Additive hypoglycemic effects may occur with concurrent use of antidiabetic agents. Close monitoring of blood-sugar control is recommended when initiating therapy with ALA.

Cisplatin: ALA antagonizes the action of cisplatin.

FOOD INTERACTIONS

The bioavailability of ALA is decreased with food.

ADVERSE REACTIONS

Nausea has been reported.

ADMINISTRATION AND DOSAGE

Adults

Diabetic neuropathy: Initiate treatment at 600mg daily in 2 or 3 divided doses. Maintenance doses range from 200mg to 600mg daily in single or divided doses.

Bromelain

EFFECTS

Bromelain is a concentrated mixture of proteolytic enzymes derived from the pineapple plant. It has anti-inflammatory, antitumor, and digestive properties. Commercial bromelain is not a chemically homogeneous substance because if the enzyme is highly purified it loses its stability and most of its physiological activity. The main ingredient is a proteolytic enzyme (a glycoprotein), but it also contains small amounts of an acid phosphatase, a peroxidase, several protease inhibitors, and organically bound calcium.

COMMON USAGE

Accepted uses: Bromelain is approved by the German Commission E as an anti-edematous agent.

Unproven uses: Bromelain may be of therapeutic value in modulating inflammation, tumor growth, blood coagulation, and debridement of third-degree burns. It could possibly enhance absorption of some drugs, including antibiotics.

CONTRAINDICATIONS

Bromelain is contraindicated in patients who have severe liver or kidney impairment or who need dialysis. The supplement should also be avoided by patients who have a coagulation disorder such as hemophilia or who have demonstrated hypersensitivity to bromelain, pineapple, or the inactive ingredients of enzyme preparations.

WARNINGS/PRECAUTIONS

Allergic reactions/hypersensitivity: Bromelain is capable of inducing IgE-mediated respiratory and gastrointestinal reactions. Cross-sensitivity reactions between bromelain and papain can occur.

Pregnancy and breastfeeding: Scientific evidence for the safe use of bromelain during pregnancy and lactation is not available.

Tachycardia: Bromelain may increase heart rate at higher doses. It should be used cautiously (doses <500mg per day) in patients with heart palpitations or tachycardia.

DRUG INTERACTIONS

Anticoagulants, low molecular weight heparins, or thrombolytic agents: Theoretically, there is an increased risk of bleeding if bromelain is used with these medications. Avoid concomitant use.

Oral antibiotics: Bromelain may alter the absorption of amoxicillin and tetracycline antibiotics.

ADVERSE REACTIONS

Mild hypersensitivity reactions such as erythema and pruritus occur infrequently. Gastrointestinal side effects are infrequent but may include stomachache and/or diarrhea.

ADMINISTRATION AND DOSAGE

Bromelain is administered orally and topically. Available preparations of bromelain tablets vary widely in their concentrations, and caution must be exercised in determining dosage regimens. Take 1 hour before or after food.

Adults

General use: 500mg to 2,000mg daily in divided doses.

Carpal tunnel syndrome: 1,000mg (with a potency of at least 3,000 microunits/gram) given 3 times/day, between meals.

Debridement: Administer a 35% topical suspension in a liquid base.

Inflammation: 500mg to 2,000mg per day. A European manufacturer recommends 450mg to 1,500 Federation Internationale Pharmaceutique (FIP) units divided into 3 daily doses and administered over 8 to 10 days.

Platelet aggregation inhibition: 160mg to 1,400mg daily.

Pediatrics

150FIP to 300FIP units daily, divided into 3 doses.

Calcium

EFFECTS

Calcium is an electrolyte, a nutrient, and a mineral that demonstrates anti-osteoporotic, antihypertensive, antihyperlipidemic, and possible anticarcinogenic properties. Calcium functions as a regulator in the release and storage of neurotransmitters and hormones, in the uptake and binding of amino acids, and in vitamin B_{12} absorption and gastrin secretion. Calcium is required to maintain the function of the nervous, muscular, and skeletal systems and cell membrane and capillary permeability. It is an activator in many enzyme reactions and is essential in the transmission of nerve impulses; contraction of cardiac, smooth, and skeletal muscles; respiration; blood coagulation; and renal function.

The scope of this monograph is limited to the oral salt formulations, including carbonate, citrate, glubionate, gluconate, lactate, phosphate, and other calcium salts.

COMMON USAGE

Accepted uses: Calcium salts are FDA-approved for the prophylaxis of calcium deficiency and osteoporosis. Calcium acetate is approved for the treatment of hyperphosphatemia related to renal failure and hemodialysis. Calcium carbonate is used alone or in combination products as an antacid to relieve symptoms of heartburn, acid indigestion, and stomach upset.

Unproven uses: Calcium supplementation may reduce premenstrual pain, total and LDL cholesterol levels, hypertension, and the occurrence of colorectal polyps. Studies show it may also reverse fluorosis in children (when combined with vitamins C and D), control age-related increases in parathyroid hormone, and reduce plasma bilirubin in patients with Crigler-Najjar syndrome (calcium phosphate only). Weaker evidence shows calcium supplementation may be helpful for leg cramps, pre-eclampsia, and prophylaxis of urinary crystallization of calcium oxalate in patients with nephrolithiasis (calcium citrate only). In clinical trials of adults with hypertension, calcium supplements lowered systolic (but not diastolic) blood pressure.

CONTRAINDICATIONS

Calcium supplements are contraindicated in patients with hypercalcemia.

WARNINGS/PRECAUTIONS

Arrhythmia: Calcium enhances the effect of cardiac glycosides on the heart and may precipitate arrhythmia.

Hypercalcemia: Oral calcium—including antacids containing calcium carbonate or other absorbable calcium salts—can cause hypercalcemia, which may result in nephrolithiasis, anorexia, nausea, vomiting, ocular toxicity, constipation, cardiac arrhythmia, nausea, nocturia, polydipsia, kidney stones, and polyuria.

Milk-alkali syndrome: Doses higher than 4g daily can result in milk-alkali syndrome. Symptoms include hypercalcemia, uremia, calcinosis, nausea, vomiting, headache, weakness, azotemia, and alterations in taste.

Pregnancy and breastfeeding: Calcium is safe in normal dietary amounts. It is FDA-rated as Pregnancy Category C.

Prostate cancer: A high intake of calcium, whether from food alone or including supplements, was associated in an epidemiological study with an increased incidence of prostate cancer, possibly due to calcium's inhibitory effect on vitamin D conversion.

DRUG INTERACTIONS

Aspirin: Concurrent use may result in decreased effectiveness of aspirin due to increased urinary pH and subsequent increased renal elimination of salicylates. Monitor for reduced aspirin effectiveness upon initiation of calcium-containing products or for possible aspirin toxicity upon withdrawal of calcium-containing products. Adjust the dose accordingly. Using buffered aspirin may limit the degree to which the urine is alkalinized.

Atenolol: Concomitant use may decrease the bioavailability of atenolol; administer atenolol 2 hours before or 6 hours after calcium-containing products.

Bismuth subcitrate: Concomitant use may result in decreased effectiveness of bismuth subcitrate. Administer at least 30 minutes apart.

Bisphosphonates: Concurrent use may interfere with the absorption of bisphosphonates such as alendronate, etidronate, tiludronate, and risedronate. Administer bisphosphonates 2 hours before or 3 to 4 hours after a dose of calcium.

Calcium channel blockers: Concomitant use can result in decreased effectiveness of calcium channel blockers. Monitor the patient and adjust dose accordingly.

Cefpodoxime: Concomitant use may result in decreased effectiveness of cefpodoxime. Concurrent administration of cefpodoxime and calcium-containing products is not recommended. If concurrent use cannot be avoided, cefpodoxime should be taken at least 2 to 3 hours before the administration of calcium. Because staggered administration may not be completely reliable, aggressively monitor patients for continued antibiotic efficacy. Alternative antibiotic therapy may need to be considered.

Diuretics: Thiazide and thiazide-like diuretics may cause hypercalcemia by decreasing renal calcium excretion. Concomitant ingestion of calcium salts and thiazide diuretics may predispose patients to developing the milk-alkali syndrome. Instruct patients to avoid excessive ingestion of calcium in any form (eg, antacids, dairy products) during thiazide diuretic therapy. Consider monitoring the patient's serum calcium level and/or parathyroid function if calcium replacement therapy is clinically necessary.

Fluoroquinolones: Concomitant use may result in decreased effectiveness of fluoroquinolones such as ciprofloxacin and enoxacin. Concurrent administration of fluoroquinolones with calcium—including calcium-fortified foods and drinks such as orange juice—should be avoided. Fluoroquinolones may be taken 2 hours before or 6 hours after taking calcium-containing products.

Hyoscyamine: Concomitant use may result in decreased absorption of hyoscyamine. Hyoscyamine should be taken prior to meals and calcium-containing products should be taken after meals.

Itraconazole: Concomitant use may result in decreased effectiveness of itraconazole. Calcium-containing products should be taken at least 1 hour before or 2 hours after itraconazole.

Ketoconazole: Concomitant use may result in decreased effectiveness of ketoconazole. Concurrent administration of ketoconazole and calcium-containing products is not recommended. If concurrent use cannot be avoided, ketoconazole should be taken at least 2 hours before calcium-containing products. Because staggered administration may not be completely reliable, aggressively monitor patients for continued antifungal efficacy.

Levothyroxine: Concurrent use with calcium carbonate may result in decreased absorption of levothyroxine. Separate the administration of levothyroxine and calcium carbonate by at least 4 hours.

Methscopolamine: Concomitant use may result in decreased absorption of methscopolamine, although the effect is minor. Monitor the patient for drug effectiveness.

Polystyrene sulfonate: Concomitant administration of calcium-containing antacids and sodium polystyrene sulfonate resin therapy has resulted in the elevation of serum carbon dioxide content levels, associated with varying degrees of metabolic alkalosis. Separate the oral administration of sodium polystyrene sulfonate and calcium-containing products by as much time as possible. Another alternative is to administer the sodium polystyrene sulfonate rectally. If concurrent oral administration cannot be avoided, monitor the patient for evidence of alkalosis.

Sucralfate: Concurrent use may result in decreased effectiveness of sucralfate. Calcium-containing products should not be taken 30 minutes before or after sucralfate administration.

Sulfasalazine: Concomitant sulfasalazine and calcium gluconate therapy has been reported to result in delayed absorption of sulfasalazine.

Tetracyclines: Concurrent use may result in decreased effectiveness of tetracyclines and is not recommended. If concurrent use cannot be avoided, tetracyclines should be taken at least 1 to 3 hours before calcium-containing products. Because staggered administration may not be completely reliable, aggressively monitor patients for continued antibiotic efficacy.

Ticlopidine: Concurrent use may result in decreased effectiveness of ticlopidine. Concurrent administration of ticlopidine and calcium-containing products is not recommended. If concurrent use cannot be avoided, ticlopidine should be taken at least 1 to 2 hours before the administration of calcium.

Zalcitabine: Concurrent use may result in decreased effectiveness of zalcitabine. Separate the administration of zalcitabine and calcium-containing products as far apart as possible.

ADVERSE REACTIONS

Constipation: Oral calcium supplementation can cause constipation.

ADMINISTRATION AND DOSAGE

Because calcium salts are bound with other molecules such as oxygen and carbon, supplements often list the percentage of elemental calcium in each tablet along with the total salt weight, usually in milligrams. The list below lists common examples.

Elemental calcium/1,000mg of salt (% and weight)
Calcium/1,000mg of salt

Carbonate 40%	(400mg)
Citrate 21%	(210mg)
Lactate 13%	(130mg)
Gluconate 9%	(90mg)

Adults

Daily Dosage: The National Institute of Medicine recommends the following Adequate Intakes (AIs) for males and females: *Adults 19 to 50 years:* 1,000mg daily; *51+ years:* 1,200mg daily. The same AIs apply to pregnant or lactating women.

Deficiency: Calcium carbonate—1g to 2g three times daily with meals; calcium citrate—950mg to 1.9g given 3 or 4 times/day after meals; calcium gluconate—15g daily in divided doses; calcium lactate—7.7g/day in divided doses with meals; calcium glubionate—15g/day in divided doses; dibasic calcium phosphate—4.4g/day in divided doses with or after meals; tribasic calcium phosphate—1.6g 2 times/day with or after meals.

Colorectal cancer prevention: 1,200mg to 2,000mg/day.

Crigler-Najjar syndrome: 4,000mg/day.

Dysmenorrhea: 1,000mg to 1,300mg/day.

Hypercholerolemia: 250mg to 400mg/day with meals.

Hyperphosphatemia: 1,334mg of calcium acetate with each meal initially. Most patients will require 2,001mg to 2,668mg with each meal. The dosage may be increased as necessary to obtain serum phosphate levels below 6mg/dL as long as hypercalcemia does not occur or, alternatively, 1g to 17g calcium carbonate daily in divided doses.

Hyperphosphatemia of renal failure and hemodialysis: 4,000mg to 8,000mg/day of calcium acetate or 2,500mg to 8,500mg/day of calcium carbonate.

Hypertension, idiopathic: 1,000mg to 2,000mg/day.

Hypertension, pregnancy-related: 1,000 to 2,000mg/day.

Nephrolithiasis, prevention: 200mg to 300mg with meals or as the citrate salt between meals.

Osteoporosis, glucocorticoid-induced, prevention of bone loss: 1,000mg/day.

Osteoporosis, idiopathic, prevention of bone loss and fractures: 500mg to 2,400mg/day.

Pre-eclampsia, prevention: 1,000mg to 2,000mg/day.

Premenstrual syndrome: 1,000mg to 1,200mg/day.

Pediatrics

Daily Dosage: The National Institute of Medicine recommends the following Adequate Intakes (AIs) for males and females:

Infants and children: 0 to 6 months: 210mg daily; *7 to 12 months:* 270mg/day; *1 to 3 years:* 500mg/day; *4 to 8 years:* 800mg/day; *9 to 18 years:* 1,300mg/day.

Bone mass accretion (adolescents): 500mg/day.

Fluorosis: 250mg/day.

Hypertension, prevention: 600mg/day.

Hypocalcemia: Calcium chloride—200mg/kg/day in divided doses every 4 to 6 hours; calcium glubionate—infants up to 1 year old should receive 1.8g calcium glubionate 5 times/day before meals; children 1 to 4 years old should receive 3.6g calcium glubionate 3 times/day before meals; children over age 4 should receive 15g/day in divided doses; calcium gluconate—200mg to 800mg/kg/day in divided doses; calcium lactate—500mg/kg/24 hours given orally in divided doses; calcium levulinate—500mg/kg/24 hours (12g/square meter/24 hours) given

orally in divided doses; dibasic calcium phosphate—200mg to 280mg/kg/day, in divided doses with or after meals.

Chondroitin Sulfate

EFFECTS

Chondroitin sulfate is a mucopolysaccharide found in most mammalian cartilaginous tissues. It has a molecular configuration similar to sodium hyaluronate, although chondroitin has a considerably shorter chain length. Chondroitin sulfate has protective effects on cartilage as well as viscoelastic effects. Preliminary evidence suggests it may also have antilipidemic, anticoagulant, and antithrombogenic properties. While ophthalmic preparations of chondroitin are FDA-approved for ophthalmic procedures, the scope of this monograph is limited to the oral preparations.

COMMON USAGE

Unproven uses: Chondroitin sulfate is used to reduce pain, improve functional capacity, and reduce the use of pain medications in patients with osteoarthritis and rheumatic disease. Results of a major follow-up trial—the Glucosamine/ Chondroitin Arthritis Intervention Trial [GAIT] failed to show superiority of chondroitin in slowing loss of cartilage in knee osteoporosis, while other studies have found positive effects. Oral chondroitin is sometimes used to treat the following: TMJ disorder, coronary heart disease, hypercholesterolemia, and nephrolithiasis. It is also used to prevent or treat disorders of connective tissue structures such as the aorta, vascular tissues, and soft tissues involved in musculoskeletal trauma.

CONTRAINDICATIONS

Patients with asthma may be at risk for symptom exacerbation.

WARNINGS/PRECAUTIONS

Pregnancy and breastfeeding: Information is not available regarding the safe use of chondroitin during pregnancy and lactation.

DRUG INTERACTIONS

Antiplatelet and anticoagulant agents: Theoretically, concurrent use with chondroitin may increase the risk of bleeding.

ADVERSE REACTIONS

Adverse reactions have not been reported with oral chondroitin.

ADMINISTRATION AND DOSAGE

Adults

Osteoarthritis: 800mg to 1200mg orally in single or divided doses.

Pediatrics

Information on pediatric dosing is not available.

Chromium

EFFECTS

Chromium is an essential trace mineral that plays a role in glucose metabolism. It is believed to potentiate the action of insulin at the cellular level. Chromium may also play a role in lipoprotein metabolism. Chromium deficiency may lead to glucose intolerance and neuropathies. Chromium is available in oral and intravenous formulations. The scope of this monograph is limited to the oral formulation.

COMMON USAGE

Accepted uses: Prevention and treatment of chromium deficiency.

Unproven uses: Chromium supplementation may aid in glycemic control in a subset of patients with type 2 diabetes and gestational diabetes. The use of chromium for glucose regulation in both hypoglycemia and diabetes has been long-standing but without uniform positive results. Chromium is not widely used in diabetics and is not endorsed by the American Diabetes Association. The optimal dose for glycemic control is not known and may exceed the estimated safe and adequate daily dietary intake of 10mcg to 200mcg, and the available studies, while of high quality, need to be expanded. Preliminary data from the diabetes studies also suggest that chromium may positively affect serum lipids. There is some interest in chromium's use in reactive hypoglycemia mostly from small clinical studies and case reports. A recent study reported that chromium supplementation (1,000mcg daily) shortened the QT interval in patients with type 2 diabetes. Popular literature touts chromium as a weight-loss and bodybuilding supplement, but there is little evidence to support chromium use for these purposes.

CONTRAINDICATIONS

Do not use in patients who have exhibited hypersensitivity to chromium.

WARNINGS/PRECAUTIONS

Diabetes: Improved glucose tolerance may affect blood glucose levels. Close monitoring of blood glucose levels is recommended.

Pregnancy and breastfeeding: Scientific evidence for the safe use of chromium in doses exceeding the recommended adequate intake is not available.

DRUG INTERACTIONS

Insulin: There is an increased risk of hypoglycemia.

Levothyroxine: Due to risk of possible reduction in levothyroxine levels, separate chromium intake by 3 to 4 hours.

ADVERSE REACTIONS

Insomnia and irritability have been reported. Genotoxicity has been documented as a risk.

ADMINISTRATION AND DOSAGE

Adults

Daily Dosage (Adequate Intakes [AI]): Males—9 to 13 years: 25mcg/day; *14 to 50 years:* 35mcg/day; *50+ years:* 30mcg/day. *Females—9 to 13 years:* 21mcg/day; *14 to 18 years:* 24mcg/ day; *19 to 50 years:* 25mcg/day; *50+ years:* 20mcg/day.

During pregnancy—up to 18 years: 29mcg/day; *19 years and older:* 30mcg/day.

During lactation—up to 18 years: 44mcg/day; *19 years and older:* 45mcg/day.

Deficiency: Treatment is individualized by the prescriber based on the severity of the deficiency.

Non-insulin dependent diabetes: 200mcg to 1,000mcg daily

Pediatrics

Daily Dosage (Adequate Intakes [AI]): Infants and children—up to 6 months: 0.2mcg/day; *7 to 12 months:* 5.5mcg/day; *1 to 3 years:* 11mcg/day; *4 to 8 years:* 15mcg/day.

Coenzyme Q10

EFFECTS

Coenzyme Q10 is a fat-soluble quinone that is synthesized intracellularly and participates in a variety of important cellular processes. It has vitamin-like characteristics and is structurally similar to vitamin K. Coenzyme Q10 is a vital component of the inner mitochondrial membrane.

Coenzyme Q10 is an antioxidant and cardiotonic. Some evidence suggests it may also have cytoprotective and neuroprotective qualities. An endogenous deficiency of coenzyme Q10 has been suggested in a variety of disorders, including cancer, congestive heart failure, hypertension, chronic hemodialysis, mitochondrial disease, and periodontal disease. Coenzyme Q10 is available for oral and parenteral administration. The scope of this monograph is limited to the oral formulation.

COMMON USAGE

Unproven uses: Coenzyme Q10 is used mainly for the treatment of various heart conditions, including congestive heart failure, hypertension, cardiomyopathy, ischemic heart disease, and angina. Studies have shown it may benefit patients having cardiovascular surgery such as cardiac valve replacement, coronary artery bypass grafting, and repair of abdominal aortic aneurysms. Coenzyme Q10 has also been used for asthenozoospermia, central nervous system problems, and muscle disorders. Athletes sometimes take it to improve performance, but current evidence does not justify this use.

CONTRAINDICATIONS

Hypersensitivity to coenzyme Q10 or its excipients.

WARNINGS/PRECAUTIONS

Hepatic failure is a precaution for use, since the primary site of metabolism is the liver. However, coenzyme Q10 has a very low toxicity profile, and higher plasma levels seem to be well-tolerated. There have been no reports of overt hepatotoxicity with coenzyme Q10.

DRUG INTERACTIONS

HMG-CoA reductase inhibitors: Use of these drugs may inhibit the natural synthesis of coenzyme Q10. Patients who have reduced levels of coenzyme Q10 may be at risk for side effects of HMG-CoA reductase inhibitors, particularly myopathy.

Oral hypoglycemic agents and insulin: Dosage adjustment may be necessary, since coenzyme Q10 could reduce insulin requirements.

Warfarin: Concurrent use could reduce anticoagulant effectiveness; monitor the INR as necessary.

ADVERSE REACTIONS

Gastrointestinal disturbances, including nausea, epigastric discomfort, diarrhea, heartburn, and appetite suppression, are the most common adverse effects, occurring in less than 1% in large studies. Insomnia, nausea, and tiredness are common side effects. Rare side effects may include skin rash, pruritus, photophobia, irritability, agitation, headache, and dizziness. Transient minor abnormalities of urinary sediment (protein, granular, and hyaline casts) were reported in patients with Parkinson's disease given doses of 400 to 800mg of coenzyme Q10 daily for 1 month. Problems resolved following discontinuation of therapy. Fatigue and increased involuntary movements were reported in patients with Huntington's chorea taking high doses.

ADMINISTRATION AND DOSAGE

For best absorption, coenzyme Q10 should be taken with food.

Adults

Angina: 150 to 600mg daily in divided doses.

Cardiac surgery: 100mg daily for 14 days before surgery, followed by 100mg daily for 30 days postoperatively.

Congestive heart failure: 50 to 150mg daily in 2 or 3 divided doses.

Migraine prevention: 150mg daily.

Neurological disease: (associated with mitochondrial ATP-producing deficiency): 150mg or more daily.

Parkinson's disease/Huntington's disease: 800 to 1,200mg daily.

Periodontal disease: 25mg twice daily; or topical solution consisting of 85mg/mL in soybean oil applied twice daily.

Pediatrics

General use: 2.4 to 3.8mg/kg daily.

Pediatric mitochondrial encephalomyopathy: 30mg daily.

Folic Acid

EFFECTS

Folic acid is a water-soluble B vitamin that has antidepressant, antiproliferative, antiteratogenic, antihomocysteinemic, and gingival anti-inflammatory effects. The coenzymes formed from folic acid are instrumental in the following intracellular metabolisms: conversion of homocysteine to methionine, conversion of serine to glycine, synthesis of thymidylate, histidine metabolism, synthesis of purines, and utilization or generation of formate.

COMMON USAGE

Accepted uses: Prevention of neural tube defects in pregnancy; treatment of megaloblastic anemias caused by folic acid deficiency; and treatment of folic acid deficiency caused by oral contraceptive or anticonvulsant therapy.

Unproven uses: Strong evidence shows that folic acid therapy can reduce high levels of homocysteine, which has been linked to coronary heart disease. Other studies have suggested that folic acid supplementation may be helpful for atherosclerosis, colon cancer prevention, coronary heart disease, depression, gingival hyperplasia, hyperhomocysteinemia, iron deficiency or sickle-cell anemia, lung cancer prevention, breast cancer prevention, methotrexate toxicity, prevention of restenosis following coronary angiography, ulcerative colitis, and vitiligo.

Weaker evidence suggests that folic acid may be of some benefit for cervical cancer prevention, aphthous ulcers, geriatric memory deficit, and the prevention of Fragile X syndrome in children. Recent evidence indicates that folic acid does not help to slow down cognitive decline in Alzheimer's disease, although some researchers have found that it may boost cognition during the natural aging process.

CONTRAINDICATIONS

Do not use in the presence of pernicious anemia and megaloblastic anemia caused by vitamin B_{12} deficiency.

WARNINGS/PRECAUTIONS

Folic acid doses above 0.1mg/day may obscure pernicious anemia.

Pregnancy and breastfeeding: FDA-rated as Pregnancy Category A (relatively safe) at doses below 0.8mg/day; doses higher than this are rated as Pregnancy Category C (effects unknown). It is safe to use during lactation.

DRUG INTERACTIONS

Barbiturates: May interfere with folate utilization, resulting in the need for folate supplementation.

Metformin: May interfere with the utilization of folate, resulting in increased need for folate supplementation.

Methotrexate: Interferes with the utilization of folate.

Pancreatic enzymes: Concurrent use may interfere with the absorption of folic acid. Patients taking pancreatin may require folic acid supplementation.

Phenytoin and fosphenytoin: Concurrent use may decrease phenytoin or fosphenytoin levels and increase seizure frequency. If folic acid is added to phenytoin therapy, monitor patients for decreased seizure control.

Pyrimethamine: Concurrent use may reduce the effectiveness of pyrimethamine. Folic acid should not be used as a folate supplement during pyrimethamine therapy as it is ineffective in preventing megaloblastic anemia. Leucovorin (folinic acid) may be added to pyrimethamine therapy to prevent hematologic toxicity without affecting pyrimethamine efficacy. However, the use of leucovorin may worsen leukemia.

Sulfasalazine: Concurrent use may decrease the absorption of folic acid; monitor patients for signs of deficiency.

Triamterene: Concurrent use may cause decreased utilization of dietary folate; monitor patient for signs of deficiency.

ADVERSE REACTIONS

Side effects of folic acid therapy include erythema, pruritus, urticaria, irritability, excitability, nausea, bloating, and flatulence. A variety of central nervous system effects have been reported following 5mg of folic acid 3 times/day, including altered sleep patterns, vivid dreaming, irritability, excitability, and overactivity. Discontinuation of the drug usually results in rapid improvement but in some cases may require 3 weeks to resolve. High-dose folic acid has been associated with zinc depletion. Evidence suggests that up to 5mg to 15mg daily of folic acid does not have significant adverse effects on zinc status in healthy, nonpregnant individuals.

ADMINISTRATION AND DOSAGE

Adults

Daily dosage: Recommended dietary allowance (RDA):

Adults and adolescents ≥14 years: 400mcg/day.

During pregnancy: 600mcg/day.

During lactation: 500mcg/day.

Deficiency: Up to 1mg/day until clinical symptoms of deficiency have resolved and blood levels have returned to normal.

Anticonvulsant-induced folate deficiency: 15mg/day.

Aphthous ulcers (canker sores): Treat as for folic acid deficiency.

Hyperhomocysteinemia: 500mcg to 5,000mcg/day.

Methotrexate toxicity: 5mg/week orally.

Oral contraceptive-induced folate deficiency: 2mg daily.

Periodontal disease: 2mg twice daily, or 5mL of 0.1% topical mouth rinse twice daily.

Prevention of birth defects: 400mcg to 4,000mcg orally daily beginning 1 month before conception.

Prevention of cerebrovascular disease: Treat as for folic acid deficiency or hyperhomocysteinemia.

Prevention of cervical cancer: 800mcg to 1,000mcg/day.

Prevention of colorectal cancer: 1mg to 5mg/day.

Prevention of lung cancer: 10mg/day.

Prevention of neural tube defects: 0.4mg/day. Doses from 0.5mg to 1mg/day are often administered during pregnancy. Patients with a previous history of neural tube defects during pregnancy should receive 4mg/day daily starting 1 month before pregnancy and throughout the first 3 months of pregnancy.

Prevention of restenosis following coronary angiography: 1mg in combination with 400mcg vitamin B_{12} and 10mg vitamin B_6 daily.

Sickle cell anemia: 1mg/day.

Ulcerative colitis: 15mg/day.

Vitiligo: 2,000mcg to 10,000mcg/day.

Pediatrics

Daily Dosage: Recommended dietary allowance (RDA):

Infants and children 0 to 6 months: 65mcg/day; *7 to 12 months:* 80mcg/day; *1 to 3 years:* 150mcg/day; *4 to 8 years:* 200mcg/day; *9 to 13 years:* 300mcg/day.

Anticonvulsant-induced folate deficiency: 5mg/day.

Folic acid deficiency: Up to 1mg/day until clinical symptoms of deficiency have resolved and blood levels have returned to normal.

Gingival hyperplasia: 5mg/day.

Hyperhomocysteinemia: 500mcg to 5,000mcg/day.

Glucosamine

EFFECTS

Glucosamine is an endogenous aminomonosaccharide synthesized from glucose and utilized for biosynthesis of two larger compounds—glycoproteins and glycosaminoglycans. These compounds are necessary for the construction and maintenance of virtually all connective tissues and lubricating fluids in the body. The sulfate salt of glucosamine forms half of the disaccharide subunit of keratan sulfate, which is decreased in osteoarthritis, and of hyaluronic acid, which is found in both articular cartilage and synovial fluid.

Supplemental glucosamine is generally used to reduce pain and immobility associated with osteoarthritis, especially in the knee joint. The supplements are usually derived from crab shells, although a corn source is also available. Most studies of osteoarthritis have used the sulfate form of glucosamine. Other forms include glucosamine hydrochloride and N-acetyl glucosamine. Glucosamine is available in oral and parenteral formulations. The scope of this monograph is limited to the oral formulations.

COMMON USAGE

Unproven uses: Glucosamine, especially the sulfate form, is a popular treatment for pain and immobility associated with osteoarthritis. Glucosamine is classified by the European League

Against Rheumatism (EULAR) as a "symptomatic slow-acting drug in osteoarthritis." This drug group is characterized by slow-onset improvement in osteoarthritis with persistent benefits after discontinuation. Whether long-term use of glucosamine can reverse the course of osteoarthritis is a theory that has yet to be investigated. Supplemental glucosamine has also been used for articular injury repair, TMJ, and cutaneous aging (wrinkles).

CONTRAINDICATIONS

Do not use in patients who have experienced hypersensitivity reactions to glucosamine.

WARNINGS/PRECAUTIONS

Allergic reactions: Glucosamine should be used with caution in patients with an allergy to shellfish and shellfish products.

Asthma: Patients with asthma may be at risk for symptom exacerbation.

Diabetes: Patients with diabetes should be cautious, since glucosamine may affect insulin sensitivity or glucose tolerance.

Pregnancy and breastfeeding: Scientific evidence for the safe use of glucosamine during pregnancy and lactation is not available.

DRUG INTERACTIONS

Antidiabetic drugs: Glucosamine may reduce their effectiveness. Glucosamine is likely safe for patients with diabetes that is well controlled with diet only or with one or two oral antidiabetic agents (HbA1c <6.5%). In patients with higher HbA1c concentrations or for those requiring insulin, closely monitor blood glucose concentrations.

Doxorubicin, etoposide, and teniposide: Glucosamine may reduce their effectiveness; avoid concomitant use.

ADVERSE REACTIONS

Most studies indicate that glucosamine is well-tolerated for periods of 30 to 90 days. The most commonly reported adverse effects are gastrointestinal disturbances, including nausea, dyspepsia, heartburn, vomiting, constipation, diarrhea, anorexia, and epigastric pain. Less than 1% of patients have reported edema, tachycardia, drowsiness, insomnia, headache, erythema, and pruritus.

ADMINISTRATION AND DOSAGE

Adults

Osteoarthritis: 1,500mg in a single dose or 3 divided doses/day.

Pediatrics

Information on pediatric dosing is not available.

Glutamine

EFFECTS

Glutamine is a nonessential amino acid; it is the most abundant amino acid in the body. Glutamine stimulates anabolism of protein and inhibits catabolism of protein. Glutamine is essential for maintaining intestinal function, the immune response, and amino acid homeostasis. Glutamine serves as a metabolic fuel for rapidly proliferating cell lines such as enterocytes, colonocytes, fibroblasts, lymphocytes, and macrophages. The body is depleted of glutamine stores during trauma, hypercatabolism, immunodeficiency, malnutrition, or extreme stress and in these states it may

be considered an essential amino acid. Human and animal studies have shown that glutamine has antioxidant, antitumor, chemoprotective, and immunostimulatory effects. Glutamine is available in oral, enteral, and parenteral formulations. The scope of this monograph is limited to the oral formulations.

COMMON USAGE

Unproven uses: Glutamine is used for a wide variety of digestive disorders such as ulcers, food allergies, leaky gut syndrome, reflux disease, and symptoms of malabsorption, including diarrhea and drug-induced diarrhea. Glutamine is used to treat environmental and multiple-chemical sensitivity and for its reported benefit in supporting Phase II liver detoxification pathways. In the practice of lifestyle and longevity medicine, glutamine is widely used to promote the release of growth hormone. Glutamine is accepted as a biomarker in determining and treating diseases of aging. In "wasting" diseases, such as cancer and AIDS, glutamine is used to support T-cell function in the immune system, to augment lean muscle mass, and to decrease cachexia. More recently, the athletic community has embraced glutamine as a muscle enhancer and recovery aid. In children with sickle cell disease, it is being used to decrease resting energy expenditure and improve nutritional status.

CONTRAINDICATIONS

Patients with liver disease should not use glutamine. This supplement is also contraindicated for patients with any condition that puts them at risk for accumulation of nitrogenous wastes in the blood—such as Reye's syndrome or cirrhosis—since it can lead to ammonia-induced encephalopathy and coma. Patients who have had a previous hypersensitivity reaction to glutamine should not use it.

WARNINGS/PRECAUTIONS

Pregnancy and breastfeeding: Scientific evidence for the safe use of glutamine during pregnancy and lactation is not available.

DRUG INTERACTIONS

No drug interaction data are available.

ADVERSE REACTIONS

Patients who are taking glutamine and have chronic renal failure should have their kidney function monitored. Extreme caution is also advised when adding glutamine to the total parenteral nutrition of cancer patients, since glutamine serves as the main substrate for many tumors. The most common side effects of supplemental glutamine are constipation, gastrointestinal upset, and bloating.

ADMINISTRATION AND DOSAGE

Adults

Cancer: 30g daily, usually taken in 3 divided doses.

Chemoprotective: 10g daily taken in 3 divided doses, or 0.5g/kg/day.

Intestinal permeability: 7g to 21g daily in single or divided doses.

Short-bowel syndrome: 0.4g/kg/day to 0.63g/kg/day.

Stomatitis (oral solution): 2g twice daily used as a mouthwash and then swallowed.

Pediatrics

Stomatitis (oral solution): 2g twice daily used as a mouthwash and then swallowed.

Iron

EFFECTS

Iron is an essential trace mineral involved in the process of respiration, including oxygen and electron transport. The function and synthesis of hemoglobin, which carries most of the oxygen in the blood, is dependent on iron. Iron is also involved in the production of cytochrome oxidase, myoglobin, L-carnitine, and aconitase, all of which are involved in energy production in the body. In addition to its fundamental role in energy production, iron is involved in DNA synthesis and may also play a role in normal brain development and immune function. Iron is involved in the synthesis of collagen and the neurotransmitters serotonin, dopamine, and norepinephrine. Iron has putative immune-enhancing, anticarcinogenic, and cognition-enhancing activities. Iron also has oxidative effects. Iron is able to catalyze reactions that produce free radical metabolites, which may damage cell membranes, cause chromosomal mutations, or oxidize low-density lipoproteins (LDL) into more atherogenic particles.

Animal studies have confirmed that atherosclerotic plaques contain a high concentration of iron, and rats given large amounts of iron have increased LDL lipid peroxidation. In human studies, atherosclerosis has been associated with increased iron levels. Supplemental iron is administered orally or by intramuscular injection. The scope of this monograph is limited to oral iron preparations.

COMMON USAGE

Accepted uses: Prophylaxis and treatment of iron-deficiency anemia.

Unproven uses: Limited research suggests that supplemental iron could be helpful for reducing the frequency of breath-holding spells in children. It may also enhance cognition in children and adolescents who have a documented iron deficiency. Likewise, iron may have some favorable effects on immunity and exercise performance—but again, these benefits are most likely limited to those with acute or borderline iron deficiency. Iron supplementation has also been used for the following: Plummer-Vinson syndrome, malaria, herpes simplex outbreaks, pediatric diarrhea, intestinal helminth infection, microcephaly prophylaxis, and decreased thyroid function in individuals consuming very-low-calorie diets.

CONTRAINDICATIONS

Iron supplementation is contraindicated in patients with hemochromatosis and hemosiderosis. It is also contraindicated for treating anemias not caused by iron deficiency, such as hemolytic anemia or thalassemia, due to the risk of excess iron storage. Sustained-release dosage forms should be avoided in patients who have conditions associated with intestinal strictures. Because levels of iron naturally rise after menopause, women of postmenopausal age may want to avoid supplemental iron at this stage and the attendant health risks.

WARNINGS/PRECAUTIONS

Toxicity: Treatment of iron-deficiency anemia must only be performed under medical supervision. Iron supplements should be used with extreme caution in those with chronic liver failure, alcoholic cirrhosis, chronic alcoholism, and pancreatic insufficiency. Iron supplements can be highly toxic or lethal to small children. Those who take iron supplements should use child-proof bottles and store them away from children.

Gastrointestinal irritation: Iron should be used cautiously in those with a history of gastritis, peptic ulcer disease, and gastrointestinal bleeding.

Elevated ferritin levels: Patients with elevated serum ferritin levels should generally avoid iron supplements.

Infection: Individuals with an active or suspected infection should generally avoid iron supplements.

Ischemic heart disease and cancer: A moderate increase in iron stores has been associated with an increased risk of ischemic heart disease and cancer.

Pregnancy and breastfeeding: FDA-rated as Pregnancy Category C. Pregnant and lactating women should not exceed the RDA unless their physician recommends it.

DRUG INTERACTIONS

Antacids: Concomitant use of aluminum- or magnesium-containing antacids may decrease the absorption of iron.

Bisphosphonates (eg, alendronate, etidronate, risedronate): Concomitant use with ferrous (II) iron supplements may decrease the absorption of bisphosphonates.

H_2 blockers (eg, cimetidine, famotidine, nizatidine, ranitidine): Concomitant use may suppress the absorption of carbonyl iron.

Levodopa: Concomitant use with iron may reduce the absorption of levodopa.

Levothyroxine: Concomitant use with iron may decrease the absorption of levothyroxine.

Penicillamine: Concomitant use with iron may decrease the absorption of penicillamine.

Proton pump inhibitors (eg, lansoprazole, omeprazole, pantoprazole, rabeprazole): Concomitant use may suppress the absorption of carbonyl iron.

Quinolones (eg, ciprofloxacin, gatifloxacin, levofloxacin, lomefloxacin, moxifloxacin, norfloxacin, ofloxacin, sparfloxacin, trovafloxacin): Concomitant use may decrease the absorption of both the quinolone and iron supplement.

Tetracyclines (eg, doxycycline, minocycline, tetracycline): Concomitant use may decrease the absorption of both the tetracycline and iron supplement.

SUPPLEMENT INTERACTIONS

Beta-carotene: Concomitant use may enhance the absorption of iron.

Calcium carbonate: Concomitant use may decrease the absorption of iron.

Copper: Concomitant use with iron supplements may decrease the copper status of tissues.

Inositol hexaphosphate: Concomitant use may decrease the absorption of iron.

L-cysteine: Concomitant use may increase the absorption of iron.

Magnesium: Concomitant use may decrease the absorption of iron.

N-acetyl-L-cysteine: Concomitant use may increase the absorption of iron.

Tocotrienols: Concomitant use of iron and tocotrienols, which are typically used in their nonesterified forms, may cause oxidation of tocotrienols.

Vanadium: Concomitant use may decrease the absorption of iron.

Vitamin C: Concomitant use may enhance the absorption of iron.

Vitamin E (eg, alpha-tocopherol, gamma-tocopherol, mixed tocopherols): Concomitant use of nonesterified tocopherols and iron may cause oxidation of the tocopherols.

Zinc: Concomitant use may decrease the absorption of iron.

FOOD INTERACTIONS

Caffeine (eg, coffee): Concomitant use may decrease the absorption of iron.

Cysteine-containing proteins (eg, meat): Concomitant use may increase the absorption of iron.

Dairy foods and eggs: Concomitant use may decrease the absorption of iron.

Oxalic acid (eg, spinach, sweet potatoes, rhubarb, beans): Concomitant use may decrease the absorption of iron.

Phytic acid (eg, unleavened bread, raw beans, seeds, nuts and grains, soy isolates): Concomitant use may decrease the absorption of iron.

Teas and tannin-containing herbs: Concomitant use may decrease the absorption of iron.

ADVERSE REACTIONS

The most common side effects of iron supplements are gastrointestinal problems, including nausea, vomiting, bloating, abdominal discomfort, black stools, diarrhea, constipation, and anorexia. Higher than recommended doses can cause serious harm. Enteric-coated iron preparations may prevent some of the gastrointestinal complaints associated with iron therapy. Temporary staining of teeth may occur from iron-containing liquids.

ADMINISTRATION AND DOSAGE

Adults

Daily Dosage: Recommended Dietary Allowance (RDA):

Adult males: 14 to 18 years: 11mg daily; *19 years and older:* 8mg daily.

Adult females: 14 to 18 years: 15mg daily; *19 to 50 years:* 18mg daily; *51 years and older:* 8mg daily.

During pregnancy (all ages): 27mg daily.

During lactation: 14 to 18 years: 10mg daily; *19 to 50 years:* 9mg daily.

Deficiency: Immediate-release dosage forms: 2mg/kg to 3 mg/kg daily in 3 divided doses; sustained-release dosage forms: 50mg to 100mg daily.

Iron deficiency in pregnancy: 60mg to 100mg daily; *prevention of:* 40mg to 100mg daily.

Decreased thyroid function during very-low-calorie diets: 9mg/day or more to bring total iron intake to 1.5 times the RDA.

Impaired athletic performance: Treat only confirmed iron deficiency.

Inflammatory bowel disease: Treat only confirmed iron deficiency.

Plummer-Vinson syndrome: 2mg/kg to 3mg/kg daily.

The following lists the elemental iron content of various forms:

Ferrous fumarate: 33%

Ferrous gluconate: 11.6%

Ferrous sulfate: 20%

Ferrous sulfate, anhydrous: 30%

Pediatrics

Daily Dosage: Recommended Dietary Allowance (RDA):

Infants and children: 0 to 6 months: 0.27mg daily; *7 to 12 months:* 11mg daily; *1 to 3 years:* 7mg daily; *4 to 8 years:* 10mg daily; *9 to 13 years:* 8mg daily.

Adolescent girls with low ferritin: 105mg to 260mg daily.

Breath-holding syndrome (ferrous sulfate solution): 5mg/kg daily.

Cognitive function: 105mg to 260mg daily.

Iron-deficiency anemia: Premature infants: 2mg to 4mg/kg/day in 2 to 4 divided doses, up to a maximum of 15mg/day; *Children:* 3mg to 6mg/kg/day in 1 to 3 divided doses.

Lutein

EFFECTS

Lutein is an antioxidant that has immunostimulant and photoprotectant properties. It is a naturally occurring carotenoid used to improve eye health, especially in people with age-related macular degeneration (AMD) and cataracts. Studies show that the retina selectively accumulates two carotenoids, lutein and its chemical cousin zeaxanthin. Within the central macula, zeaxanthin is the dominant component (up to 75%), whereas in the peripheral retina, lutein predominates (greater than 67%). The macular concentration of lutein and zeaxanthin is so high that they are visible as a dark yellow spot called the macular pigment. Because these carotenoids are powerful antioxidants and absorb blue light, researchers have hypothesized that they protect the retina. Evidence for the use of lutein to reduce the risk of age-related macular degeneration or promote eye health is mixed. While both are abundant in green and yellow fruits and vegetables, lutein is the carotenoid most often used as a supplement. Dietary intake of lutein and zeaxanthin is estimated at 1mg to 3mg daily. Sources include spinach, collard greens, corn, kiwifruit, zucchini, pumpkin, squash, peas, cucumbers, green peppers, and egg yolks.

COMMON USAGE

Unproven uses: Increased consumption of lutein may prevent, delay, or modify the course of AMD, although conclusive evidence is not available. Lutein has also been used to help prevent or treat various cancers, including breast, ovarian, endometrial, lung, and prostate. Some advocates have promoted lutein as a general anti-aging supplement.

CONTRAINDICATIONS

No data available.

WARNINGS/PRECAUTIONS

Animal studies indicate low toxicity risk from lutein supplements, although some researchers have found that smokers may be at increased risk for lung or other cancers with long-term use of the carotenoid.

DRUG INTERACTIONS

No data available.

ADVERSE REACTIONS

No data available.

ADMINISTRATION AND DOSAGE

Adults

Cancer Prevention: ≥5921mcg daily from dietary sources.

Macular degeneration prevention: 10mg daily.

Lysine

EFFECTS

Lysine is an essential amino acid involved in many biological processes, including receptor affinity, protease-cleavage points, retention of endoplasmic reticulum, nuclear structure and function, muscle elasticity, and chelation of heavy metals. Like other amino acids, the metabolism of free lysine follows two principal paths: protein synthesis and oxidative catabolism. It is required for biosynthesis of such substances as carnitine, collagen, and elastin. Lysine appears to have antiviral, anti-osteoporotic, cardiovascular, and lipid-lowering effects, although more controlled human studies are needed. The terms L-lysine and lysine are used interchangeably. The D-stereoisomer (D-lysine) is not biologically active.

COMMON USAGE

Unproven uses: The most common use of supplemental lysine is for preventing and treating episodes of herpes simplex virus. Lysine has been used in conjunction with calcium to prevent and treat osteoporosis. It has also been used for treating pain, aphthous ulcers, migraine attacks, rheumatoid arthritis, and opiate withdrawal. Many "body-building" formulations contain lysine to aid in muscle repair.

CONTRAINDICATIONS

Patients who have kidney or liver disease should not use lysine.

WARNINGS/PRECAUTIONS

Hypercholesterolemia: Patients with hypercholesterolemia should be aware that supplemental lysine has been linked to increased cholesterol levels in animal studies. However, other studies have shown lysine can also decrease cholesterol levels.

DRUG INTERACTIONS

Because lysine uses a common pathway with the amino acid arginine, high intake of arginine may lower levels of lysine.

Aminoglycoside antibiotics (eg, gentamicin, neomycin, streptomycin): Concurrent use may increase the risk of nephrotoxicity.

ADVERSE REACTIONS

Renal dysfunction, including Fanconi's syndrome and renal failure, has been reported.

ADMINISTRATION AND DOSAGE

Adults

Herpes simplex virus: 1g to 3g/day, divided and taken with meals.

Migraine headache: Oral sachet of lysine acetylsalicylate 1,620mg plus metoclopramide 10mg.

Osteoporosis prophylaxis: 400mg to 800mg daily. Take with calcium.

Pediatrics

Hyperargininemia: 250mg/kg/day. Take with ornithine 100mg/kg/day.

Magnesium

EFFECTS

Magnesium is an essential mineral said to have anti-osteoporotic, anti-arrhythmic, antihypertensive, glucose regulatory, and bronchodilating effects. It is an electrolyte, a nutrient, and a mineral. Magnesium is important as a cofactor in many enzymatic reactions in the body. There are at least 300 enzymes that are dependent upon magnesium for normal functioning. Its effects on lipoprotein lipase play an important role in reducing serum cholesterol. Magnesium is necessary for maintaining serum potassium and calcium levels due to its effect on the renal tubule. In the heart, magnesium acts as a calcium channel blocker. It also activates sodium-potassium ATPase in the cell membrane to promote resting.

Magnesium is available for oral, parenteral, and topical administration. The scope of this discussion will be limited to the oral and topical formulations.

COMMON USAGE

Accepted uses: Magnesium sulfate (Epsom salt) is approved as a laxative for the temporary relief of constipation. Magnesium sulfate is used for replacement therapy for hypomagnesemia.

Unproven uses: Magnesium is used in pregnant women to treat leg cramps and to control and prevent seizures in pre-eclampsia. Magnesium is used for migraine, bone resorption, diabetes, hypertension, arrhythmias, PMS, nephrolithiasis, and spasms. Magnesium may also be effective in treating certain cardiac arrhythmias, in asthma that is unresponsive to other treatments, during alcohol withdrawal, and for ischemic heart disease. Magnesium therapy has inconsistent effects on hypertension, but should be considered in those at risk of deficiency, including patients taking magnesium-depleting medications.

CONTRAINDICATIONS

Magnesium is not to be used in the presence of heart block, severe renal disease, or toxemia in pregnant women in the 2 hours preceding delivery.

WARNINGS/PRECAUTIONS

Administration of magnesium, especially in patients with renal impairment, may lead to loss of deep tendon reflexes, hypotension, confusion, respiratory paralysis, cardiac arrhythmias, or cardiac arrest. Increased bleeding time has been reported. Monitor to avoid magnesium toxicity.

Pregnancy and breastfeeding: Rickets in the newborn may result from prolonged magnesium sulfate administration in the second trimester of pregnancy. It is safe to use while breastfeeding.

DRUG INTERACTIONS

Aminoglycosides: Concomitant use with magnesium may precipitate neuromuscular weakness and possibly paralysis.

Calcium channel blockers: Concurrent use may enhance hypotensive effects.

Fluoroquinolones: Concomitant use with magnesium may decrease absorption and effectiveness. Fluoroquinolones should be administered at least 4 hours before magnesium or any product containing magnesium.

Labetalol: Concomitant use with magnesium may cause bradycardia and reduced cardiac output.

Levomethadyl: Concomitant use with magnesium may precipitate QT prolongation.

Neuromuscular blockers: Concomitant use with magnesium may enhance neuromuscular blocking effects.

Tetracycline: Magnesium decreases the absorption of tetracycline.

ADVERSE REACTIONS

Side effects include blurred vision, photophobia, diarrhea, hypermagnesemia, hypotension, increased bleeding times, neuromuscular blockade (in higher doses), and vasodilation.

ADMINISTRATION AND DOSAGE

Adults

Daily Dosage: Recommended Dietary Allowance (RDA):

Males—14 to 18 years: 410mg/day; *19 to 30 years:* 400mg/day; *31+ years:* 420mg/day.

Females—14 to 18 years: 360mg/day; *19 to 30 years:* 310mg/day; *31+ years:* 320mg/day.

During pregnancy—14 to 18 years: 400mg/day; *19 to 30 years:* 350mg/day; *31+ years:* 360mg/day.

During lactation: 14 to 18 years: 360mg/day; *19 to 30 years:* 310mg/day; *31+ years:* 320mg/day.

Abdominal and perineal incision wound healing: (magnesium hydroxide ointment, topical) Apply twice daily along with zinc chloride spray for 7 days.

Congestive heart failure: (enteric-coated magnesium chloride) 3,204mg/day in divided doses (equal to 15.8mmol elemental magnesium).

Detrusor instability: (magnesium hydroxide) 350mg for 4 weeks; double after 2 weeks if there is an unsatisfactory response.

Diabetes mellitus, type 2: 15.8mmol to 41.4mmol/day.

Dietary supplementation: 54mg to 483mg daily in divided doses.

Dyslipidemia: (enteric-coated magnesium chloride) Studies have used a mean dose of 17.92mmol for a mean duration of 118 days; (magnesium oxide) 15mmol/day for 3 months.

Hypertension: 360mg to 600mg/day.

Migraine prophylaxis: 360mg to 600mg/day.

Mitral valve prolapse: (magnesium carbonate capsules) During the first week of treatment, 21 mmol/day is used; then 14mmol/day is used during Weeks 2 to 5.

Nephrolithiasis prophylaxis: (magnesium hydroxide) 400mg to 500mg/day.

Osteoporosis: 250mg taken at bedtime on an empty stomach, increased to 250mg 3 times/day for 6 months, followed by 250mg daily for 18 months.

Premenstrual syndrome: 200mg to 360mg/day.

Pediatrics

Daily Dosage: Recommended Dietary Allowance (RDA):

Children—1 to 3 years: 80mg/day; *4 to 8 years:* 130mg/day; *9-13 years:* 240mg/day. There are insufficient data to establish an RDA for infants. The adequate intake (AI) for infants is 30mg/day for infants 0 to 6 months and 75mg/day for infants 7 to 12 months.

Deficiency: The oral dose of magnesium sulfate to treat hypomagnesemia in children is 100mg/day to 200mg/kg 4 times/day.

Dietary supplementation: 3mg/kg to 6mg/kg body weight per day in divided doses 3 to 4 times/day, up to a maximum of 400mg daily.

Laxative: The recommended dose of magnesium citrate for children 2 to 5 years of age is 2.7g to 6.25g daily as a single dose or as divided doses. For children 6 to 11 years of age, the dose is 5.5g to 12.5g daily in a single dose or as divided doses.

Melatonin

EFFECTS

Melatonin (N-acetyl-5-methoxytryptamine) is a neurohormone produced by pinealocytes in the pineal gland during the dark hours of the day-night cycle. Serum levels of melatonin are very low during most of the day, and it has been labeled the "hormone of darkness." The hormone serves as a messenger to the neuroendocrine system regarding environmental conditions (especially the photoperiod). Putative functions of endogenous melatonin in this regard include regulation of sleep cycles, hormonal rhythms, and body temperature. Melatonin is involved in the induction of sleep, may play a role in the internal synchronization of the mammalian circadian system, and may serve as a marker of the "biologic clock." In addition, melatonin is thought to have antioxidant and immunomodulator effects. Melatonin is administered by the oral, transdermal, transmucosal, and parenteral route. The scope of this discussion is limited to the oral formulation.

COMMON USAGE

Unproven uses: Melatonin is commonly used as a sleep aid. Evidence suggests that it is effective for the short-term treatment of delayed sleep phase syndrome. However, available data indicate that it is not effective for treating most primary or secondary sleep disorders. There is no evidence to support the claims that melatonin is effective for alleviating the sleep disturbance aspect of jet lag or shift-work disorder. Melatonin has been used in the treatment of a variety of solid tumors (in combination with interleukin-2), and to improve thrombocytopenia and other toxicities induced by cancer chemotherapy and from other conditions. In addition, melatonin is used for the treatment of cluster headaches and tinnitus; however, its efficacy is unknown.

CONTRAINDICATIONS

Hypersensitivity to melatonin or its excipients.

WARNINGS/PRECAUTIONS

Depressive symptoms: Melatonin can exacerbate dysphoria in depressed patients and cause mood swings. It can cause depressive symptoms when used with interleukin-2 in cancer therapy.

Liver disease: Increased risk of liver dysfunction.

History of neurological disorders: Increased risk of CNS effects.

Seizures: Increased risk of seizures.

DRUG INTERACTIONS

Fluvoxamine: Increased risk of CNS depression with concomitant use. Patients should be monitored for signs of CNS depression and appropriate dosage adjustments should be made.

Nifedipine: Melatonin may reduce the effectiveness of nifedipine. Close monitoring of blood pressure is advised.

Warfarin: Increased risk of bleeding with concomitant use. If both agents are taken together, monitor prothrombin time, INR, and signs and symptoms of excessive bleeding.

ADVERSE REACTIONS

Adverse effects of commercially available melatonin have generally been minimal. Drowsiness, fatigue, headache, confusion, gastrointestinal complaints, and reduced body temperature have been reported. Rarely, tachycardia, seizures, acute psychotic reactions, autoimmune hepatitis, and pruritus have been reported.

ADMINISTRATION AND DOSAGE

Adults

Cancer as combination therapy: 40mg or 50mg oral tablets given once daily at night, initiated 7 days prior to interleukin-2 and continued throughout the cycle.

Chronic insomnia: 1mg to 10mg/day orally.

Delayed sleep phase syndrome: 5mg/day orally.

Jet lag: 5mg/day orally for 3 days prior to departure, then 5mg for 4 additional days.

Sleep disorders: 5mg at bedtime.

Pediatrics

Congenital sleep disorder: 2.5mg oral tablet.

Neurological disability: 0.5mg to 10mg oral tablet at bedtime.

Sleep-wake cycle disorder: An average dose of 5.7mg, administered as a controlled-release tablet, was used in children ages 4 to 21 years who had neurodevelopmental disabilities. Doses ranged from 2mg to 12mg.

Omega-3 Fatty Acids

EFFECTS

Eicosapentaenoic acid (EPA) and docosahexaenoic acid (DHA) are nonessential omega-3 fatty acids that are synthesized in the body. The omega-3 fatty acids have anticoagulant and anti-inflammatory effects. They also lower cholesterol and triglyceride levels, and reduce blood pressure. Omega-3 fatty acids are abundant in oily fish such as salmon, tuna, and mackerel. For this reason, they are sometimes referred to as "omega-3 fish oils" or simply "fish oil." Linoleic acid is a plant-derived omega-3 fatty acid. The proven health benefits of the omega-3 fish oils have not been demonstrated in studies of linoleic acid. For the purposes of this discussion, the term "omega-3 fatty acids" refers to the omega-3 fish oils, EPA, and DHA.

COMMON USAGE

Accepted uses: The FDA has acknowledged the cardiovascular benefits of omega-3 fatty acids by granting a "qualified health claim" for foods and supplements containing fish oil. The claim states, "Supportive but not conclusive research shows that consumption of EPA and DHA omega-3 fatty acids may reduce the risk of coronary heart disease."

Unproven uses: A review of available data on omega-3 fatty acids concluded that they have mixed effects on people with inflammatory bowel disease, kidney disease, and osteoporosis and no effect on people with arthritis. Data are inconclusive regarding the effect of omega-3 fatty acids on adults and children who have asthma. In addition, omega-3 fatty acids have also been used in the following conditions: aggression, Alzheimer's disease, atopic dermatitis, cachexia, cancer, cyclosporine protectant, dementia, dermatitis, gestation prolongation, gingivitis, pediatric growth and development, hyper-

lipidemia, hypertension, inflammation, lupus erythematosus, osteoporosis, persistent antiphospholipid syndrome, platelet aggregation inhibition, psoriasis, respiratory illness, rheumatoid arthritis, and stroke.

CONTRAINDICATIONS

Hypersensitivity to EPA, DHA, or fish oils.

WARNINGS/PRECAUTIONS

Bleeding disorders: There may be an increased risk of bleeding with high doses.

Diabetics: Omega-3 fatty acids may increase blood glucose levels, decrease glucose tolerance, and decrease plasma insulin levels.

Pregnancy and breastfeeding: EPA and DHA are safe at normal doses during pregnancy and are safe for maternal use during lactation.

DRUG INTERACTIONS

Anticoagulants: Possible increased risk of bleeding with warfarin or aspirin.

ADVERSE REACTIONS

Side effects are usually minor and include abdominal pain, bloating, diarrhea, fatigue, gas, acid reflux and heartburn, increased burping, increased renal clearance, nausea, fishy aftertaste, oxidative damage in large doses, skin irritation, somnolence, thrombocytopenia, and vitamin toxicity. Vitamin E deficiency is possible with many months of omega-3 fatty acid supplementation.

ADMINISTRATION AND DOSAGE

The FDA recommends that daily consumption of fish oils be limited to 2g/day from dietary supplements and 3g/day from food sources.

Potassium

EFFECTS

Potassium is an electrolyte that plays a role in numerous cellular, neurologic, and metabolic processes. It maintains intracellular and extracellular fluid volume. It also blunts the hypertensive response to excess sodium intake. Potassium plays a role in cardiac, skeletal, and smooth muscle contraction; energy production; nerve impulse transmission; and nucleic acid synthesis. Potassium may have a protective effect against cardiovascular disease, hypertension, strokes, and possibly other degenerative diseases as well. Potassium is available for oral and intravenous administration. The intravenous use of potassium is beyond the scope of this discussion.

COMMON USAGE

Accepted uses: Potassium is FDA-approved for the prevention and treatment of hypokalemia, a life-threatening condition that can result from the use of drugs such as diuretics or from a lack of potassium in the diet.

Unproven uses: Arrhythmias, arthritis, bone turnover, hypercalciuria, fasting hyperinsulinemia, hypertension, malnutrition, myocardial infarction, nephrolithiasis, premenstrual syndrome, stroke, cardiac surgery.

CONTRAINDICATIONS

Potassium supplementation is contraindicated in patients who are experiencing acute dehydration or heat cramps. It should not be

used in patients who have adynamia episodica hereditaria. Patients who have hyperkalemia, severe renal impairment, or untreated Addison's disease should not receive potassium supplementation.

WARNINGS/PRECAUTIONS

Pregnancy and breastfeeding: Pregnant women and nursing mothers should avoid potassium supplements unless they are prescribed by their physicians.

Renal disease, diabetes: Patients with chronic renal insufficiency and diabetes are at increased risk of hyperkalemia.

DRUG INTERACTIONS

Angiotensin converting enzyme (ACE) inhibitors (eg, benazepril, captopril, enalapril, fosinopril, lisinopril, moexipril, perindopril, quinapril, ramipril, trandolapril): Increased risk of hyperkalemia.

Angiotensin receptor blockers: Increased risk of hyperkalemia.

Potassium-sparing diuretics (amiloride, triamterene, spironolactone): Increased risk of hyperkalemia.

Indomethacin: Potential for hyperkalemia, especially if the patient has underlying renal dysfunction.

HERBAL INTERACTIONS

Dandelion: Concurrent use may result in hyperkalemia due to the high potassium content of dandelion leaves and roots. Monitor serum potassium levels if the two agents are used together.

Gossypol: Gossypol may cause hypokalemia unresponsive to potassium supplementation. Monitoring of serum potassium levels is recommended if the two agents are used together.

Licorice: Hypokalemia and paralysis may result. Avoid concurrent use of licorice and potassium supplements.

ADVERSE REACTIONS

The most common adverse reactions of potassium supplements are gastrointestinal and include abdominal discomfort, diarrhea, flatulence, nausea, and vomiting. Rashes are occasionally reported. ECG changes may occur.

ADMINISTRATION AND DOSAGE

Potassium supplements are available as potassium aspartate, potassium bicarbonate, potassium chloride, potassium citrate, potassium gluconate, and potassium orotate. One milliequivalent (mEq) or millimole (mmol) of potassium is equal to 39.09 milligrams (mg).

Daily Dosage:

Because of the risks associated with hyperkalemia, potassium supplementation should be done under medical supervision. The recommended Adequate Intake (AI) of potassium from dietary sources is as follows:

Adults

Adults (19 years and older): 4.7g/day; during pregnancy: 4.7g/day; during lactation: 5.1g/day.

Deficiency: Doses are individualized and typically begin with 40mEq to 100mEq/day, with serum level monitoring.

Pediatrics

Children 0 to 6 months: 0.4g/day; *7 to 12 months:* 0.7g/day; *1 to 3 years:* 3.0g/day; *4 to 8 years:* 3.8g/day; *9 to 13 years:* 4.5g/day.

Deficiency: Doses are individualized and begin with 3mEq to 5mEq/kg/day, in divided doses, with serum level monitoring.

Probiotics

EFFECTS

Lactobacillus products are often called probiotics, translated as "for life," a popular term used to refer to bacteria in the intestine considered beneficial to health. At least 400 different species of microflora colonize the human gastrointestinal tract. The most important commercially available lactobacillus species are *L acidophilus* and *L casei* GG. Other lactobaccilli inhabiting the human gastrointestinal (GI) tract include *L brevis*, *L cellobiosus*, *L fermentum*, *L leichmannii*, *L plantarum*, and *L salivaroes*. As the intestinal flora is intimately involved in the host's nutritional status and affects immune system function, cholesterol metabolism, carcinogenesis, toxin load, and aging, lactobacillus supplementation is often used to promote overall good health.

Possible mechanisms for the effective action of lactobacilli in the treatment of various GI tract pathologies include replacement of pathogenic organisms in the GI tract by lactobacilli, elicitation of an immune response, lowering of fecal pH, and interfering with the ability of pathogenic bacteria to adhere to intestinal mucosal cells.

Commercially available lactobacillus products are designed to be taken orally with the intent to colonize the intestine and establish a balanced ecosystem. It has been proposed that lactobacilli must possess properties including adhesion, competitive exclusion, and inhibitor production to colonize a mucosal surface.

COMMON USAGE

Unproven uses: Lactobacilli are used primarily for diarrhea. Other uses include treatment of irritable bowel syndrome, urinary tract infection, vaginal candidiasis, and bacterial vaginosis.

CONTRAINDICATIONS

Lactobacillus is contraindicated in patients who have a hypersensitivity to lactose or milk.

WARNINGS/PRECAUTIONS

Infants and small children: Over-the-counter commercial preparations are not to be used in children under the age of 3 unless directed by a physician.

Liver disease: Stupor with EEG-slowing has been reported with high oral doses in patients with hepatic encephalopathy.

DRUG INTERACTIONS

Data are not available.

ADVERSE REACTIONS

Burping, diarrhea, flatulence, hiccups, increased phlegm production, rash, and vomiting have been reported infrequently with oral administration. Disagreeable sensation and burning is possible with vaginal formulations.

ADMINISTRATION AND DOSAGE

Adults

Radiation-induced diarrhea: Lactobacillus rhamnosus (Antibiophilus®) 1.5 x 109 colony-forming units 3 times/day for up to 1 week.

Uncomplicated diarrhea: 1 to 2 billion viable cells of *L acidophilus* or other *Lactobacillus* species daily.

Pediatrics

Diarrhea in undernourished children: Lactobacillus rhamnosus: GG 37 billion organisms daily 6 days/week up to 15 months.

Infantile diarrhea: Lactobacillus reuteri: 1010 CFU daily for up to 5 days or *Lactobacillus* strain GG 5 x 109 CFU daily for up to 5 days, under doctor's supervision.

Quercetin

EFFECTS

Quercetin is a bioflavonoid abundant in fruits and vegetables. It may have antioxidant, antineoplastic, anti-inflammatory, and antiviral activity. As an anticancer agent, quercetin interrupts cell cycles, ATPase activity, signal transduction, and phosphorylation. Some activity had been found against viral reverse transcriptases. Quercetin has been shown to inhibit platelet aggregation and thrombus formation. It has also been shown to stabilize the membranes of mast cells and basophils, thereby inhibiting histamine release. It has also demonstrated activity as a leukotriene inhibitor. Quercetin is available for oral and intravenous administration. The scope of this discussion will be limited to the oral formulations.

COMMON USAGE

Unproven uses: Quercetin may protect against the development of cardiovascular disease and alleviate the symptoms of prostatitis. It is used for the treatment of acute and chronic asthma symptoms, inflammation, and cancer.

CONTRAINDICATIONS

Hypersensitivity to quercetin.

WARNINGS/PRECAUTIONS

Nephrotoxicity has been a dose-limiting side effect of quercetin administration in humans.

DRUG INTERACTIONS

Cyclosporine: Concomitant use may reduce cyclosporine effectiveness; monitor cyclosporine levels.

Digoxin: Concomitant use may increase the risk of digoxin toxicity.

Fluoroquinolones: Concomitant use may reduce the effectiveness of this antibiotic class.

ADVERSE REACTIONS

Oral quercetin is well tolerated. Pain, flushing, dyspnea, and emesis have been reported after intravenous injection.

ADMINISTRATION AND DOSAGE

Daily dosage: 400mg to 500mg orally 3 times/day is recommended by practitioners of natural medicine. If the water-soluble quercetin chalcone is used, the dose is reduced to about 250mg 3 times/day.

Adults

Acute allergic symptoms: 2g every 2 hours for a maximum of 2 days.

Chronic allergies: 2g daily.

Prostatitis: 500mg twice daily.

SAMe

EFFECTS

S-Adenosylmethionine (SAMe) is a naturally occurring substance present in virtually all body tissues and fluids. SAMe is produced in the body from the amino acid methionine and adenosine triphosphate. It serves as a source of methyl groups in numerous biochemical reactions involving the synthesis, activation, and metabolism of hormones, proteins, catecholamines, nucleic acids, and phospholipids. Release of methyl groups also promotes the formation of glutathione, the chief cellular antioxidant, thereby favoring detoxification processes. SAMe is closely linked with the metabolism of folate and vitamin B_{12}, which accounts for its ability to lower excessive homocysteine serum concentrations resulting from a deficiency of one or both of these nutrients. SAMe is postulated to increase the turnover of the neurotransmitters dopamine and serotonin in the central nervous system. It has been shown to increase the levels of the serotonin metabolite 5-hydroxyindoleacetic acid in the cerebrospinal fluid.

SAMe has antidepressant action. SAMe promotes bile flow and may relieve cholestasis. It is claimed that SAMe may increase the detoxification and elimination of pharmaceuticals from the body. There is also evidence that SAMe may lessen the severity of chronic liver disease and, in animal studies, prevent liver cancer.

COMMON USAGE

Unproven uses: The clinical application of SAMe centers on the treatment of depression, pain disorders such as osteoarthritis, and liver conditions such as cholestasis.

CONTRAINDICATIONS

Hypersensitivity to SAMe.

WARNINGS/PRECAUTIONS

Bipolar disorder: Strict medical supervision is warranted when SAMe is used in individuals with bipolar disorder.

Pregnancy and breastfeeding: Data are not available.

DRUG INTERACTIONS

Tricyclic antidepressants (eg, amitriptyline, amoxapine, clomipramine, desipramine, doxepin, imipramine, nortriptyline): Concurrent use of SAMe and tricyclic antidepressants may result in an increased risk of serotonin syndrome. If SAMe and a tricyclic antidepressant are used together, use low doses of each and titrate upward slowly, while monitoring closely for early signs of serotonin syndrome such as increasing anxiety, confusion, and disorientation.

ADVERSE REACTIONS

Reported side effects are rare and include anxiety, headache, urinary frequency, pruritus, nausea, and diarrhea.

ADMINISTRATION AND DOSAGE

Tablets containing 768mg of sulfo-adenosyl-L-methionine (SAMe) sulfate-p-toluene sulfonate are equivalent to 400mg of SAMe.

Adults

Arthritis: 600mg to 800mg/day. Dosage may be reduced to 400mg, depending on response.

Depression: 200mg to 1600mg/day orally in the form of enteric-coated tablets; dosage often is graduated in increments of 200mg.

Fibromyalgia: 600mg or 800mg/day. Dosage may be reduced to 400mg daily depending on response.

Liver toxicity, estrogen-related: In one study, women treated for estrogen-related liver toxicity received 800mg of SAMe daily by the oral route. In general, the minimum recommended daily dose by mouth is 1600mg but no dose-finding studies have been done in patients with liver disease. Patients with less well-compensated disease may require larger doses.

Mood disorders, mild: Standard dosing regimens are not available. However, an open-label study (n=192) demonstrated improved mild mood disorders in subjects treated with ademetionine (SAMe) 100mg orally 2 times/day for 2 months.

Selenium

EFFECTS

Selenium is a trace mineral with antioxidant properties. Selenium is a component of the cytosolic enzyme Se-dependent glutathione peroxidase (SeGSHpx), which reduces hydrogen peroxide and thereby prevents initiation of lipid peroxidation. In platelets, SeGSHpx is required for the conversion of HPETE (L-12-hydroperoxy-5,8,14-eicosatetraenoic acid) to prostacyclin. Low SeGSHpx results in an imbalance of prostacyclin and thromboxanes, which, in cell and tissue cultures, leads to platelet aggregation and vasoconstriction. Selenium supplementation in humans has led to increased bleeding times.

COMMON USAGE

Accepted uses: Trace mineral.

Unproven uses: Selenium is often used in combination with other antioxidants as a tool in the prevention of degenerative diseases, such as cancer (although there is evidence for and against) and cardiovascular disease. No coronary disease risk intervention studies with selenium have been done, though certain cardiomyopathies appear to be related to selenium deficiency and preliminary evidence exists of post-myocardial infarction protection.

Antioxidant therapy is also considered in other chronic inflammatory or degenerative diseases, such as arthritis. Only rheumatoid arthritis has been studied, with mixed results, suggesting only milder, early disease responds to selenium supplementation. Studies concluded beneficial effects of selenium supplementation in intrinsic asthma, bronchopneumonia prevention in burn patients, erysipelas prevention in mastectomy patients, male infertility, and possibly myocardial infarction. Uncontrolled reports of success using selenium to prevent Kaschin-Beck osteoarthropathy and viral hepatitis in Chinese populations have been documented.

CONTRAINDICATIONS

Selenium hypersensitivity.

WARNINGS/PRECAUTIONS

Pregnancy and breastfeeding: Selenium is safe to use during pregnancy and lactation.

Skin cancer: There is evidence that those at high risk of non-melanoma skin cancers should avoid selenium supplements given the apparent increased risk for the development of squamous cell and other carcinomas.

Toxicity: High blood levels of selenium can lead to selenosis. Symptoms include fatigue, garlic breath odor, gastrointestinal upset, hair loss, irritability, mild nerve damage, and white, blotchy nails.

DRUG INTERACTIONS

Selenium absorption may be reduced when taken with drugs that alter stomach pH.

ADVERSE REACTIONS

Excessive selenium exposure may cause abdominal pain and cramps, diarrhea, fatigue, garlicky breath, irritability, nail and hair changes, nausea, and vomiting

ADMINISTRATION AND DOSAGE

Many forms of selenium are available and include: selenium selenite, selenomethionine, and selenium-enriched yeast. Organically bound forms may have a slight advantage.

Adults

Daily dosage: Recommended Dietary Allowance (RDA):

Females 19 years and older: 55mcg daily; *during pregnancy:* 60mcg daily; *during lactation:* 70mcg daily.

Male adults: 70 mcg daily.

Asthma: 100mcg daily.

Cancer prevention: 200mcg daily.

Erysipelas infection: 300mg to 1,000mg daily as selenium selenite.

HIV: 80mcg daily.

Male infertility: 100mcg daily.

Myocardial infarction: 100mcg daily.

Rheumatoid arthritis: 200mcg daily.

Pediatrics

Daily dosage: Adequate Intake (AI): Infants: *0 to 6 months:* 15mcg daily; *7 to 12 months:* 20mcg daily; *1 to 3 years:* 20mcg daily; *4 to 8 years:* 30mcg daily; *9 to 13 years:* 40mcg daily; *14 to 18 years:* 55mcg daily.

Vitamin A

EFFECTS

Vitamin A is a fat-soluble vitamin required for growth and bone development, vision, reproduction, and for differentiation and maintenance of epithelial tissue. The biologically active forms of vitamin A are retinol, retinal, and retinoic acid. Retinyl esters, or fatty acid esters of retinol, are the storage form of vitamin A in the body. Beta-carotene is a precursor to vitamin A. Retinol is required as a cofactor in the glycosylation of glycoproteins.

Vitamin A may enhance the function of the immune system, and some evidence indicates that it affords protection against cancer. Vitamin A may also affect membrane systems such as the mitochondria and lysosomes; however, further research is necessary to confirm this finding. Retinol is the parent compound of vitamin A, and the form that is transported within the body. Retinol is released from the liver and is bound to a serum retinol binding protein (RBP), which facilitates absorption, transport and mediation of the biological activity. Retinal is the active form required for formation of the visual pigment rhodopsin in the rods and cones of the retina.

Retinoic acid may be the active form for processes involving growth and differentiation. Although the exact mechanism of action is unknown, retinoic acid may act directly at the level of genetic transcription via a nuclear receptor to promote the synthesis of some proteins and inhibit the synthesis of others.

Vitamin A is involved in vision after conversion in the body to 11-cis-retinal. The latter interacts with opsin, a protein, to form rhodopsin, which is the light-sensitive pigment in the rods and cones of the retina. The exact mechanism of action of retinoids is not understood at the molecular level, except for their role in vision.

COMMON USAGE

Accepted uses: Treatment of vitamin A deficiency.

Unproven uses: Topical ophthalmic solutions of vitamin A have been successful in treating dry-eye syndromes. Large doses of vitamin A have shown some success in the treatment of acne with retinol therapy and in Kyrle's disease. Vitamin A in combination with vitamin E is beneficial in the treatment of abetalipoproteinemia and in Darier's disease cutaneous lesions. Studies evaluating the benefit of vitamin A therapy in conditions of cancer, Crohn's disease, cystic fibrosis, and growth promotion produced controversial results. Other studies concluded that vitamin A had no overall effect in the treatment of coronary heart disease, HIV prophylaxis, and respiratory syncytial viral infections.

CONTRAINDICATIONS

Doses above 2,500 IU are contraindicated in pregnancy; doses above 5,000 IU are contraindicated in breastfeeding. Do not use in persons who have exhibited hypersensitivity to vitamin A. Do not administer to persons with hypervitaminosis A.

WARNINGS/PRECAUTIONS

Although toxicity from vitamin A is rare, it is a fat-soluble substance and can accumulate in the body if taken in excessive doses over short or long periods of time, causing damage rather than promoting health. Oral preparations should not be used for treating vitamin A deficiency in persons with malabsorption syndromes.

Hepatotoxicity: Chronic consumption may cause liver damage.

Pregnancy and breastfeeding: Doses exceeding 2,500 IU are contraindicated during pregnancy. Retinoids, chemically synthesized analogs of vitamin A, are known to cause severe birth defects in humans. Vitamin A is excreted in human breast milk; doses above 5,000 IU are contraindicated in breastfeeding. The dangers to the nursing infant are unknown.

Toxicity: High doses can cause: blurred vision, depression, dizziness, drowsiness, headache, insomnia, irritability, lack of muscle coordination, nausea, osteoporosis, osteosclerosis, seizures, somnolence, and vomiting.

DRUG INTERACTIONS

Anticoagulants: Increased risk of bleeding.

Cholestyramine: Decreased absorption of vitamin A; separate administration times.

Colestipol: Decreased absorption of vitamin A; separate administration times.

Minocycline: Increased risk of pseudotumor cerebri.

Retinoids (eg, acitretin, bexarotene, etretinate, isotretinoin, tretinoin:): Increased risk of vitamin A toxicity.

FOOD INTERACTIONS

Carob: Caution is advised for patients who ingest large amounts of carob foods and take vitamin A supplements, due to increased bioavailability of vitamin A.

ADVERSE REACTIONS

Dermatitis and photosensitivity reactions may occur.

ADMINISTRATION AND DOSAGE

The RDAs for vitamin A are listed as Retinol Activity Equivalents (RAE) to account for the different activities of retinol and provitamin A carotenoids. 1 RAE in mcg =3.3 IU.

Adults

Daily Dosage: Recommended Dietary Allowance (RDA):

Males ≥14 years: 900mcg or 3,000IU/day.

Females ≥14 years: 700mcg or 2,310IU/day.

Pregnancy—14 to 18 years: 750mcg or 2,500 IU; *≥19 years:* 770mcg or 2,500IU/day.

Lactation: 14 to 18 years: 1,200mcg or 4,000 IU; *≥19 years:* 1,300mcg or 4,300 IU/day.

Deficiency: 100,000IU/day for 3 days, followed by 50,000IU/day for 2 weeks. Maintenance doses of 10,000 to 20,000IU/day for 2 months are recommended.

Topical use: Apply daily as needed.

Xerophthalmia: 200,000IU orally on diagnosis; repeat the following day and again at least 2 weeks later.

Pediatrics

Daily Dosage: Recommended Dietary Allowance (RDA):

Children—1 to 3 years: 300mcg or 1,000IU/day; *4 to 8 years:* 400mcg or 1,320IU/day; *9 to 13 years:* 600mcg or 2,000IU/day.

Infants—0 to 6 months (Adequate Intake [AI]): 400mcg or 1,320IU/day; *7 to 12 months:* 500mcg or 1,650IU/day.

Xerophthalmia: 110mg oral vitamin A palmitate or 55mg IM vitamin A acetate; repeat the following day and again 1 to 2 weeks later.

Vitamin C

EFFECTS

Vitamin C, also known as ascorbic acid, has antiatherogenic, anticarcinogenic, antihypertensive, antiviral, antihistamine, immunomodulatory, ophthalmoprotective, airway-protective, and heavy-metal detoxifying properties. Antioxidant effects have been demonstrated as increased resistance of red blood cells to free radical attack in elderly persons and reduced activated oxygen species in patients receiving chemotherapy and radiation. Antioxidant mechanisms have been shown in the reduction of LDL oxidation as well, though studies on the prevention of heart disease and stroke are conflicting.

COMMON USAGE

Accepted uses: FDA-approved prophylaxis of vitamin C deficiency and to increase iron absorption.

Unproven uses: Vitamin C has been used in the prevention of heart disease, pneumonia, sunburn, hyperlipidemia, cancer, muscle soreness, asthma, common cold, erythema (after CO_2 laser skin resurfacing), and for fluorosis, wound healing after severe trauma, and as an antioxidant.

CONTRAINDICATIONS

Hypersensitivity to vitamin C. High doses are contraindicated in the presence of gout, cirrhosis, and renal tubular acidosis, and other conditions exacerbated by acid loading.

WARNINGS/PRECAUTIONS

Cancer treatment: Supplemental vitamin C may reduce the effectiveness of cancer chemotherapy and its effectiveness in reducing risk from cancer and related death is unclear.

Laboratory tests: Vitamin C interferes with the results of the following laboratory tests: acetaminophen, AST (SGOT), bilirubin, carbamazepine, creatinine, glucose, LDH, stool guaiac, theophylline, and uric acid.

Medical conditions: Use cautiously in patients with preexisting kidney stone disease, erythrocyte G6PD deficiency, hemochromatosis, thalassemia, or sideroblastic anemia.

Pregnancy and breastfeeding: Vitamin C is safe at the Recommended Dietary Allowance doses.

DRUG INTERACTIONS

Antacids: Increased risk of aluminum toxicity with concomitant use. Concurrent administration is not recommended, especially in patients with renal insufficiency. If concurrent use cannot be avoided, monitor patients for possible acute aluminum toxicity (eg, encephalopathy, seizures, or coma) and adjust the doses accordingly.

Aspirin: Increased ascorbic requirements with concomitant use. Increased dietary or supplemental vitamin C intake (100mg to 200mg daily) should be considered for patients on chronic high-dose aspirin.

Cyanocobalamin: Reduced absorption and bioavailability of cyanocobalamin with concomitant use. Vitamin C should be administered 2 or more hours after a meal.

ADVERSE REACTIONS

Adverse effects of oral vitamin C include diarrhea, esophagitis (rare), and intestinal obstruction (rare).

ADMINISTRATION AND DOSAGE

Adults

Daily Dosage: Recommended Dietary Allowance (RDA):

Males—14 to 18 years: 75mg/day; *≥19 years:* 90mg/day.

Females—14 to 18 years: 65mg/day; *≥19 years:* 75mg/day.

During pregnancy—<18 years: 80mg/day; *19 to 50 years:* 85mg/day.

Lactation—18 years: 115mg/day; *19 to 50 years:* 120mg/day.

Individuals who smoke require an additional 35mg/day of vitamin C over the established RDA.

Antioxidant effects: 120mg to 450mg/day.

Asthma: 500mg to 2,000mg/day or prior to exercise.

Atherosclerosis prevention: 45mg to 1,000mg/day.

Delayed-onset muscle soreness: 3,000mg/day.

Gastric cancer: 50mg/day.

Histamine detoxification: 2,000mg/day.

Hypercholesterolemia: 300mg to 3,000mg/day.

Respiratory infection: 1,000mg to 2,000mg/day.

Scurvy: The recommended dose for the treatment of scurvy is 1g to 2g administered for the first 2 days, then 500mg/day for a week. Alternately, the AMA recommends 100mg 3 times/day for 1 week then 100mg/day for several weeks until tissue saturation is normal.

Skin erythema: Apply a topical 10% aqueous solution once daily.

Sunburn prevention: 2,000mg/day.

Urine acidification: 3g to 12g/day titrated to desired effect and given as divided doses every 4 hours.

Wound healing: 1,000mg to 1,500mg/day.

Pediatrics

Daily Dosage: Recommended Dietary Allowance (RDA):

Infants and children— 0 to 6 months: 40mg/day; *7 to 12 months:* 50mg/day; *1 to 3 years:* 15mg/day; *4 to 8 years:* 25mg/day; *9 to 13 years:* 45mg/day.

Daily Dosage: The recommended prophylactic dose for infants on formula feedings is 35mg/day orally or intramuscularly for the first few weeks of life. If the formula contains 2 to 3 times the amount of protein in human milk, the dose should be 50mg/day. Infants and children require 30 to 60mg of crystalline ascorbic acid daily. This may be taken as oral tablets or as part of the normal diet (ie, 2 to 4 oz. of orange juice).

Fluorosis: 500mg/day.

Scurvy: 100mg 3 times/day for 1 week, then 100mg daily for several weeks until tissue saturation is normal.

Vitamin D

EFFECTS

Vitamin D is both a vitamin and a steroid hormone. The vitamin can be consumed from dietary sources and the hormone synthesized in the skin with exposure to sunlight. The active metabolite operates via both nuclear receptors and nongenomic systems. However, vitamin D must first undergo a two-step metabolic process en route to the biologically active form of the drug. The first metabolic step occurs in the microsomal fraction of the liver in which vitamin D is hydroxylated at the C25 position. The compound 25-hydroxyvitamin D is the major circulating and storage form of vitamin D. Its level reflects sunlight exposure and dietary intake, and it is generally used as a clinical indicator of vitamin D stores. Next, 25-hydroxyvitamin D is bound to the same carrier protein as the parent compound and carried in the bloodstream to the kidney where it is hydroxylated at the "1" position to produce 1,25-dihydroxyvitamin D_3 (1,25D or calcitriol), the biologically active product. This final step in the production of vitamin D is dependent on the complex interaction of calcium, phosphorus, and parathyroid hormone.

Vitamin D is critical to normal bone mineralization; insufficient mineralization produces rickets in children and osteomalacia in children and adults. In addition to its effects on bone, in vitro vitamin D enhances cell differentiation and inhibits cell proliferation, actions that oppose those of cancer. Vitamin D is available for oral, topical and parenteral administration. The scope of this discussion will be limited to the oral and topical formulations.

COMMON USAGE

Accepted uses: Vitamin D is FDA-approved for the prevention and treatment of vitamin D deficiency, and for the treatment of familial hypophosphatemia, hypoparathyroidism, malabsorption syndromes, and vitamin D-resistant rickets.

Unproven uses: Vitamin D supplementation is used to prevent and treat rickets in children and osteomalacia in adults. Vitamin D prevents and treats osteopenia and osteoporosis. Patients with secondary hyperparathyroidism who are vitamin D deficient may benefit from vitamin D supplementation. Sick sinus syndrome and chronic atrial fibrillation respond successfully to vitamin D

supplementation. Supplementation with vitamin D appears to decrease symptoms associated with asthma, perhaps because of its influence on calcium metabolism. It also improves expiratory volume and decreases airway resistance.

Ingestion and topical application of vitamin D, alone or in combination with ultraviolet light, is used to treat plaque psoriasis. Localized and systemic scleroderma can be treated with oral or topical vitamin D. Supplementation with vitamin D is helpful in Crohn's disease-related osteomalacia. Supplementation with vitamin D and calcium may improve hearing. Vitamin D alleviates migraine headaches and headaches associated with menses.

CONTRAINDICATIONS

Do not use in patient with hypercalcemia or in individuals who have exhibited hypersensitivity to vitamin D. Contraindicated in patients who have systemic lupus erythematosus.

WARNINGS/PRECAUTIONS

Pregnancy and breastfeeding: Vitamin D is safe at recommended doses during pregnancy and lactation.

DRUG INTERACTIONS

Orlistat: Treatment with Orlistat has been shown to reduce serum levels of vitamin D (cholecalciferol).

ADVERSE REACTIONS

Potential adverse reactions include constipation, cardiac arrhythmia, nausea, nocturia, polydipsia, polyuria, kidney stones, and vomiting.

ADMINISTRATION AND DOSAGE

Note that 1mcg calciferol is equivalent to 40IU vitamin D. "Ergocalciferol" is vitamin D_2; "cholecalciferol" is vitamin D_3.

These values are based on the absence of adequate exposure to sunlight.

Adults

Daily Dosage: Recommended Dietary Allowance (RDA):

Adults—19 to 50 years: 5mcg/day; *50 to 70 years*: 10mcg/day; *>70 years:* 15mcg/day.

During pregnancy: 5mcg/day.

During lactation: 5mcg/day.

Epilepsy: Initial dose of Vitamin D_2 4,000IU/day for 105 days, followed by 150 days of 1,000IU/day.

Familial hypophosphatemia: Vitamin D_2 50,000IU to 75,000IU/day and phosphorus 2g/day.

Hepatic osteodystrophy: Vitamin D_2 100,000IU monthly.

Hyperparathyroidism: 50,000IU vitamin D_2/day, increased to 200,000IU/day.

Hypoparathyroidism: 2.5mg to 6.25mg vitamin D_2/day.

Osteomalacia: 36,000IU vitamin D_2/day in addition to calcium supplementation.

Osteoporosis prophylaxis: Vitamin D 400IU to 800IU/day.

Pregnancy supplementation: Vitamin D_2 given in 2 large doses of 600,000IU during the 7th and 8th months of pregnancy.

Pseudohypoparathyroidism: 2.5mg to 6.25mg vitamin D_2/day.

Psoriasis: 1mcg vitamin D_3 daily for 6 months; topical formulation consisting of 0.5mcg vitamin D_3 per gram base: Apply daily for 8 weeks.

Renal osteodystrophy: 15,000 to 20,000IU vitamin D_2/day.

Systemic scleroderma: 1.75mcg vitamin D_3 for 6 months to 3 years.

Vitamin D-resistant rickets: 50,000IU to 300,000IU vitamin D_2/day.

Pediatrics

Daily Dosage: Recommended Dietary Allowance (RDA):

Children 1 to 18 years: 5mcg/day.

Infants 0 to 12 months: 5mcg/day.

Anticonvulsant osteomalacia: 15,000IU in daily doses to 600,000IU in a single dose of vitamin D_2.

Hypoparathyroidism: 200mcg/kg of body weight (8,000IU/kg) vitamin D_2/day for 1 to 2 weeks.

Pseudohypoparathyroidism: 200mcg/kg of body weight (8,000IU/kg) vitamin D_2/day for 1 to 2 weeks.

Renal osteodystrophy: Ergocalciferol 25mcg/kg to 100mcg/kg/day.

Vitamin E

EFFECTS

Vitamin E is a powerful antioxidant that plays a role in immune function, DNA repair, and cell-membrane stabilization. Research suggests it may also have the following effects: antiplatelet, antiatherogenic, antithrombotic, anti-inflammatory, and anticarcinogenic. Vitamin E appears to have neuroprotective actions as well. Keep in mind that vitamin E is divided chemically into two groups: tocopherols and tocotrienols. The most biologically active—and the most studied—form is alpha-tocopherol. However, limited research indicates possible benefits of the other forms of vitamin E as well.

COMMON USAGE

Accepted uses: Prevention and treatment of vitamin E deficiency due to intestinal malabsorption caused by premature birth or disorders such as Crohn's disease, cystic fibrosis, and rare genetic disorders (eg, abetalipoproteinemia).

Unproven uses: Some evidence suggests supplemental vitamin E may be helpful as adjunctive treatment for type 1 diabetes, anemia in hemodialysis patients, intermittent claudication, some types of male infertility, tardive dyskinesia, osteoarthritis, rheumatoid arthritis, premenstrual syndrome, and enhanced immune function in the elderly. It may also be helpful for decreasing platelet adhesion and improving the effectiveness of antiplatelet therapy with aspirin.

Studies have reported conflicting results when vitamin E was used for preventing or treating Alzheimer's disease, heart disease, stroke, certain cancers (eg, breast, colon, prostate, and bladder), seizures, cataracts, fibrocystic breast problems, and exercise-induced tissue damage. A few small preliminary studies suggest vitamin E may be useful for sunburn protection and nitrate tolerance, but more research is needed. Currently, clinical trials have demonstrated no benefit when vitamin E was used for Huntington's chorea, ischemia reperfusion in heart surgery, lung cancer, muscular dystrophy, myotonic dystrophy, Parkinson's disease, or decreasing the rate of chronic hemolysis.

CONTRAINDICATIONS

Because of potential blood-thinning effects, supplemental vitamin E is contraindicated in patients with coagulation disorders

and during anticoagulation therapy. Topical use of vitamin E is contraindicated after a recent chemical peel or dermabrasion.

WARNINGS/PRECAUTIONS

Vitamin E is a fat-soluble substance and can accumulate in the body if taken in excessive doses over short or long periods of time, causing damage rather than promoting health.

Blood-clotting disorders: Supplementation is not advised. Monitor bleeding time in patients who decide to use vitamin E.

High doses: Research suggests a slight dose-response increase in all-cause mortality as vitamin E dosages exceed 400IU/day, although conflicting evidence indicates that dosages are unsafe only when they exceed 1,600IU. Another study reported a higher risk of hospitalization and heart failure in older patients (≥55 years) with vascular disease or diabetes who took 400IU/day, and another study indicated increased risk for gastrointestinal cancer.

Pregnancy and breastfeeding: Vitamin E is safe at RDA levels but avoid higher doses.

Thrombophlebitis: This problem has been reported in patients at risk of small-vessel disease who were taking ≥400IU/day.

DRUG INTERACTIONS

Anticoagulants: Avoid concomitant use. Vitamin E could potentiate their effects.

Colestipol: Concomitant use may reduce vitamin E absorption. Allow as much time as possible between doses.

Orlistat: Concomitant use may reduce vitamin E absorption. Allow at least 2 hours between doses.

ADVERSE REACTIONS

No side effects have been reported at recommended doses. Occasionally, doses greater than 400IU/day have been associated with diarrhea, nausea, headache, blurred vision, dizziness, and fatigue. Doses greater than 800IU/day may increase the risk of bleeding, especially in patients deficient in vitamin K.

ADMINISTRATION AND DOSAGE

Because vitamin E is fat soluble, supplements should be taken with a meal that contains fat to enhance absorption.

Daily Dosage: 1mg of alpha-tocopherol is approximately equal to 1.5 International Units (IU).

Adults

Daily Dosage: Recommended Dietary Allowance (RDA):

Adults and adolescents ≥14 years: 15mg (22.5IU)/day.

During pregnancy: 15mg (22.5IU)/day.

During lactation: 19mg (28.5IU)/day.

Deficiency: 32-50mg/day. The usual oral dose for vitamin E deficiency is 4 to 5 times the RDA. Doses as high as 300mg may be necessary.

Alzheimer's disease: 2,000IU/day.

Anemia in hemodialysis patients: 500mg/day.

Angina pectoris: 50-300IU/day.

Antioxidant effects: 100-800mg/day.

Antiplatelet effects: 200-400IU/day.

Cerebrovascular disease: 400IU/day with aspirin 325mg/day.

Colorectal cancer prevention: 50mg/day.

Coronary heart disease prevention: 100-800IU/day.

Cystic fibrosis: 50mg/day for correction of anemia.

Diabetes: 100-900IU/day for improving glucose tolerance and reducing protein glycation in insulin-dependent (and some non-insulin-dependent) patients.

Enhanced exercise performance at high altitude: 400mg/day.

Epilepsy: 400IU/day.

Exercise-induced tissue damage (prevention): 500-1,200IU/day.

Immune system support in geriatric patients: 200mg/day.

Intermittent claudication: 600-1,600mg/day.

Infertility (male): 200-300mg/day.

Nitrate tolerance: 600mg/day.

Oral leukoplakia and oropharyngeal cancer prevention: 800IU/day.

Osteoarthritis: 400-1,200IU/day.

Premenstrual symptoms: 150-600IU/day.

Prostate cancer prevention: 50mg/day.

Rheumatoid arthritis: 800-1,200IU/day.

Sunburn protection: 1,000IU of vitamin E combined with 2000mg of vitamin C daily.

Tardive dyskinesia: 1,200-1,600IU/day.

Pediatrics

Daily Dosage: Recommended Dietary Allowance (RDA):

Infants and children—0 to 6 months: 4mg (6IU)/day; *7 to 12 months:* 5mg (7.5IU)/day; *1 to 3 years:* 6mg (9IU)/day; *4 to 8 years:* 7mg (10.5IU)/day; *9 to 13 years:* 11mg (16.5IU)/day.

Malabsorption syndrome: 1 unit/kg/day of water-miscible vitamin E is given to raise plasma tocopherol to within the normal range within 2 months and for maintenance of normal plasma concentrations (1 unit=1mg alpha-tocopherol acetate).

Premature or low-birth-weight neonates: 25-50 units/day results in normal plasma tocopherol levels in 1 week (1 unit=1mg alpha-tocopherol acetate).

Zinc

EFFECTS

Zinc is an essential trace element thought to have antimicrobial, anti-sickling, cell-protective, copper-absorbing, enzyme-regulating, and growth-stimulating effects.

COMMON USAGE

Accepted uses: Zinc is approved by the FDA for the treatment of zinc deficiency.

Unproven uses: Zinc supplements are used for numerous conditions, including the following: acne vulgaris, acrodermatitis enteropathica, Alzheimer's disease, common cold, dental hygiene, diabetes mellitus, diarrhea, eczema, eye irritation, growth, Hansen's disease (leprosy), herpes simplex infection, hypertension, hypogeusia (decreased sense of taste), immunodeficiency, impotence, infertility, leg ulcers, lipid peroxidation, macular degeneration, necrolytic migratory erythema, parasites, peptic ulcer disease, psoriasis, scalp dermatoses, schistosomiasis, sepsis, sickle cell anemia, stomatitis, thalassemia major, trichomoniasis, Wilson's disease, and wound healing.

CONTRAINDICATIONS

Do not use in patients who have exhibited hypersensitivity reactions to zinc-containing products.

WARNINGS/PRECAUTIONS

Kidney disease: Use caution.

Nasal use: In 2009, the FDA issued a warning to stop using zinc nasal gels or sprays due to the risk of loss of smell.

Ophthalmic use: Zinc ophthalmic solution should be used cautiously in patients with glaucoma. Do not use zinc ophthalmic solutions that have changed color.

Pregnancy and breastfeeding: Zinc is safe at RDA doses. Zinc should not be used in doses greater than the RDA during lactation.

DRUG INTERACTIONS

Cholesterol medicines: Additive effects are possible with concurrent administration; use caution.

Copper or iron: Concurrent administration with zinc inhibits the absorption of copper and iron. Administer zinc and copper or iron as far apart as possible.

Penicillamine: Concurrent administration with zinc reduces zinc absorption.

Quinolones: Zinc decreases absorption of quinolone antibiotics (eg, ciprofloxacin, gatifloxacin, ofloxacin). Zinc salts or vitamins containing zinc should be given 2 hours after or 6 hours before antibiotics.

Tetracycline: Concurrent administration results in decreased tetracycline effectiveness. Administer tetracycline at least 2 hours before or 3 hours after zinc.

DRUG-FOOD INTERACTIONS

Concurrent administration of caffeine with zinc reduces zinc absorption. Foods containing high amounts of phosphorus, calcium (dairy), or phytates (eg, bran, brown bread) may reduce absorption.

ADVERSE REACTIONS

Side effects of high zinc intake include gastrointestinal discomfort, nausea, vomiting, headaches, drowsiness, metallic taste, and diarrhea. Daily ingestion of zinc can lower HDL levels. Ingestion of supplemental zinc for long periods of time (average 6.3 years) has been linked to a significant increase in hospitalizations for genitourinary problems. Zinc nasal products may cause tingling and burning sensations.

ADMINISTRATION AND DOSAGE

Adults

Daily Dosage: Recommended Dietary Allowance (RDA):

Males 14 and older: 11mg daily.

Females—14 to 18 years: 9 mg daily; *19 years:* 8mg daily.

During pregnancy—>18 years: 12mg daily; *19+ years:* 11mg daily.

During lactation—>18 years: 13mg daily; *19+ years:* 12mg daily.

Dietary supplement: Daily oral doses range from 9mg to 25mg.

Acne and dermatitis: A topical preparation (cream or gel) of 10mg zinc sulfate per gram or 27mg to 30mg zinc oxide per gram used several times daily.

Acne: 90mg to 135mg orally daily.

Zinc deficiency/acrodermatitis: Maximum doses up to 40mg/day orally.

Wilson's disease: 300mg to 1,200mg/day orally in divided doses.

Pediatrics

Daily Dosage: Recommended Dietary Allowance (RDA):

Infants and children—7 months to 3 years: 3 mg daily; *4 to 8 years:* 5mg daily; *9 to 13 years:* 8mg daily.

Acne: 135mg orally daily.

Zinc deficiency: Daily doses range from 1.5mg to 12mg, depending on age.

HERBAL MEDICINE PROFILES

This section covers information on commonly used herbal supplements, which are marketed under the federal Dietary Supplement Health and Education Act of 1994. The profiles are derived from clinical monographs appearing in *PDR® for Herbal Medicines* and have been updated based on recent scientific findings and reviewed by PDR's clinical staff.

Included here is information on herbs and other botanical substances intended to supplement the diet. **Note:** Herbal supplements are not regulated by the Food and Drug Administration and are not intended to diagnose, treat, cure, or prevent any disease.

Herbal Medicines

Aloe Vera

EFFECTS

Aloe gel, from the pulp of the *Aloe vera* leaf, has soothing and healing effects. A juice is made from the gel as well as from the whole leaf. A component with very different effects is taken from specialized cells of the leaf's inner lining as a liquid then dried into a yellow powder. Called aloe vera latex, this powder has powerful laxative properties.

COMMON USAGE

Accepted uses: Commission E approves of the use of aloe vera latex for constipation (the anthraquinone laxative portion of aloe is primarily used for short-term treatment of this condition) and to clear out the colon for rectal and bowel examination. *Aloe vera* gel appears to be a safe treatment for oral lichen planus.

Unproven uses: Aloe vera gel is used topically to hasten healing in mild first-degree burns (such as sunburns), wounds, and other skin infections and conditions. Its ability to treat varying degrees of more serious burns, frostbite, herpes simplex, and psoriasis remains unclear. Aloe juice and derivatives are taken for heartburn and other digestive complaints, but the effectiveness remains uncertain. Likewise unproven is its ability to help with AIDS, arthritis, asthma, cancer, diabetes, and ulcers.

CONTRAINDICATIONS

Aloe products should not be taken by mouth by people with kidney or heart disease, or with electrolyte abnormalities. In addition to hypersensitivity, contraindications to the use of aloe latex include pregnancy and breastfeeding, nausea, vomiting, symptoms of appendicitis, undiagnosed abdominal pain, and temporary paralysis of the bowel (ileus) such as bowel obstruction, fecal impaction, and acute surgical abdomen. The use of aloe latex is not recommended for children under age 12.

WARNINGS/PRECAUTIONS

Diabetes or kidney disease: Exercise caution in using aloe orally as a laxative, as electrolyte imbalances such as low potassium levels can occur, potentially causing complications such as muscle weakness or abnormal heart rhythms.

Overuse as laxative: Exercise caution in taking oral aloe formulations. More than seven consecutive days of use may cause dependency or worsening of constipation once aloe latex is stopped. Possible risk of colorectal cancer with more than 12 months of use.

Pregnancy and breastfeeding: While topical use of the gel likely poses no risk, oral use of aloe forms is contraindicated during pregnancy or breastfeeding. Compounds in aloe could, theoretically, stimulate uterine contractions. Breastfeeding women should not consume the dried juice of aloe leaves. It remains unclear whether active aloe ingredients appear in breast milk.

Wound healing: There have been cases of slowed healing and skin irritation and redness following application of aloe juice. Avoid applying prior to sun exposure. Do not apply the gel following cesarean delivery.

DRUG INTERACTIONS

Antidiabetic agents: Avoid concomitant use of oral aloe forms due to increased risk of hypoglycemia.

Digoxin: Avoid concomitant use with oral aloe forms given the theoretical risk of hypokalemia resulting in digoxin toxicity.

ADVERSE REACTIONS

Using aloe or aloe latex orally for laxative effects can cause excessive bowel activity (bloody diarrhea, nausea), cramping, and diarrhea. Oral use may lower blood sugar levels (according to a small number of human studies). In overdose, electrolyte imbalances such as low potassium levels, as well as kidney damage, are a risk. Doses of 1g/day for several days may be fatal.

Usually safe when used topically, although cases of delayed wound healing and skin irritation have been reported following application of juice to skin. Avoid applying prior to sun exposure.

Administration by injection is dangerous and linked to fatalities; more research is needed.

ADMINISTRATION AND DOSAGE

The dosing of aloe vera products is highly dependent on such varied factors as plant part used, growing and harvesting condition, and extraction methods employed.

Adults

Daily dosage: As an oral laxative, the usual (and maximum) single daily oral dose at bedtime of dried aloe extract or powdered aloe: 0.05-0.2g. Do not exceed commonly recommended dosage.

Topical use: Some sources recommend that commercial aloe gel solutions contain at least a 70% concentration of aloe to positively influence inflammation and healing. Follow directions on commercial creams and ointments for wounds or burns.

Pediatrics

Oral use is not recommended for children under age 12. Dosages for topical use are the same as those for adults.

Bilberry

EFFECTS

The fruit of the bilberry plant (*Vaccinium myrtillus*) contains potent astringent properties and antioxidant flavonoids. More than 15 different flavonoid anthocyanosides have been identified and are believed to generate much (if not all) of the plant's medicinal effects. Bilberry fruit has demonstrated the following properties: antiulcer, antineoplastic, antiplatelet, antiatherogenic, wound-healing, and antidiabetic effects. It also has shown an ability to enhance the eye's regenerative capacities.

COMMON USAGE

Accepted uses: Commission E approves of the highly nutritious bilberry fruit as an astringent and for the treatment of acute diarrhea, and topically as a gargle for mild inflammation of throat and mouth mucous membranes.

Unproven uses: Because of its high content of anthocyanins, bilberry fruit has become popular for the prevention and treatment of eye diseases (eg, cataracts, glaucoma, retinopathy, macular degeneration) in standardized extract form. Its effectiveness for

these purposes has been widely tested in Europe and attributed to the plant's antioxidant and collagen-stabilizing actions. Pilots in World War II contended that their visual acuity at night improved after consuming bilberry products, but data for the herb's value in this regard remain inconsistent.

Other uses for bilberry, though not all proven effective, include treatment of the following conditions: atherosclerosis, diabetes, hemorrhoids, inflammation, menstrual irregularities, neuralgia and neuropathy, peptic ulcer, peripheral vascular disease, pregnancy-related illnesses, varicose veins, and topically as an eyewash and compress for wounds and ulcers.

CONTRAINDICATIONS

Commission E warns against using the leaves of the bilberry plant for medicinal purposes. People with bleeding disorders or who are taking medications to thin the blood should not take very high doses of bilberry. Its use in breastfeeding is contraindicated given the historical use of bilberries for stopping lactation.

WARNINGS/PRECAUTIONS

Hypersensitivity: Hypersensitivity reactions are possible.

Pregnancy and breastfeeding: Breastfeeding is contraindicated (see above). No information is available regarding pregnancy; caution is advised.

DRUG INTERACTIONS

Anticoagulants (including low molecular weight heparins), antiplatelet agents, and thrombolytic agents: Combine with caution; bilberry could add to these drugs' blood altering effects and potentially increase their effects, promoting bleeding.

ADVERSE REACTIONS

There is potential for excessive bleeding due to decreased platelet aggregation. Nausea is possible and may abate by taking bilberry with food.

ADMINISTRATION AND DOSAGE

Only the berry (fruit, typically dried) is used; do not use the leaf for medicinal purposes. For general use, typical formulations are for bilberry fruit extract standardized for anthocyanidin content (25%): 80-160mg 3 times/day. Another common dosage for general daily use: fluid extract (1:1 concentration), 3-6mL.

Adults

Eye health: tablet/capsule (standardized to 36% anthocyanidin content): 60-160mg 3 times/day.

Mild inflammation of the mucous membranes of the mouth and throat: Decoction as a gargle (10% bilberry fruit): prepare, swish in mouth for several seconds, and spit out.

Nonspecific acute diarrhea: tablet/capsule: 20-60g/day.

Pediatrics

No information is available.

Chamomile

EFFECTS

The essential oil of chamomile has antibacterial and antifungal properties. The flowers have anti-inflammatory, antispasmodic, and sedative effects. Two species of chamomile—German chamomile (*Matricaria recutita*) and Roman chamomile (*Chamaemelum nobile* or *Anthemis nobilis*)—are commonly used.

COMMON USAGE

Accepted uses: Commission E has approved chamomile for coughs and bronchitis, fevers and colds, inflammation of the skin, mouth, and pharynx, infection, and wounds and burns.

Unproven uses: It is taken orally for tension and anxiety, insomnia, and by many women for discomforts of perimenopausal and menopausal symptoms. Its effectiveness when taken orally for diarrhea is unclear, as the data are inconclusive.

CONTRAINDICATIONS

Chamomile is contraindicated in pregnancy and in people with atopic hay fever or asthma. It also should not be taken by people with a hypersensitivity to chamomile or other members of the *Compositae* family.

WARNINGS/PRECAUTIONS

Pregnancy and breastfeeding: Internal consumption of the whole plant should be avoided during early pregnancy. No data on human teratogenicity are available. Chamomile anthemis is contraindicated throughout pregnancy due to its emmenagogic and abortifacient effects. Chamomile matricaria is contraindicated in early pregnancy due to its emmenagogic effects; it has been used during pregnancy as a weak tea for insomnia, as a diuretic, and as a carminative, with no apparent adverse effects.

Flowers can be safely consumed while breastfeeding.

Infants: Avoid chamomile tea due to risk for infant botulism.

DRUG INTERACTIONS

Anticoagulants: Caution is advised, as the coumarins present in chamomile could theoretically magnify the effect of anticoagulants, adding to the anticoagulant effect and increasing the risk of bleeding.

ADVERSE REACTIONS

Eczema (facial) has been reported with the tea. Emesis is possible when Roman chamomile is taken in high doses.

Contact dermatitis and eczema are possible with topical use.

Conjunctivitis and eyelid angioedema are possible with the use of chamomile tea as an eyewash.

Allergic reactions are possible in the presence of allergies to related plants in the *Compositae* family, such as ragweed, marigolds, and daisies.

ADMINISTRATION AND DOSAGE

Chamomile is used as a tea, essential oil, liquid extract, or as a topical cream.

Adults

Dermatitis: As a topical cream, applied 4 times/day.

Tension/anxiety: Orally, liquid extract (1:1 in 45 to 70% ethanol) 1-4mL taken 3 times/day or as a tea, 1-4 times/day in 8-oz cups, as needed.

Pediatrics

Dermatitis: A topical cream is applied 4 times daily.

Tension/anxiety: Orally, 1-4 times daily in 8-oz cups as a tea, with amount depending on age.

Cranberry

EFFECTS

Cranberry (*Vaccinium macrocarpon*) has antibacterial and antioxidant properties. Among other possible mechanisms, it is believed to inhibit the ability of bacteria to adhere to the urinary tract, thereby protecting against (and possibly resolving) urinary tract infection (UTI).

COMMON USAGE

Unproven uses: For medicinal purposes, cranberry products (primarily juices) have been used for centuries to prevent and treat urinary tract infections. Clinical trials indicate possible effectiveness for the use of cranberry for UTIs. It is possibly effective as an antioxidant in humans and in vitro. It has been used as a urine deodorant in people with incontinence. Evidence for its value in preventing the formation of dental plaque is underway. Data for treating nephrolithiasis are inconclusive.

CONTRAINDICATIONS

Cranberry is contraindicated in cases of hypersensitivity to the fruit. It should be used with caution in people with nephrolithiasis (renal colic, blood in the urine, and kidney stones).

WARNINGS/PRECAUTIONS

Pregnancy and breastfeeding: No information is available; caution is advised.

DRUG INTERACTIONS

H_2 *blockers:* Combine with caution, and avoid regular (daily) use of cranberry juice while taking this medication. Cranberry juice reduces gastric pH, and could theoretically antagonize the effect of H_2 blockers and thereby reduce their effectiveness.

Proton pump inhibitors: Combine with caution, and avoid regular (daily) use of cranberry juice while taking this medication. Cranberry juice significantly reduces gastric pH, and could theoretically reduce the effectiveness of proton pump inhibitors.

Warfarin: Avoid excess use of cranberry products while taking this medication due to the increased risk of bleeding.

ADVERSE REACTIONS

Rarely: renal colic, blood in the urine, and kidney stones.

ADMINISTRATION AND DOSAGE

Cranberry is available for oral use as a juice and in capsule and tablet forms. Juice may be difficult for women to take daily over very long periods of time. Optimum dosage or method of administration remains to be determined.

Adults

Urinary tract infection, prophylaxis: Cranberry juice: 300mL/day. *Cranberry-Lingonberry juice concentrate (7.5g cranberry concentrate and 1.7g lingonberry concentrate in 50mL water):* 50mL daily for 6 months. *Cranberry juice (unsweetened or saccharin-sweetened):* 250mL 3 times/day. *Cranberry extract (standardized) in capsule or tablet form:* 100-500mg 2-3 times/day.

Urinary tract infection, existing: Cranberry extract (standardized) in capsule or tablet form: 100-500mg 2-3 times daily.

Pediatrics

Dosing information is not available.

Echinacea

EFFECTS

Depending on the type of plant species, echinacea has demonstrated the following properties: antibacterial, anti-inflammatory, antimicrobial, antineoplastic, immunostimulating, infertility effects, radio-protectant, and wound-healing effects.

COMMON USAGE

Accepted uses: When used internally, the aerial (above-ground) parts of Echinacea purpurea—but not the root—is Commission E–approved for treating colds, flulike symptoms, fever, chronic infections of the respiratory tract (such as bronchitis), urinary tract infections, inflammation of the mouth and pharynx, and recurrent infections. It is also approved for the external treatment of superficial wounds and burns. Additionally, the root of *E pallida* is approved as supportive treatment for fevers and colds.

Unproven uses: A study funded by the National Institutes of Health concluded that extracts of *E angustifolia* root do not have clinically significant effects on rhinovirus infection. Likewise, Commission E has not approved *E angustifolia* herb or root for any indication.

CONTRAINDICATIONS

Parenteral use is contraindicated in patients with allergic tendencies, especially to members of the *Asteraceae* or *Compositae* family (eg, ragweed, chrysanthemums, marigolds, and daisies). Echinacea extract should not be used intravenously in patients with diabetes, since it could worsen their condition. Due to the possible immunostimulating effects of echinacea, Commission E cites the following contraindications based on theoretical—but not clinical—evidence: progressive systemic diseases such as tuberculosis, leukosis, collagenosis, multiple sclerosis and other autoimmune diseases, AIDS, and HIV infection.

WARNINGS/PRECAUTIONS

Fertility: In lab studies, high concentrations of *E purpurea* interfered with sperm enzymes.

Hypersensitivity: Allergic reactions—including urticaria, angioedema, asthma, and anaphylaxis—have been reported. More than half of the affected patients had a history of asthma, allergic rhinitis, rhinoconjunctivitis, or atopic dermatitis.

Pregnancy and breastfeeding: Safety has not been established; caution is advised.

DRUG INTERACTIONS

Drug interactions are unlikely but possible.

Anticancer drugs: Avoid concomitant use. Echinacea could potentially decrease their effectiveness.

Drugs metabolized by cytochrome P450: In vitro and in vivo studies found that echinacea inhibited CYP3A and CYP1A2; caution is advised when coadministering the herb with drugs dependent on CYP enzymes for their elimination.

Immunosuppressants: Avoid concomitant use. Echinacea could counteract the effects of drugs that suppress the immune system, including corticosteroids and drugs used to prevent organ rejection, such as azathioprine, basiliximab, cyclosporine, daclizumab, muromonab-CD3, mycophenolate, sirolimus, and tacrolimus.

ADVERSE REACTIONS

Oral use: Mainly allergic reactions, including breathing problems, dizziness, headache, itching, and rash.

Topical use: Rash and other skin reactions.

Parenteral use: Fever, flulike symptoms, nausea, and vomiting.

ADMINISTRATION AND DOSAGE

Adults

Therapy should not exceed 8 weeks for prophylactic treatment of recurrent infections and 1-2 weeks for acute infections. When used for extended periods, cycling is advised (eg, skipping weekend doses or taking weekly drug holidays every 4-6 weeks). Dosing schedule for the following oral forms is 3-4 times daily for short-term treatment and twice daily for long-term treatment.

Dry powdered extract: 150-300mg.

Fluid extract (1:1 preparation); 0.25-1mL.

Freeze-dried whole plant: 325-650mg.

Root extract: 300mg.

Tea: 1-2g of powdered root.

Tincture (1:5 preparation): 1-2mL.

Topical use: Dilute fluid extract in equal amount of water and apply to superficial wounds 2-3 times daily.

Pediatrics

No information is available; caution is advised.

Evening Primrose Oil

EFFECTS

The oil from the wildflower evening primrose (*Oenothera biennis*) contains gamma-linolenic acid (GLA), which the body converts to dihomo-gamma-linolenic acid and then to prostaglandins that are believed to have anti-inflammatory effects. Extracts of evening primrose oil have also shown antioxidant actions in the laboratory.

COMMON USAGE

Unproven uses: Evening primrose oil (EPO) is an omega 6 fatty acid that contains approximately 8.9% GLA. Omega 6 essential fatty acids (EFAs) are generally lacking in the standard American diet. Many chronic illnesses are said to respond to supplementation of EFAs. Placebo-controlled, randomized trials indicate possible, though not definitive, effectiveness for the treatment of rheumatoid arthritis, breast cancer, Raynaud's syndrome, diabetic neuropathy, and various types of atopic dermatitis such as eczema. Several months of use may result in relief from cyclical breast pain (mastalgia), though not all study results are positive. EPO may relieve the physical and psychological symptoms of premenstrual syndrome; however, many of the studies indicating effectiveness are inadequate in dose, length of treatment, or size of treatment/control groups. The North American Menopause Society reports that clinical trials find no benefit of EPO for menopause-associated hot flashes.

CONTRAINDICATIONS

Contraindicated in people with schizophrenia.

WARNINGS/PRECAUTIONS

Hypersensitivity: Allergic reactions to evening primrose oil have been reported.

Pregnancy and breastfeeding: Scientific evidence for the safe use of evening primrose oil is not available.

DRUG INTERACTIONS

Anticoagulants: Caution is advised when taken concomitantly with EPO due to the theoretical risk of increased bleeding.

Anticonvulsants: Avoid concomitant use due to theoretical potential for EPO to reduce the effectiveness of anticonvulsants by lowering the seizure threshold.

Antiplatelet agents, thrombolytic agents, and low molecular weight heparins: Caution is advised for concomitant use due to the theoretical risk of increased and prolonged bleeding.

Phenothiazines: Avoid concomitant use due to the risk of reduced seizure threshold. Seizures have been reported in people with schizophrenia who started taking evening primrose oil.

ADVERSE REACTIONS

Possible reactions include nausea, diarrhea, flatulence, bloating, and mild vomiting.

ADMINISTRATION AND DOSAGE

Adults

Daily Dosage: For effective treatment, EPO must be taken in substantial (gram) doses, typically 3-8g daily in divided doses. Clinical effect is often not seen until 8-12 weeks of treatment.

Eczema: 2-8g daily.

Mastalgia: 3-4g daily.

Pediatrics

Eczema: 2-4g daily.

Flaxseed

EFFECTS

The seed from the flax plant (*Linum usitatissimum*) has demonstrated anti-inflammatory, laxative, demulcent, and cholesterol-lowering properties. The oil from the seeds is the richest known plant source of omega-3 fatty acids (converted from the seeds' alpha-linolenic acid, or ALA). These compounds suppress the production of interleukin-1, tumor necrosis factor, and leukotriene B4 from monocytes and polymorphonuclear leukocytes. Flaxseed is also the richest known source of the phytoestrogen lignans.

COMMON USAGE

Accepted uses: Commission E approves of the use of flaxseed for the treatment of the colon damaged by laxative abuse, irritable colon, and diverticulitis. Flaxseed in the diet is nutritional and has medicinal benefits. It traditionally has been used as a gentle bulk laxative. The ground seeds, when presoaked or taken with large quantities of water, are palatable and valuable for relieving benign and atonic constipation. Flaxseed is also approved for use as a mucilage for gastritis and enteritis. Commission E also approves of flaxseed topically as a cataplasm for local inflammation; the mucilage from the freshly ground flower or boiled seeds is applied directly to mild rashes to pain relief. Boiled seeds also can serve as a base for enemas as part of the treatment for chronic prostatitis.

Unproven uses: Flaxseed reduces serum total and low-density lipoprotein cholesterol concentrations, reduces postprandial glucose absorption, and decreases certain markers of inflammation. The oil from flaxseed is used for its antiplatelet activity, for which there is documentation of possible effectiveness in adults.

Trials indicate that the oil decreases the tendency of platelets to aggregate. Although occasionally used for rheumatoid arthritis, . flaxseed products have shown little consistent ability to improve pain, stiffness, and other symptoms.

CONTRAINDICATIONS

Flaxseed should not be taken in cases of ileus (intestinal obstruction), thyroid insufficiency, or hypersensitivity to the seed.

WARNINGS/PRECAUTIONS

Inflammatory bowel conditions: Flaxseed should be presoaked before use in such cases.

Identification (flaxseed versus linseed): "Flaxseed" refers to products for human consumption while "linseed oil" refers to seed products that have been denatured and are unfit for human consumption. They are used in commercial products, such as paints and varnishes.

Pregnancy and breastfeeding: Scientific evidence for the safe use of flaxseed during pregnancy is not available. Dietary flaxseed oil appears to have no effect on breast milk and is likely safe for use while breastfeeding.

DRUG INTERACTIONS

Drugs of all types: Absorption may be impaired when taken concomitantly due to the mucilage and cellulose in flaxseed.

ADVERSE REACTIONS

Whole seed and oil preparations may cause gastrointestinal upset when taken daily over the course of several weeks. Flaxseed oil may increase bleeding time. Otherwise, there are no known side effects as long as flaxseed products are taken with sufficient amounts of liquid. Allergic reactions with anaphylaxis are possible, however.

ADMINISTRATION AND DOSAGE

Flaxseed is supplied as whole, crushed, or milled seeds, or as powder or oil. It is administered orally, topically, or rectally.

Adults

Constipation: Whole or ground seeds are taken orally 2-3 times/ day, 1 tablespoon with 150mL of liquid. Take with large quantities of water, or presoak seeds overnight.

As a demulcent: 1 tablespoon seeds to 1 cup water (about 30g-50g seeds to a liter of water), with liquid poured off after seeds stand in cold water for 20-30 minutes.

Hyperlipidemia: Oil and milled flaxseed are optimal forms, such as 35g-50g seeds daily in muffins or breads or 35g-50g seeds daily with adequate water.

Inflammation: 30g-50g flaxseed flour as a moist heat compress.

Prostatitis, chronic: Boiled seeds can serve as a base for enemas as part of the treatment.

Pediatrics

Dosing information is not available.

Ginseng

EFFECTS

Asian ginseng (*Panax ginseng*) is an immune system stimulant. It has demonstrated the following properties: adaptogenic (pro-vides increased resistance to physical, chemical, or biological stress), antineoplastic, antiplatelet, antiviral, gluco-regulatory, and cardiac inotropic. It also has shown the ability to stimulate enzyme reactions, hemostatic actions, hepatoprotective actions, hypoglycemic activity, platelet adhesiveness, radioprotective (radiation-protectant) actions (possible), RNA synthesis, corti-cotrophin secretion, and protein synthesis. Less information is available on the related American ginseng (*Panax quinquefolium*; also commonly referred to as western ginseng and North American ginseng), which is reported to have antidiabetic, anti-oxidant and possible hypotensive and liver-protective actions.

COMMON USAGE

Accepted uses: Commission E gives ginseng a positive evaluation for use as a tonic for fatigue, debility, and declining concentration, and for use during convalescence. It has been used medicinally in China for millennia and is in the pharmacopoeia of many countries (Australia, China, France, Germany, Japan, Switzerland). It is used widely to enhance mental and physical well-being. Some trials in humans show positive results for ginseng to improve blood alcohol levels, lower serum cholesterol levels and blood glucose, and control hemoglobin A1c in non-insulin dependent diabetes.

Unproven uses: Ginseng may alleviate postmenopausal symptoms. Some studies show improved endurance, stamina, and mental ability, and possible effectiveness for enhanced cognitive function, immune system stimulation, and male infertility. Possible tumor-preventive properties have been identified. However, numerous analyses in the West fail to consistently find effectiveness of ginseng for most uses. There is no Commission E monograph for American ginseng, which is commonly used for many of the same purposes as *Panax ginseng*. It was long used by Native Americans and others to increase physical and mental endurance, for stress relief, for its hypoglycemic effects, and to ease menopausal symptoms. A preliminary open-label study indicated some subjective improvement in children with attention deficit hyperactivity disorder (ADHD).

CONTRAINDICATIONS

Ginseng is contraindicated in people with hypersensitivity to the herb, in people with hypertension, diabetes, or those predisposed to hypoglycemia.

WARNINGS/PRECAUTIONS

Blood pressure: Ginseng may increase blood pressure and alter control in patients with hypertension.

Diabetes: Ginseng may lower blood glucose levels in diabetic as well as nondiabetic individuals; caution is advised in people with diabetes or those predisposed to hypoglycemia.

Ginseng abuse syndrome: A constellation of symptoms consisting of hypertension, nervousness, insomnia, morning diarrhea, and skin eruptions may occur after 1 to 3 weeks of ingestion of 3g/day of *Panax ginseng* root.

Hyperactivity: Ginseng should be used with caution in patients who are hyperactive or are taking stimulants such as caffeine.

Laboratory modifications: Ginseng may have the potential to generate false increases in digoxin concentrations. Alert clinician to potential for this interaction.

Prior to surgery: Ginseng may interfere with blood coagulation; discontinue use 1 to 2 weeks prior to elective surgery.

Pregnancy and breastfeeding: Scientific evidence for the safe use of ginseng during pregnancy or while breastfeeding is not available.

DRUG INTERACTIONS

Albendazole: Exercise caution in combining with ginseng due to reduced intestinal concentration of drug.

Anticoagulants: Avoid concomitant use of ginseng due to risk of decreased drug efficacy. A recent study in healthy individuals found that American ginseng reduced the effect of the anticoagulant warfarin.

Antidiabetic agents: Exercise caution in concomitant use with ginseng given the (theoretical) risk of increased hypoglycemia.

Drugs metabolized by CYP450 or CYP34A: Herb-mediated modulation of CYP450 activity may underlie interactions with Panax ginseng and medications metabolized in this way. CYP activity may decrease in older individuals, many of whom take numerous medications; caution is advised. Also see nifedipine, below.

Estrogen (topical or oral): Avoid concomitant use with any type of ginseng given the (theoretical) risk of additive estrogenic effects.

Loop diuretics: Avoid concomitant use due to increased risk of diuretic resistance.

Monoamine oxidase inhibitors: Avoid concomitant use of ginseng with phenelzine and other drugs in this class due to increased risk of insomnia, tremor, headache, agitation, and worsening of depression. Separate use by several weeks.

Nifedipine: Exercise caution in combining with ginseng due to increased risk of drug side effects. Other drugs metabolized in a similar way (by CYP34A) may be similarly affected.

Opioid analgesics: Exercise caution in combining with ginseng due to potential for reduced drug effectiveness.

ADVERSE REACTIONS

Possible adverse effects include nervousness, gastrointestinal upset or diarrhea, insomnia, headache, nausea, vomiting, edema, euphoria, vaginal bleeding, skin eruptions and ulcerations, blood pressure problems, and a so-called "Ginseng abuse syndrome." Estrogenic effects have been observed with ginseng products, though the exact type of ginseng (ie, American, Asian [*Panax*], Siberian) was unclear.

ADMINISTRATION AND DOSAGE

Commission E recommends that *Panax ginseng* generally be used for up to 3 months. American ginseng is taken for longer periods of time to generate an effect. For *Panax ginseng*, a 2-week break should be observed between all ginseng courses. Dosing can be challenging because commercial ginseng preparations can vary widely in their contents. *Panax ginseng* is available in capsule, powdered root, tablet, tea, and tincture forms for oral use. American ginseng is available in several forms, including capsule, leaf, powdered root, tablet, tea, and tincture forms for oral use. It is not typically used for its short-term effects but instead for long-term actions.

Adults

Daily dosage (Panax ginseng): 500mg-2g dry root in 2 divided doses; 200mg-600mg. Solid extract; 1 cup tea up to 3 times/day for 3-4 weeks; 3 cups/day decoction from powder (to prepare put 1/2 tsp powdered root in a cup of water, bring to a boil, and simmer gently 10 minutes, cool slightly).

Emotional or physical stress (American ginseng): 2-4oz cold infusion 3 times/day; 10-20 drops alcoholic extract 3 times/day; 20-40 drops cultivated roots 3 times/day; 30-60 drops leaf preparations 3 times/day.

Hyperglycemia: 3g/day (capsule).

Pediatrics

No information is available.

Grape Seed Extract

EFFECTS

Grape seed extract has demonstrated powerful antioxidant activity; the membrane of the seed is a rich source of proanthyocyanidins (also known as procyanidins or procyanidolic oligomers, or PCOs), a highly beneficial group of plant flavonoids. Grape seed extract has shown vascular, cytotoxic, chemopreventative, and cytoprotective effects. In experimental models, the antioxidant activity of PCOs from grape seed extract is approximately 50 times greater than that of vitamins C and E.

COMMON USAGE

Unproven uses: Most studies of grape seed extract have been in vitro or in animals. Based on the handful of small but relatively good human trials, there is possible benefit with grape seed extract for venous and capillary disorders such as venous insufficiency and varicose veins. Grape seed extract also is used for eye conditions such as retina disorders, macular degeneration, and diabetic retinopathy. Excellent antioxidant effects of grape seed extract may also help to protect against chronic degenerative diseases such as atherosclerosis and certain cancers. It may improve resistance to glare and promote recovery from exposure to eye strain such as bright light and ocular stress, according to data of fair quality. PCOs from grape seeds (and pine bark) have been marketed and promoted in France for decades to improve retinopathies, venous insufficiency, and vascular fragility.

CONTRAINDICATIONS

Grape seed extract is contraindicated in people with hypersensitivity to it.

WARNINGS/PRECAUTIONS

Pregnancy and breastfeeding: Scientific evidence for the safe use of grape seed extract during pregnancy and while breastfeeding is not available.

DRUG INTERACTIONS

No human interaction data are available.

ADVERSE REACTIONS

Information on adverse reactions is not available.

ADMINISTRATION AND DOSAGE

Grape seed extract is taken orally in extract, capsule, or geltab forms. The extract typically contains up to 95% PCOs, and PCO content is often indicated on dosing forms.

Adults

Daily Dosage: 50mg for preventative antioxidant effect and 150mg-300mg for therapeutic antioxidant effect.

Pediatrics

No information is available.

Hawthorn

EFFECTS

Hawthorn (*Crataegus oxyacantha*) is an inotropic agent. It has vasodilator, cardiotonic, and antilipidemic effects. Extracts are useful in treating mild forms of cardiac insufficiency by generating positive inotropy, prolonging the myocardial refractory period, and vasodilating coronary and skeletal muscle vessels. The compounds in hawthorn are believed to reduce blood cholesterol concentration and lessen myocardial oxygen consumption due in part to antioxidant effects. It is listed as a flavonoid drug in Germany (its flowers and leaves contain up to 2.5% flavonoids). Much of its action on the cardiovascular system is attributed to flavonoid constituents. Certain extracts prevent elevation of such plasma lipids as total cholesterol, triglycerides, and LDL and VLDL fractions, and upregulate LDL receptors in the liver.

COMMON USAGE

Approved uses: Commission E approves of hawthorn leaf with flowers for treatment of heart failure (Stage II NYHA). This herb is well-studied for cardiovascular disease and is commonly used in combination with cardiac glycosides to potentiate their effects and thereby lessen the dose of cardiac glycoside drugs. Most clinical trials support its use for mild to moderate congestive heart failure. A 2008 Cochrane Database System Review found evidence for its value as an adjunctive treatment in controlling symptoms and the physiologic outcome of chronic heart failure.

Unproven uses: More research is needed to determine hawthorn's value in treating hypertension, atherosclerosis, hyperlipidemia, asthma, arrhythmia in the elderly, and orthostatic hypertension. Due to its high flavonoid content, it may be used to decrease capillary fragility, lessen inflammation, and prevent collagen destruction of joints. The herb has been used as a coffee substitute and to flavor cigarettes.

CONTRAINDICATIONS

Hawthorn is contraindicated in cases of hypersensitivity or a history of allergic reaction to *Crataegus* or any of its components. It is also contraindicated in children under age 12.

WARNINGS/PRECAUTIONS

Hawthorn is widely considered safe when used appropriately, for short periods of time and in usual doses, for most conditions.

Pregnancy and breastfeeding: No information is available; caution is advised both for use in pregnancy and while breastfeeding.

DRUG INTERACTIONS

Antiplatelet agents: Caution is advised when taking hawthorn with antiplatelet agents due to the theoretical risk of increased bleeding. Signs and symptoms of excessive bleeding should be monitored.

Digoxin: Caution is advised in combining hawthorn with digoxin due to the theoretical risk of increased pharmacodynamic effect of digoxin. One trial showed reduced digoxin bioavailability.

ADVERSE REACTIONS

Infrequently, hot flushes and gastrointestinal upset occur. Also possible are palpitations, dyspnea, headache, epistaxis, and dizziness.

ADMINISTRATION AND DOSAGE

Oral forms include capsules, tablets, teas, tinctures, and solutions. Dosage depends upon the preparation used.

Adults

Cardiac insufficiency: 160mg-900mg dried extract in 3 divided doses daily for at least 6 weeks. Tincture (standardized 1:5): 4mL-5mL 3 times/day.

Pediatrics

Not recommended for children under age 12.

Milk Thistle

EFFECTS

Milk thistle (Silybum marianum) has renal and hepatoprotective properties due to antioxidant effects and free radical elimination. Hepatoprotective actions against chemical, environmental, and infectious toxins have been demonstrated.

COMMON USAGE

Accepted uses: Commission E gives milk thistle seeds a positive evaluation for dyspepsia (when used as a crude drug), toxic liver damage, and hepatic cirrhosis. It is also approved as a supportive treatment in chronic inflammatory liver disease when using a standardized extract of at least 70% silymarin plus silibinin, silydianin, and silychristin. The active agent in milk thistle is silymarin. It has been used to treat acute and chronic liver problems and bile problems for more than 2,000 years.

Unproven uses: Many but not all clinical studies indicate that it has a positive hepatoprotective effect in the treatment of liver cirrhosis associated with chronic alcohol abuse or viruses (such as hepatitis B or C). Results for treatment of mushroom poisoning with silymarin are positive overall, although its true effectiveness for this purpose is difficult to determine given variations in treatment protocols in studies with adults and animals. It is commonly used for preventing gallstones. Studies are examining effectiveness for protecting against various cancers, including skin cancer, and also for its value in controlling thalassemia.

CONTRAINDICATIONS

Use of milk thistle is contraindicated in people with a known hypersensitivity to it or any of its components.

WARNINGS/PRECAUTIONS

Pregnancy and breastfeeding: Milk thistle has been used for as long as 3 weeks to treat intrahepatic cholestasis of pregnancy; however, overall safety has not been determined.

DRUG INTERACTIONS

Metronidazole: Concomitant use is not recommended; in a clinical trial of healthy volunteers, the extract silymarin reduced metronidazole and active metabolite exposure. If concomitant use is necessary, metronidazole dose may need to be increased.

ADVERSE REACTIONS

A 2007 Cochrane Database Systematic Review reported no significantly increased risk of adverse events with the use of milk thistle. Urticaria and other allergic reactions are rare.

ADMINISTRATION AND DOSAGE

Milk thistle is available in capsule, tablet, and tincture forms for oral use. (Intravenous solutions are not available in the U.S.) Note that silymarin concentrations may vary considerably.

Adults

Hepatoprotection: 420mg/day of extract (standardized to 70%-80% silymarin), divided into three doses for 6-8 weeks, followed by a maintenance dose of 280mg/day.

Cyclopeptide mushroom poisoning: Intravenous solution for parenteral administration (or oral formulation if no intravenous preparation is available) for approximately 33mg/kg/day for a mean duration of 81.67 hours.

Pediatrics

No information is available.

Saw Palmetto

EFFECTS

Saw palmetto (*Serenoa repens*) has demonstrated genitourinary effects due to its testosterone-altering properties (antiandrogenic, antiestrogenic, estrogenic). Also, as demonstrated in animal and tissue studies: anti-inflammatory, antineoplastic, cholesterol-blocking, enzyme inhibition, platelet inhibition, and protein synthesis inhibition actions.

COMMON USAGE

Approved uses: Commission E approves of saw palmetto (typically, the extract *Serenoa repens*) for the treatment of urinary problems of benign prostatic hyperplasia (BPH) stage I (abnormal frequent urination, nocturia, delayed onset of urination, and weak urinary stream) and stage II (urge to urinate and residual urine). Documentation for its use in BPH includes numerous controlled clinical trials. In one study, a *Serenoa repens* extract of 320mg a day for periods of 30 days to 12 months resulted in significant improvement in urine flow, dysuria, nocturia, residual urine, urgency, prostate volume, and subjective complaints. But a 2009 Cochrane Database Systematic Review failed to find *Serenoa repens* more effective than placebo for urinary symptoms of BPH.

Unproven uses: Evidence for saw palmetto's effectiveness in prostate cancer treatment is inconclusive. Other historical uses of the herb include treatment for chronic cystitis and as a mild diuretic, although the main use always has been for a variety of urinary tract conditions. Topically, saw palmetto has been used for androgen-induced acne.

CONTRAINDICATIONS

The use of saw palmetto is contraindicated in cases of hypersensitivity to it or any of its components.

WARNINGS/PRECAUTIONS

Hormone-dependent cancer: Saw palmetto has shown anti-androgenic, antiestrogenic, and estrogenic actions in animals. Caution is warranted, as no information is available about the action of this herb in people with breast cancer, prostate cancer, or other hormone-related diseases.

Pregnancy and breastfeeding: Scientific evidence for the safe use of saw palmetto during pregnancy and lactation is not available.

DRUG INTERACTIONS

An extensive 2009 review of *Serenoa repens* found no evidence for drug interactions with the herb.

Warfarin: Caution is advised due to the increased risk of bleeding likely due to the cyclooxygenase inhibition by saw palmetto.

ADVERSE REACTIONS

A detailed 2008 assessment of *Serenoa repens* extract for lower urinary tract symptoms documented no evidence for serious toxicity concerns. Other studies have documented pruritus, headache, dizziness, fatigue, asthenia, dry mouth, postural hypotension, nausea, abdominal pain, and other mild gastrointestinal effects. Rarely: ejaculation disorders, erectile dysfunction, and reduced libido. Estrogenic effects have been reported following treatment with the multi-ingredient PC-SPES.

ADMINISTRATION AND DOSAGE

Saw palmetto is available for oral use in capsule and tablet forms, and for topical use in ointment form. For BPH, look . for extracts with proven pharmacological activity and clinical efficacy.

Adults

Daily Dosage: 320mg of lipophilic extract produced with lipophilic solvents (90% v/v) or super-critical fluid extraction from carbon dioxide.

Pediatrics

No information is available.

Siberian Ginseng

EFFECTS

Siberian ginseng (*Eleutherococcus senticosus*) has demonstrated immunostimulant effects, as well as some antibacterial, antineoplastic, and antioxidant properties. Hormonal effects may occur, but human studies are lacking. Some, but not all, studies demonstrate blood sugar-reducing effects.

COMMON USAGE

Approved uses: Commission E approves of Siberian ginseng as a tonic for invigoration and fortification during times of fatigue, debility, or declining capacity for work and concentration. It is also approved for use during convalescence.

Unproven uses: Siberian ginseng is most often used for its adaptogenic effects to improve physical stamina and enhance immune states. It is used worldwide to increase endurance, immunity, and resistance to stress. Although not proven in studies, other clinical uses include treatment for cancer, hypotension, immune system depression, and infertility. Its use for Familial Mediterranean Fever is inconclusive. Topically, an extract may slow the manifestation of skin aging, although study results are inconclusive.

CONTRAINDICATIONS

Siberian ginseng is contraindicated in people with hypertension or in those with known hypersensitivity to the herb or any of its extracts. It is also not recommended for use in people with diabetes or those with cardiac conditions such as myocardial infarction.

WARNINGS/PRECAUTIONS

Drug-lab interactions: Possible false increase in digoxin concentrations when Siberian ginseng is taken. The herb has been shown to falsely increase serum digoxin levels using the fluorescence polarization immunoassay (FPIA) and falsely decrease levels using the microparticle enzyme immunoassay (MEIA) ex vivo. Patients should be asked about their use of Siberian

ginseng when unanticipated serum digoxin concentrations are obtained.

Pregnancy and breastfeeding: Scientific evidence for the safe use of Siberian ginseng during pregnancy is not available.

Stimulant use: Siberian ginseng is not recommended for patients using stimulants, even mild ones such as caffeine.

DRUG INTERACTIONS

Antidiabetic agents and insulin: The herb may alter the effects of insulin or other medications.

ADVERSE REACTIONS

In rare cases, the herb may cause altered heart rhythm, elevated blood pressure, palpitations, pericardial pain, tachycardia, and neuropathy. Slight drowsiness immediately after taking the extract has been reported, as has insomnia.

ADMINISTRATION AND DOSAGE

Available in capsule, ethanolic extract, powder, tablet, and tincture forms. Therapy should not exceed 3 months, although a repeat course is feasible. When used for extended periods, extract-free periods of 2-3 weeks are recommended between courses of therapy.

Adults

Daily Dosage: 2g-3g tea of powdered or cut root daily or aqueous alcoholic extracts (for internal use) daily for up to 3 months; 2g-3g infusion daily in 150mL water. 2mL-3mL fluid extract (1:1g/mL preparation) daily; 10mL-15mL tincture (1:5g/mL preparation) daily.

Pediatrics

No information is available.

St. John's Wort

EFFECTS

St. John's wort (*Hypericum perforatum*) has demonstrated antidepressant properties as well as anxiolytic, anti-inflammatory, analgesic, and antimicrobial actions.

COMMON USAGE

Accepted uses: Commission E approves of St. John's wort for oral use to treat depressive moods, post-vegetative disturbances, anxiety or nervous unrest, and dyspeptic complaints (oily preparation only). St. John's wort is used primarily for mild to moderate depression. Multiple controlled clinical trials demonstrate the effectiveness of extracts for this use, including for major depression. It may reduce symptoms of seasonal affective disorder. Commission E approves of its use topically (oily preparations) for acute injuries and bruises, myalgias, and first-degree burns.

Unproven uses: St John's wort is often used as an antiviral, an antibacterial (internally and in eardrops for otitis media), and as a topical analgesic or for wound healing. A cream containing *Hypericum* is used to treat mild to moderate atopic dermatitis. It appears to be ineffective as an antiviral agent for people with AIDS. Primarily positive results have been reported from clinical trials using St. John's wort in the treatment of acute otitis media, menopausal symptoms, obesity, fatigue, premenstrual syndrome, and to improve sleep quality and cognitive function.

CONTRAINDICATIONS

St. John's wort is contraindicated in cases of hypersensitivity or allergy to the herb or any of its constituents, as well as in people with a history of photosensitivity.

WARNINGS/PRECAUTIONS

Drug and herb interactions: St. John's wort interacts with numerous medications (see below). Caution is advised.

Fertility: Genotoxic actions are suggested but not proven. The herb is mutagenic to sperm.

Photosensitivity: Avoid direct sun exposure while taking St. John's wort in cases of previous photosensitization to any chemicals.

Pregnancy and breastfeeding: Contraindicated during pregnancy. Scientific evidence for the safe use of St. John's wort during lactation is not available.

DRUG INTERACTIONS

St. John's wort appears to act in clinically significant ways with numerous medicines, in some cases decreasing the effect or concentration of the drug. No other supplement has as many documented drug interactions.

Acitretin: Avoid concomitant use due to the theoretically increased risk of unplanned pregnancy and birth defects.

Aminolevulinic acid: Avoid concomitant use due to potentially increased risk of phototoxic reaction.

Amiodarone: Avoid concomitant use due to the theoretically increased risk of reduced drug levels.

Amsacrine: Avoid concomitant use due to possible reduced drug efficacy, as indicated by in vitro studies.

Anesthetics: Avoid concomitant use due to increased risk of cardiovascular collapse or delayed emergence from anesthesia.

Anticoagulants: Avoid concomitant use due to possible risk of reduced anticoagulant efficacy.

Antidiabetic agents: Avoid concomitant use due to the risk of hypoglycemia.

Barbiturates: Avoid concomitant use due to the risk of decreased central nervous system depressant effect with the drug.

Benzodiazepines: Avoid concomitant use due to the risk for reduced drug efficacy.

Beta-adrenergic blockers: Avoid concomitant use due to the (theoretical) risk of reduced drug efficacy.

Buspirone: Avoid concomitant use due to the increased risk for serotonin syndrome.

Calcium channel blockers: Avoid concomitant use due to the risk of decreased drug efficacy.

Carbamazepine: Avoid concomitant use due to the risk for altered drug blood concentrations.

Chlorzoxazone: Avoid concomitant use due to the risk of reduced drug efficacy.

Clozapine: Avoid concomitant use due to the theoretically increased risk of reduced drug efficacy.

Contraceptives (combination): Avoid concomitant use due to the risk of decreased contraceptive efficacy.

Cyclophosphamide: Avoid concomitant use due to the theoretically increased risk of reduced drug efficacy.

Cyclosporine: Avoid concomitant use due to the risk of decreased drug levels and risk for acute transplant rejection.

Debrisoquin: Avoid concomitant use due to the risk of reduced drug efficacy.

Digoxin: Avoid concomitant use due to the risk of reduced drug efficacy.

Drugs metabolized by CYP450 3A4, 1A2, or 2E1: Avoid concomitant use. St. John's wort could potentially decrease drug concentrations and lessen drug effectiveness.

Erlotinib: Avoid concomitant use due to the theoretically increased risk for reduced drug plasma concentrations and clinical efficacy.

Estrogens: Avoid concomitant use due to the theoretically increased risk of reduced drug efficacy.

Etoposide: Avoid concomitant use due to the risk for reduced drug efficacy.

Fenfluramine: Avoid concomitant use due to the increased risk of serotonin syndrome.

Ginkgo biloba: Avoid concomitant use given the increased risk for changes in mental status.

HMG CoA reductase inhibitors (statins): Avoid concomitant use due to the risk for reduced drug efficacy.

Imatinib: Avoid concomitant use due to the risk for elevated drug clearance.

Irinotecan: Avoid concomitant use due to the risk for reduced drug effectiveness and treatment failure.

Loperamide: Avoid concomitant use due to the risk for delirium with symptoms of confusion, agitation, and disorientation.

Methadone: Avoid concomitant use due to the risk for reduced drug levels and increased risk for withdrawal symptoms.

Monoamine oxidase inhibitors: Avoid concomitant use due to the theoretically increased risk for serotonin syndrome or hypertensive crisis.

Nefazodone: Avoid concomitant use due to the increased risk for serotonin syndrome.

Non-nucleoside reverse transcriptase inhibitors: Avoid concomitant use due to the risk for decreased drug concentrations and the increased risk for antiretroviral resistance, and treatment failure.

Opioid analgesics: Avoid concomitant use due to the risk for increased sedation.

Paclitaxel: Avoid concomitant use due to the theoretically increased risk for reduced drug effectiveness.

Phenytoin: Avoid concomitant use due to the theoretically increased risk for reduced drug effectiveness.

Photosensitization drugs: Avoid concomitant use due to the theoretically increased risk for a photosensitivity reaction.

Protease inhibitors: Avoid concomitant use due to the risk for decreased drug concentrations and greater risk for antiretroviral resistance, and treatment failure.

Reserpine: Avoid concomitant use due to the risk for reduced drug effectiveness.

Selective serotonin reuptake inhibitors: Avoid concomitant use due to the increased risk for serotonin syndrome.

Serotonin agonists: Avoid concomitant use due to the theoretically increased risk for additive serotonergic effects and cerebral vasoconstriction disorders.

Sirolimus: Avoid concomitant use due to the theoretically increased risk for subtherapeutic drug levels, resulting in possible transplant rejection.

Tacrolimus: Avoid concomitant use due to the theoretically increased risk for subtherapeutic drug levels, resulting in possible transplant rejection.

Tamoxifen: Avoid concomitant use due to the theoretically increased risk for reduced drug efficacy.

Theophylline: Avoid concomitant use due to the risk for reduced drug efficacy.

Trazodone: Avoid concomitant use due to the increased risk of serotonin syndrome.

Tricyclic antidepressants: Avoid concomitant use due to the increased risk for serotonin syndrome.

Venlafaxine: Avoid concomitant use due to the theoretically increased risk for serotonin syndrome.

Verapamil: Avoid concomitant use due to the risk for decreased drug bioavailability.

ADVERSE REACTIONS

Common side effects include dry mouth, dizziness, diarrhea, nausea, fatigue, and increased sensitivity to the sun. Also possible: skin rash, frequent urination, edema, anorgasmia, hypersensitivity, neuropathy, anxiety, and hypomania. St. John's wort may elevate thyroid-stimulating hormone levels and precipitate hypothyroidism.

ADMINISTRATION AND DOSAGE

St. John's wort is available in capsule, liquid extract, tablet, and tea forms. Preparations are often standardized to hypericin (0.3%) and/or hyperforin (3%) content; marker compounds may not reflect content of other potentially biologically important compounds.

Adults

Daily Dosage: The common dose for most conditions is 300mg of standardized extract (0.3% hypericin content) 3 times/day, or 200mcg-1,000mcg daily of hypericin.

Depression: 300mg standardized extract (0.3% hypericin content 3 times/day; 2g-4g dried herb 3 times/day; 2mL liquid extract (1:1 in 25% ethanol) 3 times/day; 2g-3g dried herb for tea in boiling water as single dose; 2mL-4mL tincture (1:1 in 45% ethanol) 3 times/day.

Premenstrual syndrome: 300mg capsule/tablet (standardized to 900mcg hypericin) daily.

Seasonal affective disorder: 300mg 3 times/day.

Topical use: Various creams and oily preparations are available; use as directed. Note they may only stay stable for a limited time (a few weeks to 6 months).

Pediatrics

Under medical supervision only, oral extract 200mg-400mg in divided doses for children 6-12 years old.

PRODUCT COMPARISON TABLES

This section provides a quick comparison of the ingredients and dosages of common OTC brand-name drugs. The tables are organized alphabetically and include the following:

- Acne Products
- Allergic Rhinitis Products
- Analgesic Products
- Antacid and Heartburn Products
- Antidiarrheal Products
- Antiflatulent Products
- Antifungal Products
- Anitpyretic Products
- Antiseborrheal Products
- Artificial Tear Products
- Canker and Cold Sore Products
- Contact Dermatitis Products
- Cough-Cold-Flu Products
- Dandruff Products

- Diaper Rash Products
- Dry Skin Products
- Headache/Migraine Products
- Hemorrhoidal Products
- Insomnia Products
- Is It a Cold, the Flu, or an Allergy?
- Laxative Products
- Nasal Decongestant/Moisturizing Products
- Ophthalmic Decongestant/Antihistamine Products
- Psoriasis Products
- Smoking Cessation Products
- Weight Management Products
- Wound Care Products

TABLE 1. ACNE PRODUCTS

Brand Name	Ingredient/Strength	Dose
BENZOYL PEROXIDE		
Clean & Clear Continuous Control Acne Cleanser	Benzoyl Peroxide 10%	**Adults & Peds:** Use bid.
Clean & Clear Persa-Gel 10, Maximum Strength	Benzoyl Peroxide 10%	**Adults & Peds:** Use qd-tid.
Clearasil Stay Clear Vanishing Acne Treatment Cream	Benzoyl Peroxide 10%	**Adults & Peds:** Use qd-tid.
Clearasil Total Acne Control	Benzoyl Peroxide 10%	**Adults & Peds:** Use qd-tid.
Clearasil Acne Treatment Tinted Cream	Benzoyl Peroxide 10%	**Adults & Peds:** Use up to tid.
Clearasil Ultra Acne Rapid Action Treatment Vanishing Cream	Benzoyl Peroxide 10%	**Adults & Peds:** Use up to tid.
Neutrogena Clear Pore Cleanser Mask	Benzoyl Peroxide 3.5%	**Adults & Peds:** Use biw-tiw.
Neutrogena On-the-Spot Acne Treatment Vanishing Formula	Benzoyl Peroxide 2.5%	**Adults & Peds:** Apply qd initially, then bid-tid.
Oxy Chill Factor Daily Wash	Benzoyl Peroxide 10%	**Adults & Peds:** Use bid-tid.
Oxy Maximum Daily Wash	Benzoyl Peroxide 10%	**Adults & Peds:** Use bid-tid.
Oxy Spot Treatment	Benzoyl Peroxide 10%	**Adults & Peds:** Use qd-tid.
PanOxyl Aqua Gel Maximum Strength Gel	Benzoyl Peroxide 10%	**Adults & Peds:** Apply qd initially, then bid-tid.
PanOxyl Bar 10% Maximum Strength	Benzoyl Peroxide 10%	**Adults & Peds:** Apply qd initially, then bid-tid.
PanOxyl Facial Bar 5%	Benzoyl Peroxide 5%	**Adults & Peds:** Use qd initially, then bid-tid.
ZAPZYT Maximum Strength Acne Treatment Gel	Benzoyl Peroxide 10%	**Adults & Peds:** Use up to tid. If dryness occurs, use qd or qod.
ZAPZYT Treatment Bar	Benzoyl Peroxide 10%	**Adults & Peds:** Use qd initially, then bid-tid. If dryness occurs, use qd or qod.
SALICYLIC ACID		
Aveeno Clear Complexion Cleansing Bar	Salicylic Acid 0.5%	**Adults & Peds:** Use daily.
Aveeno Clear Complexion Foaming Cleanser	Salicylic Acid 0.5%	**Adults & Peds:** Use daily.
Biore Blemish Fighting Ice Cleanser	Salicylic Acid 2%	**Adults & Peds:** Use qd.
Clean & Clear Advantage Acne Spot Treatment	Salicylic Acid 2%	**Adults & Peds:** Use qd-tid.
Clean & Clear Blackhead Clearing Daily Cleansing Pads	Salicylic Acid 1%	**Adults & Peds:** Use qd.
Clean & Clear Blackhead Clearing Scrub	Salicylic Acid 2%	**Adults & Peds:** Use qd.
Clean & Clear Advantage Oil-Free Acne Moisturizer	Salicylic Acid 0.5%	**Adults & Peds:** Use qd.
Clean & Clear Continuous Control Acne Wash, Oil Free	Salicylic Acid 2%	**Adults & Peds:** Use qd-tid.
Clearasil Stay Clear Acne Fighting Cleansing Wipes	Salicylic Acid 2%	**Adults & Peds:** Use qd-tid.
Clearasil Stay Clear Skin Perfecting Wash	Salicylic Acid 2%	**Adults & Peds:** Use bid.
Clearasil Stay Clear Oil Free Gel Wash	Salicylic Acid 2%	**Adults & Peds:** Use bid.
Clearasil Stay Clear Daily Pore Cleansing Pads	Salicylic Acid 2%	**Adults & Peds:** Use qd-tid.

(Continued)

TABLE 1. ACNE PRODUCTS (cont.)

BRAND NAME	INGREDIENT/STRENGTH	DOSE
Clearasil Stay Clear Daily Facial Scrub	Salicylic Acid 2%	**Adults & Peds:** Use qd.
Clearasil Ultra Acne Clearing Gel Wash	Salicylic Acid 2%	**Adults & Peds:** Use qd.
Clearasil Ultra Daily Face Wash	Salicylic Acid 2%	**Adults & Peds:** Use qd.
Clearasil Ultra Acne Clearing Scrub	Salicylic Acid 2%	**Adults & Peds:** Use qd.
Clearasil Ultra Deep Pore Cleansing Pads	Salicylic Acid 2%	**Adults & Peds:** Use qd-tid.
Neutrogena Advanced Solutions Acne Mark Fading Peel with CelluZyme	Salicylic Acid 2%	**Adults & Peds:** Use biw-tiw.
Neutrogena Blackhead Eliminating Daily Scrub	Salicylic Acid 2%	**Adults & Peds:** Use bid.
Neutrogena Blackhead Eliminating Foaming Pads	Salicylic Acid 0.5%	**Adults & Peds:** Use qd.
Neutrogena Body Clear Body Scrub	Salicylic Acid 2%	**Adults & Peds:** Use qd.
Neutrogena Oil Free Acne Wash Foam Cleanser	Salicylic Acid 2%	**Adults & Peds:** Use bid.
Neutrogena Clear Pore Oil-Eliminating Astringent	Salicylic Acid 2%	**Adults & Peds:** Use qd-tid.
Neutrogena Oil Free Acne Stress Control Power Clear Scrub	Salicylic Acid 2%	**Adults & Peds:** Use qd.
Neutrogena Acne Stress Control 3-in-1 Hydrating Acne Treatment	Salicylic Acid 2%	**Adults & Peds:** Use qd-tid.
Neutrogena Oil Free Acne Wash Cleansing Cloths	Salicylic Acid 2%	**Adults & Peds:** Use qd.
Neutrogena Oil Free Acne Wash Cream Cleanser	Salicylic Acid 2%	**Adults & Peds:** Use qd-bid.
Neutrogena Rapid Clear Acne Defense Face Lotion	Salicylic Acid 2%	**Adults & Peds:** Use qd-tid.
Neutrogena Rapid Clear Acne Eliminating Spot Gel	Salicylic Acid 2%	**Adults & Peds:** Use qd-tid.
Neutrogena Oil-Free Anti-Acne Moisturizer	Salicylic Acid 0.5%	**Adults & Peds:** Use qd initially, then bid-tid. If dryness occurs, use qd or qod.
Noxzema Triple Clean Anti-Blemish Astringent	Salicylic Acid 2%	**Adults & Peds:** Use qd-tid. If dryness occurs, use qd or qod.
Noxzema Triple Clean Anti-Blemish Pads	Salicylic Acid 2%	**Adults & Peds:** Use qd-tid.
Olay Daily Facials Lathering Cleansing Cloths-Clarifying for Combination/Oily Skin	Salicylic Acid (strength NA)	**Adults & Peds:** Apply qd.
Olay Regenerist Daily Regenerating Cleanser	Salicylic Acid	**Adults & Peds:** Use qd.
Olay Total Effects Plus Blemish Control Moisturizer	Salicylic Acid 1.5%	**Adults & Peds:** Apply qd-tid.
Oxy Chill Factor Cleansing Pads	Salicylic Acid 0.2%	**Adults & Peds:** Use qd-tid.
Oxy Maximum Face Scrub	Salicylic Acid 2%	**Adults & Peds:** Use qd-tid.
Oxy Maximum Daily Cleansing Pads	Salicylic Acid 2%	**Adults & Peds:** Use qd-tid.
Oxy Body Wash	Salicylic Acid 2%	**Adults & Peds:** Use qd.

TABLE 1. ACNE PRODUCTS (cont.)

BRAND NAME	INGREDIENT/STRENGTH	DOSE
Phisoderm Anti-Blemish Body Wash	Salicylic Acid 2%	**Adults & Peds:** Use qd.
St. Ives Medicated Apricot Scrub	Salicylic Acid 2%	**Adults & Peds:** Use qd.
Stridex Facewipes to Go with Acne Medication	Salicylic Acid 0.5%	**Adults & Peds:** Use qd-tid.
Stridex Maximum Strength, Alcohol Free	Salicylic Acid 2%	**Adults & Peds:** Use qd-tid.
Stridex Essential Pads with Salicylic Acid	Salicylic Acid 1%	**Adults & Peds:** Use qd-tid.
Stridex Sensitive Skin Pads, Alcohol Free	Salicylic Acid 0.5%	**Adults & Peds:** Use qd-tid.
ZAPZYT Acne Wash Treatment For Face & Body	Salicylic Acid 2%	**Adults & Peds:** Use bid.
ZAPZYT Pore Treatment Gel	Salicylic Acid 2%	**Adults & Peds:** Use qd-tid.
TRICLOSAN		
Noxzema Triple Clean Anti-Bacterial Lathering Cleanser	Triclosan 0.3%	**Adults & Peds ≥6 months:** Use qd each time skin is cleansed.

TABLE 2. ALLERGIC RHINITIS PRODUCTS

BRAND NAME	INGREDIENT/STRENGTH	DOSE
ANTIHISTAMINE		
Alavert Oral Disintegrating Tablets	Loratadine 10mg	**Adults & Peds ≥6 yrs:** 1 tab qd. **Max:** 1 tab q24h.
Alavert 24-Hour Allergy Tablets	Loratadine 10mg	**Adults & Peds ≥6 yrs:** 1 tab qd. **Max:** 1 tab q24h.
Benadryl Allergy Quick Dissolve Strips	Diphenhydramine HCl 25mg	**Adults & Peds ≥12 yrs:** Dissolve 1-2 strips on tongue q4-6h. **Max:** 6 doses q24h.
Benadryl Allergy Kapgels	Diphenhydramine HCl 25mg	**Adults & Peds ≥12 yrs:** 1-2 caps q4-6h. **Peds 6-<12 yrs:** 1 cap q4-6h. **Max:** 6 doses q24h.
Benadryl Allergy Ultratab	Diphenhydramine HCl 25mg	**Adults & Peds ≥12 yrs:** 1-2 tabs q4-6h. **Peds 6-<12 yrs:** 1 tab q4-6h. **Max:** 6 doses q24h.
Benadryl Liqui-Gels	Diphenhydramine HCl 25mg	**Adults & Peds ≥12 yrs:** 1-2 softgels q4-6h. **6-<12 yrs:** 1 softgel q4-6h. **Max:** 6 doses q24h.
Children's Benadryl Allergy Liquid	Diphenhydramine HCl 12.5mg/5mL	**Peds 6-12 yrs:** 1-2 tsp (5-10mL) q4-6h. **Max:** 6 doses q24h.
Chlor-Trimeton 4-Hour Allergy Tablets	Chlorpheniramine Maleate 4mg	**Adults & Peds ≥12 yrs:** 1 tab q4-6h. **Max:** 6 tabs q24h. **Peds 6-<12 yrs:** ½ tab q4-6h. **Max:** 3 tabs q24h.
Claritin 24 Hour Allergy Tablets	Loratadine 10mg	**Adults & Peds ≥6 yrs:** 1 tab qd. **Max:** 1 tab q24h.
Claritin Children's Chewables	Loratadine 5mg	**Adults & Peds ≥6 yrs:** 2 tabs qd. **Max:** 2 tabs q24h. **Peds 2-<6 yrs:** 1 tab qd. **Max:** 1 tab q24h.
Claritin Children's Syrup	Loratadine 5mg/5mL	**Adults & Peds ≥6 yrs:** 2 tsp qd. **Max:** 2 tsp q24h. **Peds 2-<6 yrs:** 1 tsp qd. **Max:** 1 tsp q24h.
Claritin RediTabs	Loratadine 10mg	**Adults & Peds ≥6 yrs:** 1 tab qd. **Max:** 1 tab q24h.
Zyrtec Tablets	Cetirizine 10mg	**Adults 18-64 yrs & Peds ≥6 yrs:** 1 tab q24h. **Max:** 1 tab q24h.
Zyrtec Children's Syrup	Cetirizine 5mg/5mL	**Adults & Peds 6-64 yrs:** 1-2 tsp qd. **Max:** 2 tsp q24h. **Adults ≥65 yrs:** 1 tsp qd. **Max:** 1 tsp q24h. **Peds 2-<6 yrs:** ½ tsp qd-bid. **Max:** 1 tsp q24h.
Zyrtec Children's Chewables 5mg	Cetirizine 5mg	**Adults & Peds 6-64 yrs:** 1-2 tabs q24h. **Max:** 2 tabs q24h. **Adults ≥65 yrs:** 1 tab q24h. **Max:** 1 tab q24h.
Zyrtec Children's Chewables 10mg	Cetirizine 10mg	**Adults & Peds ≥6 yrs:** 1 tab q24h. **Adults ≥65 yrs:** Ask doctor. **Max:** 1 tab qd.
Zyrtec Children's Hive Relief Syrup	Cetirizine 5mg/5mL	**Adults & Peds 6-64yrs:** 1-2 tsp (5-10mL) q24h. **Max:** 2 tsp (10mL) q24h. **Adults ≥65:** 1 tsp q24h. **Max:** 1 tsp (5mL) q24h.
ANTIHISTAMINE COMBINATIONS		
Advil Allergy Sinus Caplets	Chlorpheniramine Maleate/ Ibuprofen/Pseudoephedrine 2mg-200mg-30mg	**Adults & Peds ≥12 yrs:** 1 tab q4-6h. **Max:** 6 tabs q24h.
Alavert D-12 Hour Allergy and Sinus Tablets	Loratadine/Pseudoephedrine Sulfate 5mg-120mg	**Adults & Peds ≥12 yrs:** 1 tab q12h. **Max:** 2 tabs q24h.
Benadryl Severe Allergy & Sinus Headache Caplets	Diphenhydramine HCl/ Acetaminophen/Phenylephrine HCl 25mg-325mg-5mg	**Adults & Peds ≥12 yrs:** 2 tabs q4h. **Max:** 12 tabs q24h.
Benadryl-D Allergy & Sinus Tablets	Diphenhydramine/Phenylephrine HCl 25mg-10mg	**Adults & Peds ≥12 yrs:** 1 tab q4h. **Max:** 6 doses q24h.
Children's Benadryl-D Allergy & Sinus Liquid	Diphenhydramine HCl/ Phenylephrine 12.5mg-5mg/5mL	**Adults & Peds ≥12 yrs:** 2 tsp q4h. **Peds 6-<12 yrs:** 1 tsp q4h. **Max:** 6 doses q24h.

(Continued)

TABLE 2. ALLERGIC RHINITIS PRODUCTS (cont.)

Brand Name	Ingredient/Strength	Dose
Claritin-D 12 Hour Allergy & Congestion Tablets	Loratadine/Pseudoephedrine Sulfate 5mg-120mg	**Adults & Peds ≥12 yrs:** 1 tab q12h. **Max:** 2 tabs q24h.
Claritin-D 24 Hour Allergy & Congestion Tablets	Loratadine/Pseudoephedrine Sulfate 10mg-240mg	**Adults & Peds ≥12 yrs:** 1 tab qd. **Max:** 1 tab q24h.
Dimetapp Elixir Cold & Allergy	Brompheniramine/Phenylephrine 1mg-2.5mg/5mL	**Adults & Peds ≥12 yrs:** 4 tsp (20mL) q4h. **Peds 6-<12 yrs:** 2 tsp (10mL) q4h. **Max:** 6 doses q24h.
Dimetapp Children's Chewable Tablets	Brompheniramine/Phenylephrine 1mg-2.5mg	**Peds 6-<12 yrs:** 2 tabs q4h. **Max:** 6 doses q24h.
Sudafed PE Sinus & Allergy Tablets	Chlorpheniramine/Phenylephrine HCl 4mg-10mg	**Adults ≥12 yrs:** 1 tab q4h. **Max:** 6 tabs q24h.
Tylenol Allergy Complete Multi-Symptom Cool Burst Caplets	Chlorpheniramine Maleate/ Acetaminophen/Phenylephrine HCl 2mg-325mg-5mg	**Adults & Peds ≥12 yrs:** 2 tabs q4h. **Max:** 12 tabs q24h.
Tylenol Allergy Complete Nighttime Cool Burst Caplets	Diphenhydramine HCl/ Acetaminophen/Phenylephrine HCl 25mg-325mg-5mg	**Adults & Peds ≥12 yrs:** 2 tabs q4h. **Max:** 12 tabs q24h.
Tylenol Severe Allergy Caplets	Diphenhydramine HCl/ Acetaminophen 12.5mg-500mg	**Adults & Peds ≥12 yrs:** 2 tabs q4-6h. **Max:** 8 tabs q24h.
Zyrtec-D	Cetirizine/Pseudoephedrine HCl 5mg-120mg	**Adults 12-65 yrs:** 1 tab q12h. **Max:** 2 tabs q24h.
TOPICAL NASAL DECONGESTANTS		
4-Way Fast Acting Nasal Decongestant Spray	Phenylephrine HCl 1%	**Adults & Peds ≥12 yrs:** Instill 2-3 sprays per nostril q4h.
4-Way Mentholated Nasal Decongestant Spray	Phenylephrine HCl 1%	**Adults & Peds ≥12 yrs:** Instill 2-3 sprays per nostril q4h.
Afrin No Drip Extra Moisturizing Nasal Spray	Oxymetazoline HCl 0.05%	**Adults & Peds ≥6 yrs:** Instill 2-3 sprays per nostril q10-12h. **Max:** 2 doses q24h.
Afrin No Drip Sinus Nasal Spray	Oxymetazoline HCl 0.05%	**Adults & Peds ≥6 yrs:** Instill 2-3 sprays per nostril q10-12h. **Max:** 2 doses q24h.
Afrin No Drip Original Pump Mist Nasal Spray	Oxymetazoline HCl 0.05%	**Adults & Peds ≥6 yrs:** Instill 2-3 sprays per nostril q10-12h. **Max:** 2 doses q24h.
Afrin No Drip All Night 12 Hour Pump Mist	Oxymetazoline HCl 0.05%	**Adults & Peds ≥6 yrs:** Instill 2-3 sprays per nostril q10-12h. **Max:** 2 doses q24h.
Afrin No Drip Severe Congestion Nasal Spray	Oxymetazoline HCl 0.05%	**Adults & Peds ≥6 yrs:** Instill 2-3 sprays per nostril q10-12h. **Max:** 2 doses q24h.
Benzedrex Inhaler	Propylhexedrine 250mg	**Adults & Peds ≥6 yrs:** Inhale 2 sprays per nostril q2h.
Dristan 12 Hour Nasal Spray	Oxymetazoline HCl 0.05%	**Adults & Peds ≥12 yrs:** Instill 2-3 sprays per nostril q10-12h. **Max:** 2 doses q24h.
Mucinex Full Force Nasal Spray	Oxymetazoline HCl 0.05%	**Adults & Peds ≥6 yrs:** Instill 2-3 sprays per nostril q10-12h. **Max:** 2 doses q24h.
Neo-Synephrine Nasal Spray Nighttime Spray	Oxymetazoline HCl 0.05%	**Adults & Peds ≥6 yrs:** Instill 2-3 sprays per nostril q10-12h. **Max:** 2 doses per 24 hours.
Neo-Synephrine Extra Strength Nasal Spray	Phenylephrine HCl 1%	**Adults & Peds ≥12 yrs:** Instill 2-3 sprays per nostril q4h.
Neo-Synephrine Mild Formula Nasal Spray	Phenylephrine HCl 0.25%	**Adults & Peds ≥6 yrs:** Instill 2-3 sprays per nostril q4h.
Neo-Synephrine Regular Strength Nasal Decongestant Spray	Phenylephrine HCl 0.5%	**Adults & Peds ≥12 yrs:** Instill 2-3 sprays per nostril q4h.
Nostrilla Original Fast Relief	Oxymetazoline HCl 0.05%	**Adults & Peds ≥6 yrs:** Instill 2-3 sprays per nostril q10-12h. **Max:** 2 doses q24h.

TABLE 2. ALLERGIC RHINITIS PRODUCTS (cont.)

Brand Name	Ingredient/Strength	Dose
Nostrilla Complete Congestion Relief	Oxymetazoline HCl 0.05%	**Adults & Peds ≥6 yrs:** Instill 2-3 sprays per nostril q10-12h. **Max:** 2 doses q24h.
Sudafed Sinus Congestion 12 Hour Nasal Spray	Oxymetazoline HCl 0.05%	**Adults & Peds ≥6 yrs:** Instill 2-3 sprays per nostril q10-12h. **Max:** 2 doses q24h.
Sudafed Sinus Cold 12 Hour Nasal Spray	Oxymetazoline HCl 0.05%	**Adults & Peds ≥6 yrs:** Instill 2-3 sprays per nostril q10-12h. **Max:** 2 doses q24h.
Vicks Sinex 12 Hour Ultra Fine Mist For Sinus Relief	Oxymetazoline HCl 0.05%	**Adults & Peds ≥6 yrs:** Instill 2-3 sprays per nostril q10-12h. **Max:** 2 doses q24h.
Vicks Sinex 12 Hour Nasal Spray	Oxymetazoline HCl 0.05%	**Adults & Peds ≥6 yrs:** Instill 2-3 sprays per nostril q10-12h. **Max:** 2 doses per day.
Vicks Sinex Nasal Spray For Sinus Relief	Phenylephrine HCl 0.5%	**Adults & Peds ≥12 yrs:** Instill 2-3 sprays per nostril q4h.
Zicam Extreme Congestion Relief	Oxymetazoline HCl 0.05%	**Adults & Peds ≥6 yrs:** Instill 2-3 sprays per nostril q10-12h. **Max:** 2 doses q24h.
Zicam Intense Sinus Relief	Oxymetazoline HCl 0.05%	**Adults & Peds ≥6 yrs:** Instill 2-3 sprays per nostril q10-12h. **Max:** 2 doses q24h.

TOPICAL NASAL MOISTURIZERS

Brand Name	Ingredient/Strength	Dose
4-Way Saline Moisturizing Mist	Water, Boric Acid, Glycerin, Sodium Chloride, Sodium Borate, Eucalyptol, Menthol, Polysorbate 80, Benzalkonium Chloride	**Adults & Peds ≥2 yrs:** Instill 2-3 sprays per nostril prn.
Ayr Allergy & Sinus Nasal Mist	Sodium Chloride 2.65%	**Adults & Peds:** Spray bid-tid prn.
Ayr Baby's Saline Nose Spray, Drops	Sodium Chloride 0.65%	**Peds:** Instill 2-6 drops in each nostril.
Ayr Saline Nasal Gel With Soothing Aloe	Water, Methyl Gluceth 10, Propylene Glycol, Glycerin, Glyceryl Polymethacrylate, Triethanolamine, Aloe Barbadensis Leaf Juice (Aloe Vera Gel), PEG/PPG 18/18 Dimethicone, Carbomer, Poloxamer 184, Sodium Chloride, Xanthan Gum, Diazolidinyl Urea, Methyl-paraben, Propylparaben, Glycine Soja Oil (Soybean), Geranium Maculatum Oil, Tocopheryl Acetate, Blue 1	**Adults & Peds:** Apply to nostril prn.
Ayr Saline Nasal Gel, No-Drip Sinus Spray	Water, Sodium Carbomethyl Starch, Propylene Glycol, Glycerin, Aloe Barbadensis Leaf Juice (Aloe Vera Gel), Sodium Chloride, Cetyl Pyridinium Chloride, Citric Acid, Disodium EDTA, Glycine Soja (Soybean Oil), Tocopheryl Acetate, Benzyl Alcohol, Benzalkonium Chloride, Geranium Maculatum Oil	**Adults & Peds:** Instill 1 spray in each nostril prn.
Ayr Saline Nasal Mist	Sodium Chloride 0.65%	**Adults & Peds:** Instill 2 sprays per nostril prn.
ENTSOL Mist, Buffered Hypertonic Nasal Irrigation Mist	Purified Water, Sodium Chloride, Sodium Phosphate Dibasic Edetate Disodium, Potassium Phosphate Monobasic, Benzalkonium Chloride	**Adults & Peds:** Instill 1-2 sprays per nostril prn.
ENTSOL Spray, Buffered Hypertonic Saline Nasal Spray	Purified Water, Sodium Chloride Phosphate Dibasic, Potassium Phosphate Monobasic	**Adults & Peds:** Instill 1 spray per nostril 2-6 times daily.
ENTSOL Nasal Gel with Aloe and Vitamin E	Water (Purified), Propylene Glycol, Aloe, Glycerin, Dimethicone Copolyol, Poloxamer 184, Methyl Gluceth 10, Triethanolamine, Carbomer, Sodium Chloride, Vitamin E, Disodium EDTA, Xanthan Gum, Benzalkonium Chloride	**Adults & Peds:** Use prn.

(Continued)

TABLE 2. ALLERGIC RHINITIS PRODUCTS (cont.)

Brand Name	Ingredient/Strength	Dose
Little Noses Saline Spray/Drops, Non-Medicated	Sodium Chloride 0.65%	**Peds:** 2-6 drops or sprays per nostril as directed.
Nostrilla Conditioning Double Moisture	Benzalkonium Chloride Solution, Carboxymethylcellulose Sodium, Eucalyptol, Glycine, Hyaluronic Acid Sodium, Polyethylene Glycol, Povidone, Propylene Glycol, Sodium Chloride (as 1.9% saline solution), Spearmint Oil, Wintergreen Oil, Water	**Adults & Peds:** Spray once per nostril prn.
Ocean Premium Saline Nasal Spray	Sodium Chloride 0.65%	**Adults & Peds ≥6 yrs:** Instill 2 sprays per nostril prn.
Simply Saline Sterile Saline Nasal Mist	Sodium Chloride 0.9%	**Adults & Peds:** Use prn as directed.
SinoFresh Nasal & Sinus Care	Eucalyptus Globules 20x, Kalium Bichromicum 30x, Benzalkonium Chloride, Cetylpyridium Chloride, Dibasic Sodium Phosphate, Essential Oil Blend (wintergreen, spearmint, peppermint, and eucalyptus oils), Monobasic Sodium Phosphate, Polysorbate 80, Propylene Glycol, Purified Water, Sodium Chloride, Sorbitol Solution	**Adults & Peds:** Instill 1-2 sprays per nostril bid.
MISCELLANEOUS		
NasalCrom Nasal Allergy Symptom Prevention and Controller, Nasal Spray	Cromolyn Sodium 5.2mg	**Adults & Peds ≥2 yrs:** Instill 1 spray per nostril q4-6h. **Max:** 6 doses q24h.
Similasan Hay Fever Relief, Non-Drowsy Formula, Nasal Spray	Cardiospermum HPUS 6X, Galphimia Glauca HPUS 6X, Luffa Operculata HPUS 6X, Sabadilla HPUS 6x	**Adults & Peds:** Instill 1 to 3 sprays in each nostril prn.
Zicam Allergy Relief, Homeopathic Nasal Solution, Pump	Luffa Operculata 4x, 12x, 30x, Galphimia Glauca 12x, 30x, Histaminum Hydrochloricum 12x, 30x, 200x, Sulphur 12x, 30x, 200x	**Adults & Peds ≥6 yrs:** Instill 1 spray per nostril q4h.

TABLE 3. ANALGESIC PRODUCTS

BRAND NAME	INGREDIENT/STRENGTH	DOSE
ACETAMINOPHEN		
Anacin Extra Strength Aspirin Free Tablets	Acetaminophen 500mg	**Adults & Peds ≥12 yrs:** 2 tabs q6h. **Max:** 8 tabs q24h.
FeverAll Childrens' Suppositories	Acetaminophen 120mg	**Peds 3-6 yrs:** 1 supp. q4-6h. **Max:** 6 supp. q24h.
FeverAll Infants' Suppositories	Acetaminophen 80mg	**Peds 3-11 months:** 1 supp. q6h. **12-36 months:** 1 supp. q4h. **Max:** 6 supp. q24h.
FeverAll Jr. Strength Suppositories	Acetaminophen 325mg	**Peds 6-12 yrs:** 1 supp. q4-6h. **Max:** 6 supp. q24h.
Tylenol 8 Hour Caplets	Acetaminophen 650mg	**Adults & Peds ≥12 yrs:** 2 tabs q8h prn. **Max:** 6 tabs q24h.
Tylenol Arthritis Caplets	Acetaminophen 650mg	**Adults:** 2 tabs q8h prn. **Max:** 6 tabs q24h.
Tylenol Arthritis Geltabs	Acetaminophen 650mg	**Adults:** 2 tabs q8h prn. **Max:** 6 tabs q24h.
Tylenol Children's Meltaways Tablets	Acetaminophen 80mg	**Peds 2-3 yrs (24-35 lbs):** 2 tabs. **4-5 yrs (36-47 lbs):** 3 tabs. **6-8 yrs (48-59 lbs):** 4 tabs. **9-10 yrs (60-71 lbs):** 5 tabs. **11 yrs (72-95 lbs):** 6 tabs.
Tylenol Children's Suspension	Acetaminophen 160mg/5mL	**Peds 2-3 yrs (24-35 lbs):** 1 tsp (5mL). **4-5 yrs (36-47 lbs):** 1.5 tsp (7.5mL). **6-8 yrs (48-59 lbs):** 2 tsp (10mL). **9-10 yrs (60-71 lbs):** 2.5 tsp (12.5mL). **11 yrs (72-95 lbs):** 3 tsp (15mL). May repeat q4h. **Max:** 5 doses q24h.
Tylenol Extra Strength Caplets	Acetaminophen 500mg	**Adults & Peds ≥12 yrs:** 2 tabs q4-6h prn. **Max:** 8 tabs q24h.
Tylenol Extra Strength Cool Caplets	Acetaminophen 500mg	**Adults & Peds ≥12 yrs:** 2 tabs q4-6h prn. **Max:** 8 tabs q24h.
Tylenol Extra Strength Rapid Release Gelcaps	Acetaminophen 500mg	**Adults & Peds ≥ 12 yrs:** 2 caps q4-6h prn. **Max:** 8 caps q24h.
Tylenol Extra Strength Rapid Blast Liquid	Acetaminophen 1000mg/30mL	**Adults & Peds ≥12 yrs:** 2 tbl (30mL) q4-6h prn. **Max:** 8 tbl (120mL) q24h.
Tylenol Extra Strength EZ Tablets	Acetaminophen 500mg	**Adults & Peds ≥12 yrs:** 2 tabs q4-6h prn. **Max:** 8 tabs q24h.
Tylenol Infants' Drops	Acetaminophen 80mg/0.8mL	**Peds 2-3 yrs (24-35 lbs):** 1.6 mL q4h prn. **Max:** 5 doses (8mL) q24h.
Tylenol Junior Meltaways Tablets	Acetaminophen 160mg	**Peds 6-8 yrs (48-59 lbs):** 2 tabs. **9-10 yrs (60-71 lbs):** 2.5 tabs. **11 yrs (72-95 lbs):** 3 tabs. **12 yrs (≥96 lbs):** 4 tabs. May repeat q4h. **Max:** 5 doses q24h.
Tylenol Regular Strength Tablets	Acetaminophen 325mg	**Adults & Peds ≥12 yrs:** 2 tabs q4-6h prn. **Max:** 12 tabs q24h. **Peds 6-11 yrs:** 1 tab q4-6h. **Max:** 5 tabs q24h.
ACETAMINOPHEN COMBINATIONS		
Anacin Advanced Headache Tablets	Acetaminophen/Aspirin/Caffeine 250mg-250mg-65mg	**Adults & Peds ≥12 yrs:** 2 tabs q6h. **Max:** 8 tabs q24h.
Excedrin Back & Body Caplets	Acetaminophen/Aspirin Buffered 250mg-250mg	**Adults & Peds ≥12 yrs:** 2 tabs q6h. **Max:** 8 tabs q24h.
Excedrin Extra Strength Caplets	Acetaminophen/Aspirin/Caffeine 250mg-250mg-65mg	**Adults & Peds ≥12 yrs:** 2 tabs q6h. **Max:** 8 tabs q24h.
Excedrin Extra Strength Geltabs	Acetaminophen/Aspirin/Caffeine 250mg-250mg-65mg	**Adults & Peds ≥12 yrs:** 2 tabs q6h. **Max:** 8 tabs q24h.
Excedrin Extra Strength Express Gels	Acetaminophen/Aspirin/Caffeine 250mg-250mg-65mg	**Adults & Peds ≥12 yrs:** 2 tabs q6h. **Max:** 8 tabs q24h.

(Continued)

TABLE 3. ANALGESIC PRODUCTS (cont.)

Brand Name	Ingredient/Strength	Dose
Excedrin Extra Strength Tablets	Acetaminophen/Aspirin/Caffeine 250mg-250mg-65mg	**Adults & Peds ≥12 yrs:** 2 tabs q6h. **Max:** 8 tabs q24h.
Excedrin Migraine Caplets	Acetaminophen/Aspirin/Caffeine 250mg-250mg-65mg	**Adults:** 2 tabs prn. **Max:** 2 tabs q24h.
Excedrin Migraine Geltabs	Acetaminophen/Aspirin/Caffeine 250mg-250mg-65mg	**Adults:** 2 tabs prn. **Max:** 2 tabs q24h.
Excedrin Migraine Tablets	Acetaminophen/Aspirin/Caffeine 250mg-250mg-65mg	**Adults:** 2 tabs prn. **Max:** 2 tabs q24h.
Excedrin Sinus Headache Caplets	Acetaminophen/Phenylephrine HCl 325mg-5mg	**Adults & Peds ≥12 yrs:** 2 tabs q4h. **Max:** 12 tabs q24h.
Excedrin Tension Headache Caplets	Acetaminophen/Caffeine 500mg-65mg	**Adults & Peds ≥12 yrs:** 2 tabs q6h. **Max:** 8 tabs q24h.
Excedrin Tension Headache Express Gels	Acetaminophen/Caffeine 500mg-65mg	**Adults & Peds ≥12 yrs:** 2 tabs q6h. **Max:** 8 tabs q24h.
Excedrin Tension Headache Geltabs	Acetaminophen/Caffeine 500mg-65mg	**Adults & Peds ≥12 yrs:** 2 tabs q6h. **Max:** 8 tabs q24h.
Goody's Body Pain Powder	Acetaminophen/Aspirin 325mg-500mg	**Adults & Peds ≥12 yrs:** 1 powder q4-6h. **Max:** 4 powders q24h.
Goody's Cool Orange	Acetaminophen/Aspirin/Caffeine 325mg-500mg-65mg	**Adults & Peds ≥12 yrs:** 1 powder q6h. **Max:** 4 powders q24h.
Goody's Extra Strength Headache Powders	Acetaminophen/Aspirin/Caffeine 260mg-520mg-32.5mg	**Adults & Peds ≥12 yrs:** 1 powder q4-6h. **Max:** 4 powders q24h.
Midol Menstrual Complete Caplets	Acetaminophen/Caffeine/Pyrilamine Maleate 500mg-60mg-15mg	**Adults & Peds ≥12 yrs:** 2 tabs q6h. **Max:** 8 tabs q24h.
Midol Menstrual Complete Gelcaps	Acetaminophen/Caffeine/Pyrilamine Maleate 500mg-60mg-15mg	**Adults & Peds ≥12 yrs:** 2 caps q6h. **Max:** 8 caps q24h.
Midol Teen Formula Caplets	Acetaminophen/Pamabrom 500mg-25mg	**Adults & Peds ≥12 yrs:** 2 tabs q6h. **Max:** 8 tabs q24h.
Pamprin Cramp Caplets	Acetaminophen/Magnesium Salicylate/Pamabrom 250mg-250mg-25mg	**Adults & Peds ≥12 yrs:** 2 tabs q4-6h. **Max:** 8 tabs q24h.
Pamprin Max Caplets	Acetaminophen/Aspirin/Caffeine 250mg-250mg-65mg	**Adults & Peds ≥12 yrs:** 2 tabs q4-6h. **Max:** 8 tabs q24h.
Pamprin Multi-Symptom Caplets	Acetaminophen/Pamabrom/Pyrilamine 500mg-25mg-15mg	**Adults & Peds ≥12 yrs:** 2 tabs q4-6h. **Max:** 8 tabs q24h.
Premsyn PMS Caplets	Acetaminophen/Pamabrom/Pyrilamine 500mg-25mg-15mg	**Adults & Peds ≥12 yrs:** 2 tabs q4-6h. **Max:** 8 tabs q24h.
Vanquish Caplets	Acetaminophen/Aspirin/Caffeine 194mg-227mg-33mg	**Adults & Peds ≥12 yrs:** 2 tabs q6h. **Max:** 8 tabs q24h.
ACETAMINOPHEN/SLEEP AIDS		
Excedrin PM Caplets	Acetaminophen/Diphenhydramine 500mg-38mg	**Adults & Peds ≥12 yrs:** 2 tabs qhs.
Excedrin PM Tablets	Acetaminophen/Diphenhydramine Citrate 500mg-38mg	**Adults & Peds ≥12 yrs:** 2 tabs qhs.
Goody's PM Powder	Acetaminophen/Diphenhydramine 1000mg-76mg/dose	**Adults & Peds ≥12 yrs:** 1 packet (2 powders) qhs.
Tylenol PM Caplets	Acetaminophen/Diphenhydramine 500mg-25mg	**Adults & Peds ≥12 yrs:** 2 tabs qhs.
Tylenol PM Rapid Release Gels	Acetaminophen/Diphenhydramine 500mg-25mg	**Adults & Peds ≥12 yrs:** 2 caps qhs.

TABLE 3. ANALGESIC PRODUCTS (cont.)

BRAND NAME	INGREDIENT/STRENGTH	DOSE
Tylenol PM Geltabs	Acetaminophen/Diphenhydramine 500mg-25mg	**Adults & Peds ≥12 yrs:** 2 tabs qhs.
Tylenol PM Vanilla Liquid	Acetaminophen/Diphenhydramine 1000mg-50mg/30mL	**Adults & Peds ≥12 yrs:** 2 tbl (30mL) qhs. **Max:** 8 tbl (120mL) q24h.
NSAIDS		
Advil Caplets	Ibuprofen 200mg	**Adults & Peds ≥12 yrs:** 1-2 tabs q4-6h. **Max:** 6 tabs q24h.
Advil Children's Suspension	Ibuprofen 100mg/5mL	**Peds 2-3 yrs (24-35 lbs):** 1 tsp (5mL). **4-5 yrs (36-47 lbs):** 1.5 tsp (7.5mL). **6-8 yrs (48-59 lbs):** 2 tsp (10mL). **9-10 yrs (60-71 lbs):** 2.5 tsp (12.5mL). **11 yrs (72-95 lbs):** 3 tsp (15mL). May repeat q6-8h. **Max:** 4 doses q24h.
Advil Gel Caplets	Ibuprofen 200mg	**Adults & Peds ≥12 yrs:** 1-2 tabs q4-6h. **Max:** 6 tabs q24h.
Advil Infants' Concentrated Drops	Ibuprofen 50mg/1.25mL	**Peds 6-11 months (12-17 lbs):** 1.25mL. **12-23 months (18-23 lbs):** 1.875mL. May repeat q6-8h. **Max:** 4 doses q24h.
Advil Liqui-Gels	Ibuprofen 200mg	**Adults & Peds ≥12 yrs:** 1-2 caps q4-6h. **Max:** 6 caps q24h.
Advil Migraine Capsules	Ibuprofen 200mg	**Adults:** 2 caps prn. **Max:** 2 caps q24h.
Advil Tablets	Ibuprofen 200mg	**Adults & Peds ≥12 yrs:** 1-2 tabs q4-6h. **Max:** 6 tabs q24h.
Aleve Caplets	Naproxen Sodium 220mg	**Adults & Peds ≥12 yrs:** 1 tab q8-12h. May take 1 additional tab within 1h of first dose. **Max:** 2 tabs q8-12h or 3 tabs q24h.
Aleve Liquid Gels	Naproxen Sodium 220mg	**Adults & Peds ≥12 yrs:** 1 cap q8-12h. May take 1 additional cap within 1 hour of first dose. **Max:** 2 caps q8-12h or 3 caps q24h.
Aleve Smooth Gels	Naproxen Sodium 220mg	**Adults & Peds ≥12 yrs:** 1 cap q8-12h. May take 1 additional cap within 1 hour of first dose. **Max:** 2 caps q8-12h or 3 caps q24h.
Aleve Tablets	Naproxen Sodium 220mg	**Adults & Peds ≥12 yrs:** 1 tab q8-12h. May take 1 additional tab within 1 hour of first dose. **Max:** 2 tabs q8-12h or 3 tabs q24h.
Midol Cramps and Body Aches Tablets	Ibuprofen 200mg	**Adults & Peds ≥12 yrs:** 1-2 tabs q4-6h. **Max:** 6 tabs q24h.
Midol Extended Relief Caplets	Naproxen Sodium 220mg	**Adults & Peds ≥12 yrs:** 1-2 tabs q8-12h. **Max:** 2 tabs q8-12h or 3 tabs q24h.
Motrin Children's Suspension	Ibuprofen 100mg/5mL	**Peds 2-3 yrs (24-35 lbs):** 1 tsp (5mL). **4-5 yrs (36-47 lbs):** 1.5 tsp (7.5mL). **6-8 yrs (48-59 lbs):** 2 tsp (10mL). **9-10 yrs (60-71 lbs):** 2.5 tsp (12.5mL). **11 yrs (72-95 lbs):** 3 tsp (15mL).
Motrin IB Caplets	Ibuprofen 200mg	**Adults & Peds ≥12 yrs:** 1-2 tabs q4-6h. **Max:** 6 tabs q24h.
Motrin IB Tablets	Ibuprofen 200mg	**Adults & Peds ≥12 yrs:** 1-2 tabs q4-6h. **Max:** 6 tabs q24h.
Motrin Infants' Drops	Ibuprofen 50mg/1.25mL	**Peds 6-11 months (12-17 lbs):** 1.25mL. **12-23 months (18-23 lbs):** 1.875mL. May repeat q6-8h. **Max:** 4 doses q24h.
Motrin Junior Strength Caplets	Ibuprofen 100mg	**Peds 6-8 yrs (48-59 lbs):** 2 tabs. **9-10 yrs (60-71 lbs):** 2.5 tabs. **11 yrs (72-95 lbs):** 3 tabs. May repeat q6-8h. **Max:** 4 doses q24h.

(Continued)

TABLE 3. ANALGESIC PRODUCTS (cont.)

BRAND NAME	INGREDIENT/STRENGTH	DOSE
Motrin Junior Strength Chewable Tablets	Ibuprofen 100mg	**Peds 2-3 yrs (24-35 lbs):** 1 tab. **4-5 yrs (36-47 lbs):** 1.5 tabs. **6-8 yrs (48-59 lbs):** 2 tabs. **9-10 yrs (60-71 lbs):** 2.5 tabs. **11 yrs (72-95 lbs):** 3 tabs. May repeat q6-8h. **Max:** 4 doses q24h.
Pamprin All Day Caplets	Naproxen Sodium 220mg	**Adults & Peds ≥12 yrs:** 1-2 tabs q8-12h. **Max:** 3 tabs q24h.

NSAID SLEEP AIDS

Advil PM Caplets	Ibuprofen/Diphenhydramine Citrate 200mg-38mg	**Adults & Peds ≥12 yrs:** 2 tabs qhs. **Max:** 2 tabs q24h.
Advil PM Liqui-Gels	Ibuprofen/Diphenhydramine Citrate 200mg-25mg	**Adults & Peds ≥12 yrs:** 2 caps qhs. **Max:** 2 tabs q24h.

SALICYLATES

Anacin 81 Tablets	Aspirin 81mg	**Adults & Peds ≥12 yrs:** 2 tabs q6h. **Max:** 8 tabs q24h.
Bayer Aspirin Extra Strength Caplets	Aspirin 500mg	**Adults & Peds ≥12 yrs:** 1-2 tabs q4-6h. **Max:** 8 tabs q24h.
Bayer Aspirin Safety Coated Caplets	Aspirin 325mg	**Adults & Peds ≥12 yrs:** 1-2 tabs q4h. **Max:** 12 tabs q24h.
Bayer Low Dose Aspirin Chewable Tablets	Aspirin 81mg	**Adults & Peds ≥12 yrs:** 4-8 tabs q4h. **Max:** 48 tabs q24h.
Bayer Low Dose Aspirin Safety Coated Tablets	Aspirin 81mg	**Adults & Peds ≥12 yrs:** 4-8 tabs q4h. **Max:** 48 tabs q24h.
Bayer Genuine Aspirin Tablets	Aspirin 325mg	**Adults & Peds ≥12 yrs:** 1-2 tabs q4h or 3 tabs q6h. **Max:** 12 tabs q24h.
Doan's Extra Strength Caplets	Magnesium Salicylate Tetrahydrate 580mg	**Adults & Peds ≥12 yrs:** 2 tabs q6h. **Max:** 8 tabs q24h.
Ecotrin Low Strength Tablets	Aspirin 81mg	**Adults:** 4-8 tabs q4h. **Max:** 48 tabs q24h.
Ecotrin Regular Strength Tablets	Aspirin 325mg	**Adults & Peds ≥12 yrs:** 1-2 tabs q4h. **Max:** 12 tabs q24h.
Halfprin 162mg Tablets	Aspirin 162mg	**Adults & Peds ≥12 yrs:** 2-4 tabs q4h. **Max:** 24 tabs q24h.
Halfprin 81mg Tablets	Aspirin 81mg	**Adults & Peds ≥12 yrs:** 4-8 tabs q4h. **Max:** 48 tabs q24h.
St. Joseph Chewable Aspirin Tablets	Aspirin 81mg	**Adults & Peds ≥12 yrs:** 4-8 tabs q4h. **Max:** 48 tabs q24h.
St. Joseph Enteric Safety-Coated Tablets	Aspirin 81mg	**Adults & Peds ≥12 yrs:** 4-8 tabs q4h. **Max:** 48 tabs q24h.

SALICYLATES, BUFFERED

Alka-Seltzer Original Effervescent Tablets	Aspirin/Citric Acid/Sodium Bicarbonate 325mg-1000mg-1916mg	**Adults & Peds ≥12 yrs:** 2 tabs q4h. **Max:** 8 tabs q24h. **≥60 yrs: Max:** 4 tabs q24h.
Alka-Seltzer Extra Strength Effervescent Tablets	Aspirin/Citric Acid/Sodium Bicarbonate 500mg-1000mg-1985mg	**Adults & Peds ≥12 yrs:** 2 tabs q6h. **Max:** 7 tabs q24h. **≥60 yrs: Max:** 3 tabs q24h.
Ascriptin Maximum Strength Tablets	Aspirin 500mg Buffered with Aluminum Hydroxide/Calcium Carbonate/Magnesium Hydroxide	**Adults:** 2 tabs q6h. **Max:** 8 tabs q24h.
Ascriptin Regular Strength Tablets	Aspirin 325mg Buffered with Aluminum Hydroxide/Calcium Carbonate/Magnesium Hydroxide	**Adults:** 2 tabs q4h. **Max:** 12 tabs q24h.
Bayer Extra Strength Plus Caplets	Aspirin 500mg Buffered with Calcium Carbonate	**Adults & Peds ≥12 yrs:** 1-2 tabs q4-6h. **Max:** 8 tabs q24h.

TABLE 3. ANALGESIC PRODUCTS (cont.)

Brand Name	Ingredient/Strength	Dose
Bayer Women's Low Dose Aspirin Caplets	Aspirin 81mg Buffered with Calcium Carbonate	**Adults & Peds ≥12 yrs:** 4-8 tabs q4h. **Max:** 10 tabs q24h.
Bufferin Extra Strength Tablets	Aspirin 500mg Buffered with Calcium Carbonate/Magnesium Oxide/Magnesium Carbonate	**Adults & Peds ≥12 yrs:** 2 tabs q6h. **Max:** 8 tabs q24h.
Bufferin Tablets	Aspirin 325mg Buffered with Calcium Carbonate/Magnesium Oxide/Magnesium Carbonate	**Adults & Peds ≥12 yrs:** 2 tabs q4h. **Max:** 12 tabs q24h.
SALICYLATE COMBINATIONS		
Alka-Seltzer Wake-Up Call	Aspirin/Caffeine 500mg-65mg	**Adults & Peds ≥12 yrs:** 2 tabs q6h. **Max:** 8 tabs q24h. **≥60 yrs: Max:** 4 tabs q24h.
Anacin Max Strength Tablets	Aspirin/Caffeine 500mg-32mg	**Adults & Peds ≥12 yrs:** 2 tabs q6h. **Max:** 8 tabs q24h.
Anacin Tablets	Aspirin/Caffeine 400mg-32mg	**Adults & Peds ≥12 yrs:** 2 tabs q6h. **Max:** 8 tabs q24h.
Bayer Back & Body Pain Caplets	Aspirin/Caffeine 500mg-32.5mg	**Adults & Peds ≥12 yrs:** 2 tabs q6h. **Max:** 8 tabs q24h.
BC Arthritis Strength Powders	Aspirin/Caffeine/Salicylamide 742mg-38mg-222mg	**Adults & Peds ≥12 yrs:** 1 powder q3-4h. **Max:** 4 powders q24h.
BC Original Formula Powders	Aspirin/Caffeine/Salicylamide 650mg-33.3mg-195mg	**Adults & Peds ≥12 yrs:** 1 powder q3-4h. **Max:** 4 powders q24h.
SALICYLATE/SLEEP AID		
Alka-Seltzer PM Effervescent Tablets	Aspirin/Diphenhydramine Citrate 325mg-38mg	**Adults & Peds ≥12 yrs:** 2 tabs qhs.
Bayer PM Caplets	Aspirin/Diphenhydramine 500mg-38.3mg	**Adults & Peds ≥12 yrs:** 2 tabs qhs.
Doan's Extra Strength PM Caplets	Magnesium Salicylate Tetrahydrate/Diphenhydramine 580mg-25mg	**Adults & Peds ≥12 yrs:** 2 tabs qhs.

TABLE 4. ANTACID AND HEARTBURN PRODUCTS

Brand Name	Ingredient/Strength	Dose
ANTACID		
Alka-Seltzer Gold Tablets	Citric Acid/Potassium Bicarbonate/Sodium Bicarbonate 1000mg-344mg-1050mg	**Adults ≥60 yrs:** 2 tabs q4h prn. **Max:** 6 tabs q24h. **Adults & Peds ≥12 yrs:** 2 tabs q4h prn. **Max:** 8 tabs q24h. **Peds ≤12 yrs:** 1 tab q4h prn. **Max:** 4 tabs q24h.
Alka-Seltzer Heartburn Relief Tablets	Citric Acid/Sodium Bicarbonate 1000mg-1940mg	**Adults ≥60 yrs:** 2 tabs q4h prn. **Max:** 4 tabs q24h. **Adults & Peds ≥12 yrs:** 2 tabs q4h prn. **Max:** 8 tabs q24h.
Alka-Seltzer Lemon Lime Tablets	Aspirin/Citric Acid/Sodium Bicarbonate 325mg-1000mg-1700mg	**Adults ≥60 yrs:** 2 tabs q4h prn. **Max:** 4 tabs/24h. **Adults & Peds ≥12 yrs:** 2 tabs q4h prn. **Max:** 8 tabs q24h.
Alka-Seltzer Tablets, Original	Aspirin/Citric Acid/Sodium Bicarbonate 325mg-1000mg-1916mg	**Adults ≥60 yrs:** 2 tabs q4h prn. **Max:** 4 tabs q24h. **Adults & Peds ≥12 yrs:** 2 tabs q4h prn. **Max:** 8 tabs q24h.
Alka-Seltzer Tablets, Extra-Strength	Aspirin/Citric Acid/Sodium Bicarbonate 500mg-1000mg-1985mg	**Adults ≥60 yrs:** 2 tabs q6h prn. **Max:** 3 tabs q24h. **Adults & Peds ≥12 yrs:** 2 tabs q6h prn. **Max:** 7 tabs q24h.
Brioschi Powder	Sodium Bicarbonate/Tartaric Acid 2.69g-2.43g/dose	**Adults & Peds ≥12 yrs:** 1-2 capfuls (6g) dissolved in 4-6 oz water q1h. **Max:** 6 doses q24h. **Adults ≥60 yrs:** Use half of maximum dose.
Gaviscon Extra Strength Liquid	Aluminum Hydroxide/Magnesium Carbonate 254mg-237.5mg/5mL	**Adults:** 2-4 tsp (10-20mL) qid.
Gaviscon Extra Strength Tablets	Aluminum Hydroxide/Magnesium Carbonate 160mg-105mg	**Adults:** 2-4 tabs qid. **Max:** 16 doses q24h.
Gaviscon Regular Strength Tablets	Aluminum Hydroxide/Magnesium Trisilicate 80mg-14.2mg	**Adults:** 2-4 tabs qid. **Max:** 16 tabs q24h.
Gaviscon Regular Strength Liquid	Aluminum Hydroxide/Magnesium Carbonate 95mg-358mg/15mL	**Adults:** 1-2 tbl (15-30mL) qid. **Max:** 8 tbl q24h.
Maalox Children's Relief Chewables	Calcium Carbonate 400mg	**Peds 2-5 yrs (24-47 lbs):** 1 tab prn. **Max:** 3 tabs q24h. **Peds 6-11 yrs (48-95 lbs):** 2 tabs prn. **Max:** 6 tabs q24h.
Maalox Regular Strength Chewable Tablets	Calcium Carbonate 600mg	**Adults:** 1-2 tabs prn. **Max:** 12 tabs q24h.
Mylanta, Children's	Calcium Carbonate 400mg	**Peds 6-11 yrs (48-95 lbs):** Take 2 tab prn. **Max:** 6 tabs q24h. **Peds 2-5 yrs (24-47 lbs):** Take 1 tab prn. **Max:** 3 tabs q24h.
Mylanta Ultimate Strength Liquid	Aluminum Hydroxide/Magnesium Hydroxide 500mg-500mg/5mL	**Adults & Peds ≥12 yrs:** 2-4 tsp (10-20mL) qid (between meals & hs). **Max:** 9 tsp (45mL) q24h for ≤2 weeks.
Mylanta Supreme Antacid Liquid	Calcium Carbonate/Magnesium Hydroxide 400mg-135mg/5mL	**Adults:** 2-4 tsp (10-20mL) qid (between meals & hs). **Max:** 18 tsp (90mL) q24h.
Mylanta Ultimate Strength Chewable Tablets	Calcium Carbonate/Magnesium Hydroxide 700mg-300mg	**Adults:** 2-4 tabs qid (between meals & hs). **Max:** 10 tabs q24h for ≤2 weeks.
Rolaids Extra Strength Softchews	Calcium Carbonate 1177mg	**Adults:** 2-3 chews q1h prn. **Max:** 6 chews q24h.
Rolaids Extra Strength Tablets	Calcium Carbonate/Magnesium Hydroxide 675mg-135mg	**Adults:** 2-4 tabs q1h prn. **Max:** 10 tabs q24h.
Rolaids Tablets	Calcium Carbonate/Magnesium Hydroxide 550mg-110mg	**Adults:** 2-4 tabs q1h prn. **Max:** 12 tabs q24h.
Titralac Chewable Tablets	Calcium Carbonate 420mg	**Adults:** 2 tabs q2-3h prn. **Max:** 19 tabs q24h.
Tums Chewable Tablets	Calcium Carbonate 500mg	**Adults:** 2-4 tabs q1h prn. **Max:** 15 tabs q24h.
Tums E-X 750 Chewable Tablets	Calcium Carbonate 750mg	**Adults:** 2-4 tabs prn. **Max:** 10 tabs q24h.
Tums E-X 750 Sugar Free Chewable Tablets	Calcium Carbonate 750mg	**Adults:** 2-4 tabs prn. **Max:** 9 tabs q24h.

(Continued)

TABLE 4. ANTACID AND HEARTBURN PRODUCTS (cont.)

BRAND NAME	INGREDIENT/STRENGTH	DOSE
Tums Kids Chewable Tablets	Calcium Carbonate 750mg	**Peds >4 yrs (>49 lbs):** Take 1 tab tid. **Max:** 4 tabs q24h. **Peds 2-4 yrs (24-47 lbs):** Take ½-1 tab bid. **Max:** 2 tabs q24h.
Tums Smoothies Tablets	Calcium Carbonate 750mg	**Adults:** 2-4 tabs prn. **Max:** 10 tabs q24h.
Tums Ultra 1000 Chewable Tablets	Calcium Carbonate 1000mg	**Adults:** 2-3 tabs prn. **Max:** 7 tabs q24h for ≤2 weeks.

ANTACID/ANTIFLATULENT

BRAND NAME	INGREDIENT/STRENGTH	DOSE
Gelusil Chewable Tablets	Aluminum Hydroxide/Magnesium Hydroxide/Simethicone 200mg-200mg-25mg	**Adults:** 2-4 tabs qid. **Max:** 12 tabs q24h.
Maalox Advanced Maximum Strength Liquid	Aluminum Hydroxide/Magnesium Hydroxide/Simethicone 400mg-400mg-40mg/5mL	**Adults & Peds ≥12 yrs:** 2-4 tsp (10-20mL) bid. **Max:** 8 tsp (40mL) q24h.
Maalox Advanced Maximum Strength Chewable Tablets	Calcium Carbonate/Simethicone 1000mg-60mg	**Adults & Peds ≥12 yrs:** 1-2 tabs prn. **Max:** 8 tabs q24h.
Maalox Junior Relief Chewables	Calcium Carbonate/Simethicone 400mg-24mg	**Peds 6–11 yrs:** 2 tabs prn. **Max:** 6 tabs q24h.
Maalox Advanced Regular Strength Liquid	Aluminum Hydroxide/Magnesium Hydroxide/Simethicone 200mg-200mg-20mg/5mL	**Adults & Peds ≥12 yrs:** 2-4 tsp (10-20mL) qid. **Max:** 16 tsp (80mL) q24h.
Mylanta Maximum Strength Liquid	Aluminum Hydroxide/Magnesium Hydroxide/Simethicone 400mg-400mg-40mg/5mL	**Adults & Peds ≥12 yrs:** 2-4 tsp (between meals and hs) (10-20mL) qid. **Max:** 12 tsp (60mL) q24h.
Mylanta Regular Strength Liquid	Aluminum Hydroxide/Magnesium Hydroxide/Simethicone 200mg-200mg-20mg/5mL	**Adults & Peds ≥12 yrs:** 2-4 tsp (between meals and hs) (10-20mL) qid. **Max:** 24 tsp (120mL) q24h.
Rolaids Multi-Symptom Chewable Tablets	Calcium Carbonate/Magnesium Hydroxide/Simethicone 675mg-135mg-60mg	**Adults:** 2-4 tabs q1h prn. **Max:** 8 tabs q24h.
Rolaids Extra Strength Plus Gas Soft Chews	Calcium Carbonate/Simethicone 1177mg-80mg	**Adults:** 2-3 chews q1h prn. **Max:** 6 chews q24h.
Titralac Plus Chewable Tablets	Calcium Carbonate/Simethicone 420mg-21mg	**Adults:** 2 tabs q2-3h prn. **Max:** 19 tabs q24h.

BISMUTH SUBSALICYLATE

BRAND NAME	INGREDIENT/STRENGTH	DOSE
Maalox Total Relief Maximum Strength Liquid	Bismuth Subsalicylate 525mg/15mL	**Adults & Peds ≥12 yrs:** 2 tbl (30mL) q1h prn. **Max:** 8 tbl (120mL) q24h.
Pepto Bismol Chewable Tablets	Bismuth Subsalicylate 262mg	**Adults & Peds ≥12 yrs:** 2 tabs q1/2-1h prn. **Max:** 8 doses q24h.
Pepto Bismol Caplets	Bismuth Subsalicylate 262mg	**Adults & Peds ≥12 yrs:** 2 tabs q1/2-1h prn. **Max:** 8 doses q24h.
Pepto Bismol Liquid	Bismuth Subsalicylate 262mg/15mL	**Adults & Peds ≥12 yrs:** 2 tbl (30mL) q1/2-1h prn. **Max:** 8 doses (240mL) q24h.
Pepto Bismol Maximum Strength Liquid	Bismuth Subsalicylate 525mg/15mL	**Adults & Peds ≥12 yrs:** 2 tbl (30mL) q1h prn. **Max:** 4 doses (120mL) q24h.

TABLE 4. ANTACID AND HEARTBURN PRODUCTS (cont.)

Brand Name	Ingredient/Strength	Dose
H$_2$-RECEPTOR ANTAGONIST		
Pepcid AC Gelcaps	Famotidine 10mg	**Adults & Peds ≥12 yrs:** 1 cap qd. **Max:** 2 caps q24h.
Pepcid AC Maximum Strength EZ Chews	Famotidine 20mg	**Adults & Peds ≥12 yrs:** 1 tab qd. **Max:** 2 tabs q24h.
Pepcid AC Maximum Strength Tablets	Famotidine 20mg	**Adults & Peds ≥12 yrs:** 1 tab qd. **Max:** 2 tabs q24h.
Pepcid AC Tablets	Famotidine 10mg	**Adults & Peds ≥12 yrs:** 1 tab qd. **Max:** 2 tabs q24h.
Tagamet HB Tablets	Cimetidine 200mg	**Adults & Peds ≥12 yrs:** 1 tab qd. **Max:** 2 tabs q24h.
Zantac 150 Tablets	Ranitidine 150mg	**Adults & Peds ≥12 yrs:** 1 tab qd. **Max:** 2 tabs q24h.
Zantac 75 Tablets	Ranitidine 75mg	**Adults & Peds ≥12 yrs:** 1 tab qd. **Max:** 2 tabs q24h.
H$_2$-RECEPTOR ANTAGONIST/ANTACID		
Pepcid Complete Chewable Tablets	Famotidine/Calcium Carbonate/ Magnesium Hydroxide 10mg-800mg-165mg	**Adults & Peds ≥12 yrs:** 1 tab qd. **Max:** 2 tabs q24h.
PROTON PUMP INHIBITOR		
Prilosec OTC Tablets	Omeprazole 20mg	**Adults:** 1 tab qd x 14 days. May repeat 14 day course q4 months.

TABLE 5. ANTIDIARRHEAL PRODUCTS

BRAND NAME	INGREDIENT/STRENGTH	DOSE
ABSORBENT AGENTS		
Equalactin Chewable Tablets	Calcium Polycarbophil 625mg	**Adults & Peds ≥12 yrs:** 2 tabs/dose. **Max:** 8 tabs q24h. **Peds 6-12 yrs:** 1 tab/dose. **Max:** 4 tabs q24h. **Peds 2 to ≤6 yrs:** 1 tab/dose. **Max:** 2 tabs q24h.
Fibercon Caplets	Calcium Polycarbophil 625mg	**Adults & Peds ≥12 yrs:** 2 tabs qd. **Max:** 8 tabs q24h.
Konsyl Fiber Caplets	Calcium Polycarbophil 625mg	**Adults & Peds ≥12 yrs:** 2 tabs qd-qid. **Peds 6-12 yrs:** 1 tab qd-tid. **Max:** 8 tabs q24h.
ANTIPERISTALTIC AGENTS		
Imodium A-D Caplets	Loperamide HCl 2mg	**Adults & Peds ≥12 yrs:** 2 tabs after first loose stool; 1 tab after each subsequent loose stool. **Max:** 4 tabs q24h. **Peds 9-11 yrs (60-95 lbs):** 1 tab after first loose stool; ½ tab after each subsequent loose stool. **Max:** 3 tabs q24h. **Peds 6-8 yrs (48-59 lbs):** 1 tab after first loose stool; ½ tab after each subsequent loose stool. **Max:** 2 tabs q24h.
Imodium A-D E-Z Chews	Loperamide HCl 2mg	**Adults & Peds ≥12 yrs:** 2 tabs after first loose stool; 1 tab after each subsequent loose stool. **Max:** 4 tabs q24h. **Peds 9-11 yrs (60-95 lbs):** 1 tab after first loose stool; ½ tab after each subsequent loose stool. **Max:** 3 tabs q24h. **Peds 6-8 yrs (48-59 lbs):** 1 tab after first loose stool; ½ tab after each subsequent loose stool. **Max:** 2 tabs q24h.
Imodium A-D Liquid	Loperamide HCl 1mg/7.5mL	**Adults & Peds ≥12 yrs:** 4 tsp (20mL) after first loose stool; 2 tsp (10mL) after each subsequent loose stool. **Max:** 8 tsp (40mL) q24h. **Peds 9-11 yrs (60-95 lbs):** 2 tsp (10mL) after the first loose stool; 1 tsp (5mL) after each subsequent loose stool. **Max:** 6 tsp (30mL) q24h. **Peds 6-8 yrs (48-59 lbs):** 2 tsp (10mL) after the first loose stool; 1 tsp (5mL) after each subsequent loose stool. **Max:** 4 tsp (20mL) q24h.
Imodium A-D Liquid For Use In Children (Mint Flavor)	Loperamide HCl 1mg/7.5mL	**Adults & Peds ≥12 yrs:** 6 tsp (30mL) after first loose stool; 3 tsp (15mL) after each subsequent loose stool. **Max:** 12 tsp (60mL) q24h. **Peds 9-11 yrs (60-95 lbs):** 3 tsp (15mL) after the first loose stool; 1½ tsp (7.5mL) after each subsequent loose stool. **Max:** 9 tsp (45mL) q24h. **Peds 6-8 yrs (48-59 lbs):** 3 tsp (15mL) after first loose stool; 1½ tsp (7.5mL) after each subsequent loose stool. **Max:** 6 tsp (30mL) q24h.
ANTIPERISTALTIC/ANTIFLATULENT AGENTS		
Imodium Multi-Symptom Relief Caplets	Loperamide HCl/Simethicone 2mg-125mg	**Adults & Peds ≥12 yrs:** 2 tabs after first loose stool; 1 tab after each subsequent loose stool. **Max:** 4 tabs q24h. **Peds 9-11 yrs (60-95 lbs):** 1 tab after first loose stool; ½ tab after each subsequent loose stool. **Max:** 3 tabs q24h. **6-8 yrs (48-59 lbs):** 1 tab after first loose stool; ½ tab after each subsequent loose stool. **Max:** 2 tabs q24h.
Imodium Multi-Symptom Relief Chewable Tablets	Loperamide HCl/Simethicone 2mg-125mg	**Adults & Peds ≥12 yrs:** 2 tabs with 4-8 oz water after first loose stool; 1 tab with 4-8 oz water after each subsequent loose stool. **Max:** 4 tabs q24h. **Peds 9-11 yrs (60-95 lbs):** 1 tab with 4-8 oz water after first loose stool; ½ tab after each subsequent loose stool. **Max:** 3 tabs q24h. **Peds 6-8 yrs (48-59 lbs):** 1 tab with 4-8 oz water after first loose stool; ½ tab with 4-8 oz water after each subsequent loose stool. **Max:** 2 tabs q24h.

(Continued)

TABLE 5. ANTIDIARRHEAL PRODUCTS (cont.)

Brand Name	Ingredient/Strength	Dose
BISMUTH SUBSALICYLATE		
Kaopectate Extra Strength Liquid	Bismuth Subsalicylate 525mg/15mL	**Adults & Peds ≥12 yrs:** 2 tbl (30mL) q1h prn. **Max:** 4 doses (8 tbl) q24h.
Kaopectate Liquid	Bismuth Subsalicylate 262mg/15mL	**Adults & Peds ≥12 yrs:** 2 tbl (30mL) q½-1h prn. **Max:** 8 doses (16 tbl) q24h.
Maalox Total Relief Liquid	Bismuth Subsalicylate 525mg/15mL	**Adults & Peds ≥12 yrs:** 2 tbl (30mL) q1h prn. **Max:** 4 doses (8 tbl) q24h.
Pepto Bismol Caplets	Bismuth Subsalicylate 262mg	**Adults & Peds ≥12 yrs:** 2 tabs q½-1h. **Max:** 8 doses (16 tabs) q24h.
Pepto Bismol Chewable Tablets	Bismuth Subsalicylate 262mg	**Adults & Peds ≥12 yrs:** 2 tabs q½-1h. **Max:** 8 doses (16 tabs) q24h.
Pepto Bismol Liquid	Bismuth Subsalicylate 262mg/15mL	**Adults & Peds ≥12 yrs:** 2 tbl (30mL) q½-1h prn. **Max:** 8 doses (16 tbl) q24h.
Pepto Bismol Liquid Max	Bismuth Subsalicylate 525mg/15mL	**Adults & Peds ≥12 yrs:** 2 tbl (30mL) q1h prn. **Max:** 4 doses (8 tbl) q24h.

TABLE 6. ANTIFLATULENT PRODUCTS

Brand Name	Ingredient/Strength	Dose
ALPHA-GALACTOSIDASE		
Beano Food Enzyme Dietary Supplement Drops	Alpha-Galactosidase Enzyme 150 GalU (per 5 drops)	**Adults:** Add 5 drops to first bite of food serving.
Beano Food Enzyme Dietary Supplement Tablets	Alpha-Galactosidase Enzyme 150 GalU	**Adults:** Take 3 tabs before meals.
ANTACID/ANTIFLATULENT		
Gas-X Extra Strength with Maalox Chewable Tablets	Calcium Carbonate/Simethicone 500mg-125mg	**Adults:** 1-2 tabs prn. **Max:** 4 tabs q24h.
Gelusil Chewable Tablets	Aluminum Hydroxide/Magnesium Hydroxide/Simethicone 200mg-200mg-25mg	**Adults:** 2-4 tabs q1h prn. **Max:** 12 tabs q24h.
Maalox Advanced Maximum Strength Liquid	Aluminum Hydroxide/Magnesium Hydroxide/Simethicone 400mg-400mg-40mg/5mL	**Adults & Peds ≥12 yrs:** 2-4 tsp (10-20mL) bid. **Max:** 8 tsp (40mL) q24h.
Maalox Advanced Maximum Strength Chewable Tablets	Calcium Carbonate/Simethicone 1000mg-60mg	**Adults & Peds ≥12 yrs:** 1-2 tabs prn. **Max:** 8 tabs q24h.
Maalox Advanced Regular Strength Liquid	Aluminum Hydroxide/Magnesium Hydroxide/Simethicone 200mg-200mg-20mg/5mL	**Adults & Peds ≥12 yrs:** 2-4 tsp (10-20mL) qid. **Max:** 16 tsp (80mL) q24h.
Mylanta Maximum Strength Liquid	Aluminum Hydroxide/Magnesium Hydroxide/Simethicone 400mg-400mg-40mg/5mL	**Adults & Peds ≥12 yrs:** 2-4 tsp (10-20mL) between meals & hs. **Max:** 12 tsp (60mL) q24h.
Mylanta Regular Strength Liquid	Aluminum Hydroxide/Magnesium Hydroxide/Simethicone 200mg-200mg-20mg/5mL	**Adults & Peds ≥12 yrs:** 2-4 tsp (10-20mL) between meals & hs. **Max:** 24 tsp (120mL) q24h.
Rolaids Antacid & Antigas Soft Chews	Calcium Carbonate/Simethicone 1177mg-80mg	**Adults:** 2-3 chews hourly prn.
Titralac Plus Chewable Tablets	Calcium Carbonate/Simethicone 420mg-21mg	**Adults:** 2 tabs q2-3h prn. **Max:** 19 tabs q24h.
SIMETHICONE		
GasAid Maximum Strength Anti-Gas Softgels	Simethicone 125mg	**Adults & Peds ≥12 yrs:** Take 1-2 caps prn and qhs. **Max:** 4 caps q24h.
Baby Gas-X Infant Drops	Simethicone 20mg/0.3mL	**Peds ≥2 yrs (≥24 lbs):** 0.6mL prn. **Peds <2 yrs (<24 lbs):** 0.3mL prn. **Max:** 6 doses q24h.
Gas-X Children's Thin Strips	Simethicone 40mg	**Peds 2-12 yrs:** 1 strip prn and hs. **Max:** 6 strips q24h.
Gas-X Thin Strips	Simethicone 62.5mg	**Adults:** Allow 2-4 strips to dissolve prn after meals and hs. **Max:** 8 strips q24h.
Gas-X Antigas Chewable Tablets	Simethicone 80mg	**Adults:** Chew 1-2 tabs prn and qhs. **Max:** 6 tabs q24h.
Gas-X Extra Strength Antigas Softgels	Simethicone 125mg	**Adults:** Take 1-2 caps prn and qhs. **Max:** 4 caps q24h.
Gas-X Ultra Strength Softgels	Simethicone 180mg	**Adults:** Take 1-2 caps prn after meals and qhs. **Max:** 2 caps q24h.
Little Tummys Gas Relief Drops	Simethicone 20mg/0.3mL	**Peds ≥2 yrs (≥24 lbs):** 0.6mL prn (after meals & hs). **Peds <2 yrs (<24 lbs):** 0.3mL prn (after meals & hs). **Max:** 12 doses q24h.
Mylanta Gas Maximum Strength Softgels	Simethicone 125mg	**Adults:** Take 1-2 caps (after meals & hs). **Max:** 4 caps q24h.
Mylanta Gas Maximum Strength Chewable Tablets	Simethicone 125mg	**Adults:** Chew 1-2 tabs (after meals & hs). **Max:** 4 tabs q24h.
Mylicon Infant's Gas Relief Drops	Simethicone 20mg/0.3mL	**Peds ≥2 yrs (≥24 lbs):** 0.6mL (after meals & hs). **Peds <2 yrs (<24 lbs):** 0.3mL (after meals & hs). **Max:** 12 doses q24h.

TABLE 7. ANTIFUNGAL PRODUCTS

BRAND NAME	INGREDIENT/STRENGTH	DOSE
BUTENAFINE		
Lotrimin Ultra Antifungal Cream	Butenafine HCl 1%	**Adults & Peds ≥12 yrs:** Use qd or bid.
CLOTRIMAZOLE		
Clearly Confident Triple Action Fungus Treatment	Clotrimazole 1%	**Adults:** Apply to affected area qd.
FungiCure Maximum Strength Anti-Fungal Liquid Spray	Clotrimazole 1%	**Adults & Peds:** Use bid.
FungiCure Intensive Spray	Clotrimazole 1%	**Adults & Peds ≥2 yrs:** Use bid.
FungiCure Manicure/Pedicure Formula Liquid	Clotrimazole 1%	**Adults & Peds ≥2 yrs:** Use bid.
Lotrimin AF Antifungal Athlete's Foot Cream	Clotrimazole 1%	**Adults & Peds ≥2 yrs:** Use bid.
Lotrimin AF For Her Antifungal Cream	Clotrimazole 1%	**Adults & Peds ≥2 yrs:** Use bid.
MICONAZOLE		
Desenex Antifungal Liquid Spray	Miconazole Nitrate 2%	**Adults & Peds ≥2 yrs:** Use bid.
Desenex Antifungal Powder	Miconazole Nitrate 2%	**Adults & Peds ≥2 yrs:** Use bid.
Desenex Antifungal Spray	Miconazole Nitrate 2%	**Adults & Peds ≥2 yrs:** Use bid.
Lotrimin AF Antifungal Aerosol Liquid Spray	Miconazole Nitrate 2%	**Adults & Peds ≥2 yrs:** Use qd-bid.
Lotrimin AF Antifungal Jock Itch Aerosol Powder Spray	Miconazole Nitrate 2%	**Adults & Peds ≥2 yrs:** Use bid.
Lotrimin AF Antifungal Powder	Miconazole Nitrate 2%	**Adults & Peds ≥2 yrs:** Use bid.
Micatin Cream	Miconazole Nitrate 2%	**Adults:** Use bid.
Neosporin AF Athlete's Foot Cream	Miconazole Nitrate 2%	**Adults & Peds ≥12 yrs:** Use bid.
Neosporin AF Athlete's Foot Antifungal Spray Liquid	Miconazole Nitrate 2%	**Adults & Peds ≥12 yrs:** Use bid.
Neosporin AF Athlete's Foot Antifungal Spray Powder	Miconazole Nitrate 2%	**Adults & Peds ≥12 yrs:** Use bid.
Neosporin AF Jock Itch Antifungal Cream	Miconazole Nitrate 2%	**Adults & Peds ≥12 yrs:** Use bid.
Zeasorb Super Absorbent Antifungal Powder	Miconazole Nitrate 2%	**Adults & Peds:** Use bid.
TERBINAFINE		
Lamisil AT Continuous Spray	Terbinafine HCl 1%	**Adults & Peds ≥12 yrs:** Use qd or bid.
Lamisil AT Cream	Terbinafine HCl 1%	**Adults & Peds ≥12 yrs:** Use qd-bid.
Lamisil AT Gel	Terbinafine HCl 1%	**Adults & Peds ≥12 yrs:** Use qd.
TOLNAFTATE		
FungiCure Anti-Fungal Gel	Tolnaftate 1%	**Adults & Peds ≥2 yrs:** Use bid.
Miracle of Aloe Miracure Anti-Fungal	Tolnaftate 1%	**Adults & Peds ≥12 yrs:** Use bid.
Tinactin Antifungal Deodorant Powder Spray	Tolnaftate 1%	**Adults & Peds:** Use qd or bid.
Tinactin Antifungal Liquid Spray	Tolnaftate 1%	**Adults & Peds:** Use qd or bid.
Tinactin Antifungal Powder Spray	Tolnaftate 1%	**Adults & Peds:** Use qd or bid.

(Continued)

TABLE 7. ANTIFUNGAL PRODUCTS (cont.)

Brand Name	Ingredient/Strength	Dose
Tinactin Antifungal Cream	Tolnaftate 1%	**Adults & Peds:** Use qd or bid.
Tinactin Antifungal Absorbent Powder	Tolnaftate 1%	**Adults & Peds:** Use qd or bid.
Tinactin Antifungal Jock Itch Powder Spray	Tolnaftate 1%	**Adults & Peds:** Use qd or bid.
UNDECYLENIC ACID		
Fungi Nail Anti-fungal Solution	Undecylenic Acid 25%	**Adults & Peds ≥2 yrs:** Use bid.
FungiCure Anti-fungal Liquid	Undecylenic Acid 12.5%	**Adults & Peds ≥2 yrs:** Use bid.
FungiCure Professional Formula Liquid	Undecylenic Acid 15%	**Adults & Peds ≥2 yrs:** Use bid.
Tineacide Antifungal Cream	Undecylenic Acid 10%	**Adults & Peds ≥12 yrs:** Use bid.

TABLE 8. ANTIPYRETIC PRODUCTS

BRAND NAME	INGREDIENT/STRENGTH	DOSE
ACETAMINOPHEN		
Anacin Aspirin Free Extra Strength Tablets	Acetaminophen 500mg	**Adults & Peds ≥12 yrs:** 2 tabs q6h. **Max:** 8 tabs q24h.
FeverAll Childrens' Suppositories	Acetaminophen 120mg	**Peds 3-6 yrs:** 1 supp. q4-6h. **Max:** 6 supp q24h.
FeverAll Infants' Suppositories	Acetaminophen 80mg	**Peds 3-11 months:** 1 supp q6h. **12-36 months:** 1 supp q4h. **Max:** 6 supp q24h.
FeverAll Jr. Strength Suppositories	Acetaminophen 325mg	**Peds 6-12 yrs:** 1 supp q4-6h. **Max:** 6 supp q24h.
Tylenol 8 Hour Caplets	Acetaminophen 650mg	**Adults & Peds ≥12 yrs:** 2 tabs q8h prn. **Max:** 6 tabs q24h.
Tylenol Arthritis Caplets	Acetaminophen 650mg	**Adults:** 2 tabs q8h prn. **Max:** 6 tabs q24h.
Tylenol Arthritis Geltabs	Acetaminophen 650mg	**Adults:** 2 tabs q8h prn. **Max:** 6 tabs q24h.
Tylenol Children's Meltaways Tablets	Acetaminophen 80mg	**Peds 2-3 yrs (24-35 lbs):** 2 tabs. **4-5 yrs (36-47 lbs):** 3 tabs. **6-8 yrs (48-59 lbs):** 4 tabs. **9-10 yrs (60-71 lbs):** 5 tabs. **11 yrs (72-95 lbs):** 6 tabs. **Max:** 5 doses q24h.
Tylenol Children's Suspension	Acetaminophen 160mg/5mL	**Peds 2-3 yrs (24-35 lbs):** 1 tsp (5mL). **4-5 yrs (36-47 lbs):** 1.5 tsp (7.5mL). **6-8 yrs (48-59 lbs):** 2 tsp (10mL). **9-10 yrs (60-71 lbs):** 2.5 tsp (12.5mL). **11 yrs (72-95 lbs):** 3 tsp (15mL). May repeat q4h. **Max:** 5 doses q24h.
Tylenol Extra Strength Caplets	Acetaminophen 500mg	**Adults & Peds ≥12 yrs:** 2 tabs q4-6h prn. **Max:** 8 tabs q24h.
Tylenol Extra Strength Cool Caplets	Acetaminophen 500mg	**Adults & Peds ≥12 yrs:** 2 tabs q4-6h prn. **Max:** 8 tabs q24h.
Tylenol Extra Strength Rapid Release Gelcaps	Acetaminophen 500mg	**Adults & Peds ≥12 yrs:** 2 caps q4-6h prn. **Max:** 8 caps q24h.
Tylenol Extra Strength Rapid Blast Liquid	Acetaminophen 1000mg/30mL	**Adults & Peds ≥12 yrs:** 2 tbl (30mL) q4-6h prn. **Max:** 8 tbl (120mL) q24h.
Tylenol Extra Strength EZ Tablets	Acetaminophen 500mg	**Adults & Peds ≥12 yrs:** 2 tabs q4-6h prn. **Max:** 8 tabs q24h.
Tylenol Infants' Drops	Acetaminophen 80mg/0.8mL	**Peds 2-3 yrs (24-35 lbs):** 1.6 mL q4h prn. **Max:** 5 doses (8mL) q24h.
Tylenol Junior Meltaways Tablets	Acetaminophen 160mg	**Peds 6-8 yrs (48-59 lbs):** 2 tabs. **9-10 yrs (60-71 lbs):** 2.5 tabs. **11 yrs (72-95 lbs):** 3 tabs. **12 yrs (≥96 lbs):** 4 tabs. May repeat q4h. **Max:** 5 doses q24h.
Tylenol Regular Strength Tablets	Acetaminophen 325mg	**Adults & Peds ≥12 yrs:** 2 tabs q4-6h prn. **Max:** 12 tabs q24h. **Peds 6-11 yrs:** 1 tab q4-6h. **Max:** 5 doses q24h.
NONSTEROIDAL ANTI-INFLAMMATORY DRUGS (NSAIDs)		
Advil Caplets	Ibuprofen 200mg	**Adults & Peds ≥12 yrs:** 1-2 tabs q4-6h. **Max:** 6 tabs q24h.
Advil Children's Suspension	Ibuprofen 100mg/5mL	**Peds 2-3 yrs (24-35 lbs):** 1 tsp (5mL). **4-5 yrs (36-47 lbs):** 1.5 tsp (7.5mL). **6-8 yrs (48-59 lbs):** 2 tsp (10mL). **9-10 yrs (60-71 lbs):** 2.5 tsp (12.5mL). **11 yrs (72-95 lbs):** 3 tsp (15mL). May repeat q6-8h. **Max:** 4 doses q24h.
Advil Gel Caplets	Ibuprofen 200mg	**Adults & Peds ≥12 yrs:** 1-2 tabs q4-6h. **Max:** 6 tabs q24h.
Advil Infants' Concentrated Drops	Ibuprofen 50mg/1.25mL	**Peds 6-11 months (12-17 lbs):** 1.25mL. **12-23 months (18-23 lbs):** 1.875mL. May repeat q6-8h. **Max:** 4 doses q24h.

(Continued)

TABLE 8. ANTIPYRETIC PRODUCTS (cont.)

BRAND NAME	INGREDIENT/STRENGTH	DOSE
Advil Liqui-Gels	Ibuprofen 200mg	**Adults & Peds ≥12 yrs:** 1-2 caps q4-6h. **Max:** 6 caps q24h.
Advil Tablets	Ibuprofen 200mg	**Adults & Peds ≥12 yrs:** 1-2 tabs q4-6h. **Max:** 6 tabs q24h.
Aleve Caplets	Naproxen Sodium 220mg	**Adults & Peds ≥12 yrs:** 1 tab q8-12h. May take 1 additional tab within 1 hour of first dose. **Max:** 2 tabs q8-12h or 3 tabs q24h.
Aleve Liquid Gels	Naproxen Sodium 220mg	**Adults & Peds ≥12 yrs:** 1 cap q8-12h. May take 1 additional cap within 1 hour of first dose. **Max:** 2 caps q8-12h or 3 caps q24h.
Aleve Smooth Gels	Naproxen Sodium 220mg	**Adults & Peds ≥12 yrs:** 1 cap q8-12h. May take 1 additional cap within 1 hour of first dose. **Max:** 2 caps q8-12h or 3 caps q24h.
Aleve Tablets	Naproxen Sodium 220mg	**Adults & Peds ≥12 yrs:** 1 tab q8-12h. May take 1 additional tab within 1 hour of first dose. **Max:** 2 tabs q8-12h or 3 tabs q24h.
Motrin Children's Suspension	Ibuprofen 100mg/5mL	**Peds 2-5 yrs (24-47 lbs):** 1 tsp (5mL). **6-11 yrs (48-95 lbs):** 2 tsp (10mL). May repeat q6h. **Max:** 4 doses q24h.
Motrin IB Caplets	Ibuprofen 200mg	**Adults & Peds ≥12 yrs:** 1-2 tabs q4-6h. **Max:** 6 tabs q24h.
Motrin IB Tablets	Ibuprofen 200mg	**Adults & Peds ≥12 yrs:** 1-2 tabs q4-6h. **Max:** 6 tabs q24h.
Motrin Infants' Drops	Ibuprofen 50mg/1.25mL	**Peds 6-11 months (12-17 lbs):** 1.25mL. **12-23 months (18-23 lbs):** 1.875mL. May repeat q6-8h. **Max:** 4 doses q24h.
Motrin Junior Strength Caplets	Ibuprofen 100mg	**Peds 6-8 yrs (48-59 lbs):** 2 tabs. **9-10 yrs (60-71 lbs):** 2.5 tabs. **11 yrs (72-95 lbs):** 3 tabs. May repeat q6-8h. **Max:** 4 doses q24h.
Motrin Junior Strength Chewable Tablets	Ibuprofen 100mg	**Peds 2-3 yrs (24-35 lbs):** 1 tab. **4-5 yrs (36-47 lbs):** 1.5 tabs. **6-8 yrs (48-59 lbs):** 2 tabs. **9-10 yrs (60-71 lbs):** 2.5 tabs. **11 yrs (72-95 lbs):** 3 tabs. May repeat q6-8h. **Max:** 4 doses q24h.
SALICYLATES		
Anacin 81 Tablets	Aspirin 81mg	**Adults & Peds ≥12 yrs:** 2 tabs q6h. **Max:** 8 tabs q24h.
Bayer Aspirin Extra Strength Caplets	Aspirin 500mg	**Adults & Peds ≥12 yrs:** 1-2 tabs q4-6h. **Max:** 8 tabs q24h.
Bayer Aspirin Safety Coated Caplets	Aspirin 325mg	**Adults & Peds ≥12 yrs:** 1-2 tabs q4h. **Max:** 12 tabs q24h.
Bayer Genuine Aspirin Tablets	Aspirin 325mg	**Adults & Peds ≥12 yrs:** 1-2 tabs q4h or 3 tabs q6h. **Max:** 12 tabs q24h.
Bayer Low-Dose Aspirin Chewable Tablets	Aspirin 81mg	**Adults & Peds ≥12 yrs:** 4-8 tabs q4h. **Max:** 48 tabs q24h.
Bayer Low-Dose Aspirin Safety Coated Tablets	Aspirin 81mg	**Adults & Peds ≥12 yrs:** 4-8 tabs q4h. **Max:** 48 tabs q24h.
Ecotrin Low Strength Tablets	Aspirin 81mg	**Adults:** 4-8 tabs q4h. **Max:** 48 tabs q24h.
Ecotrin Regular Strength Tablets	Aspirin 325mg	**Adults & Peds ≥12 yrs:** 1-2 tabs q4h. **Max:** 12 tabs q24h.
Halfprin 162mg Tablets	Aspirin 162mg	**Adults & Peds ≥12 yrs:** 2-4 tabs q4h. **Max:** 24 tabs q24h.
Halfprin 81mg Tablets	Aspirin 81mg	**Adults & Peds ≥12 yrs:** 4-8 tabs q4h. **Max:** 48 tabs q24h.

TABLE 8. ANTIPYRETIC PRODUCTS (cont.)

Brand Name	Ingredient/Strength	Dose
St. Joseph Aspirin Chewable Tablets	Aspirin 81mg	**Adults & Peds ≥12 yrs:** 4-8 tabs q4h. **Max:** 48 tabs q24h.
St. Joseph Enteric Safety-Coated Tablets	Aspirin 81mg	**Adults & Peds ≥12 yrs:** 4-8 tabs q4h. **Max:** 48 tabs q24h.
SALICYLATES, BUFFERED		
Bayer Extra Strength Plus Caplets	Aspirin 500mg Buffered with Calcium Carbonate	**Adults & Peds ≥12 yrs:** 1-2 tabs q4-6h. **Max:** 8 tabs q24h.
Bayer Women's Low Dose Aspirin Caplets	Aspirin 81mg Buffered with Calcium Carbonate 777mg	**Adults & Peds ≥12 yrs:** 4-8 tabs q4h. **Max:** 10 tabs q24h.
Bufferin Extra Strength Tablets	Aspirin 500mg Buffered with Calcium Carbonate/Magnesium Oxide/Magnesium Carbonate	**Adults & Peds ≥12 yrs:** 2 tabs q6h. **Max:** 8 tabs q24h.
Bufferin Tablets	Aspirin 325mg Buffered with Benzoic Acid/ Citric Acid	**Adults & Peds ≥12 yrs:** 2 tabs q4h. **Max:** 12 tabs q24h.

TABLE 9. ANTISEBORRHEAL PRODUCTS

Brand Name	Ingredient/Strength	Dose
COAL TAR		
Denorex Therapeutic Protection 2-in-1 Shampoo	Coal Tar 2.5%	**Adults & Peds:** Use at least biw.
Denorex Therapeutic Protection Shampoo	Coal Tar 2.5%	**Adults & Peds:** Use at least biw.
DHS Tar Dermatological Hair & Scalp Shampoo	Coal Tar 0.5%	**Adults & Peds:** Use tiw.
Ionil-T Plus Shampoo	Coal Tar 2%	**Adults & Peds:** Use at least biw.
Ionil-T Shampoo	Coal Tar 2%	**Adults & Peds:** Use at least biw.
MG217 Ointment	Coal Tar 2%	**Adults & Peds:** Apply to affected area qd-qid.
MG217 Tar Shampoo	Coal Tar 3%	**Adults & Peds:** Use at least biw.
Neutrogena T/Gel Shampoo Extra Strength	Coal Tar 1%	**Adults & Peds:** Use at least biw.
Neutrogena T/Gel Shampoo Original Formula	Coal Tar 0.5%	**Adults & Peds:** Use at least biw.
Neutrogena T/Gel Stubborn Itch Shampoo	Coal Tar 0.5%	**Adults & Peds:** Use at least biw.
Psoriasin Gel	Coal Tar 1.25%	**Adults:** Apply to affected area qd-qid.
Psoriasin Liquid Dab-on	Coal Tar 0.66%	**Adults:** Apply to affected area qd-qid.
CORTICOSTEROIDS		
Aveeno Hydrocortisone 1% Anti-Itch Cream	Hydrocortisone 1%	**Adults & Peds ≥2 yrs:** Apply to affected area tid-qid.
Cortaid Advanced 12-Hour Anti-Itch Cream	Hydrocortisone 1%	**Adults & Peds ≥2 yrs:** Apply to affected area tid-qid.
Cortaid Intensive Therapy Cooling Spray	Hydrocortisone 1%	**Adults & Peds ≥2 yrs:** Apply to affected area tid-qid.
Cortaid Intensive Therapy Moisturizing Cream	Hydrocortisone 1%	**Adults & Peds ≥2 yrs:** Apply to affected area tid-qid.
Cortaid Maximum Strength Cream	Hydrocortisone 1%	**Adults & Peds ≥2 yrs:** Apply to affected area tid-qid.
Cortaid Maximum Strength Ointment	Hydrocortisone 1%	**Adults & Peds ≥2 yrs:** Apply to affected area tid-qid.
Cortizone-10 Creme Plus	Hydrocortisone 1%	**Adults & Peds ≥2 yrs:** Apply to affected area tid-qid.
Cortizone-10 Maximum Strength Anti-Itch Ointment	Hydrocortisone 1%	**Adults & Peds ≥2 yrs:** Apply to affected area tid-qid.
Cortizone-10 Ointment	Hydrocortisone 1%	**Adults & Peds ≥2 yrs:** Apply to affected area tid-qid.
Cortizone-10 Intensive Healing Formula	Hydrocortisone 1%	**Adults & Peds ≥2 yrs:** Apply to affected area tid-qid.
PYRITHIONE ZINC		
Denorex Dandruff Shampoo, Daily Protection	Pyrithione Zinc 2%	**Adults & Peds:** Use biw.
Head & Shoulders Dry Scalp Care Dandruff Shampoo Plus Conditioner; Shampoo; Conditioner	Pyrithione Zinc 1%	**Adults & Peds:** Use biw.
Head & Shoulders Smooth & Silky Dandruff Shampoo Plus Conditioner; Shampoo; Conditioner	Pyrithione Zinc 1%	**Adults & Peds:** Use biw.
Head & Shoulders Citrus Breeze Dandruff Shampoo Plus Conditioner; Shampoo	Pyrithione Zinc 1%	**Adults & Peds:** Use biw.
Head & Shoulders Classic Clean Dandruff Shampoo Plus Conditioner; Shampoo; Conditioner	Pyrithione Zinc 1%	**Adults & Peds:** Use biw.

(Continued)

TABLE 9. ANTISEBORRHEAL PRODUCTS (cont.)

Brand Name	Ingredient/Strength	Dose
Head & Shoulders Extra Volume Dandruff Shampoo	Pyrithione Zinc 1%	**Adults & Peds:** Use biw.
Head & Shoulders Ocean Lift Dandruff Shampoo Plus Conditioner; Shampoo	Pyrithione Zinc 1%	**Adults & Peds:** Use biw.
Head & Shoulders Dandruff Refresh Shampoo Plus Conditioner; Shampoo	Pyrithione Zinc 1%	**Adults & Peds:** Use biw.
Head & Shoulders Restoring Shine - Dandruff Shampoo Plus Conditioner; Shampoo	Pyrithione Zinc 1%	**Adults & Peds:** Use biw.
Head & Shoulders Sensitive Care Dandruff Shampoo Plus Conditioner; Shampoo	Pyrithione Zinc 1%	**Adults & Peds:** Use biw.
Head & Shoulders Intensive Solutions Dandruff Shampoo and Conditioner; Shampoo	Pyrithione Zinc 1%	**Adults & Peds:** Use biw.
L'Oreal VIVE Pro Anti-Dandruff for Men Shampoo and Conditioner	Pyrithione Zinc 1%	**Adults & Peds:** Use biw.
Neutrogena T-Gel Daily Control Dandruff Shampoo	Pyrithione Zinc 1%	**Adults & Peds:** Use biw.
Pantene Pro-V Shampoo + Conditioner, Anti-Dandruff	Pyrithione Zinc 1%	**Adults & Peds:** Use biw.
Pert Plus Dandruff Away Shampoo Plus Conditioner	Pyrithione Zinc 0.45%	**Adults & Peds:** Use at least biw.
Pert Plus for Men Daily Dandruff 2-in-1 Shampoo Plus Conditioner	Pyrithione Zinc 1%	**Adults & Peds:** Use qd.
Selsun Salon Shampoo Plus Conditioner	Pyrithione Zinc 1%	**Adults & Peds:** Use at least biw.
Suave for Men 2 in 1 Shampoo/ Conditioner, Dandruff	Pyrithione Zinc 0.5%	**Adults & Peds:** Use biw.
SALICYLIC ACID		
Neutrogena T/Gel Conditioner	Salicylic Acid 2%	**Adults & Peds:** Use at least tiw.
Neutrogena T/Sal Shampoo, Scalp Build-up Control	Salicylic Acid 3%	**Adults & Peds:** Use biw.
Psoriasin Therapeutic Shampoo and Body Wash	Salicylic Acid 3%	**Adults & Peds:** Use biw.
Scalpicin Anti-Itch Liquid Scalp Treatment (Combe)	Salicylic Acid 3%	**Adults:** Apply to affected area qd-qid.
SELENIUM SULFIDE		
Head & Shoulders Dandruff Shampoo, Intensive Treatment	Selenium Sulfide 1%	**Adults & Peds:** Use biw.
Selsun Blue Dandruff Shampoo, Medicated Treatment	Selenium Sulfide 1%	**Adults & Peds:** Use biw.
Selsun Blue Dandruff Shampoo Plus Conditioner	Selenium Sulfide 1%	**Adults & Peds:** Use biw.
Selsun Blue Dandruff Shampoo	Selenium Sulfide 1%	**Adults & Peds:** Use biw.
Selsun Blue Dandruff Shampoo, Moisturizing Treatment	Selenium Sulfide 1%	**Adults & Peds:** Use biw.
SULFUR/SALICYLIC ACID		
Sebulex Medicated Dandruff Shampoo	Sulfur/Salicylic Acid 2%-2%	**Adults & Peds:** Use qd.

TABLE 10. ARTIFICIAL TEAR PRODUCTS

Brand Name	Ingredient/Strength	Dose
Akwa Tears Lubricant Eye Drops	Polyvinyl Alcohol/Benzalkonium Chloride 1.4%-0.005%	**Adults:** Instill 1-2 drops to affected eye prn.
Akwa Tears Lubricant Ophthalmic Ointment	White Petrolatum/Mineral Oil/ Lanolin 83%-15%-2%	**Adults:** Place ¼ in oint inside eyelid one or more times daily.
Allergan Optive Lubricant Eye Drops	Carboxymethylcellulose Sodium/Glycerin 0.5%-0.9%	**Adults:** Instill 1-2 drops to affected eye prn.
Allergan Lacri-Lube S.O.P. Lubricant Eye Ointment	Mineral Oil/White Petrolatum 42.5%-56.8%	**Adults:** Place ¼ in oint inside eyelid qd.
Allergan Refresh Celluvisc Lubricant Eye Drops	Carboxymethylcellulose Sodium 1%	**Adults:** Instill 1-2 drops to affected eye prn.
Allergan Refresh Liquigel Lubricant Eye Drops	Carboxymethylcellulose Sodium 1%	**Adults:** Instill 1-2 drops to affected eye prn.
Allergan Refresh Plus Lubricant Eye Drops	Carboxymethylcellulose Sodium 0.5%	**Adults:** Instill 1-2 drops to affected eye prn.
Allergan Refresh PM Sensitive Lubricant Eye Ointment	White Petrolatum/Mineral Oil 57.3%-42.5%	**Adults:** Place ¼ in oint inside eyelid.
Allergan Refresh Tears Lubricant Eye Drops	Carboxymethylcellulose Sodium 0.5%	**Adults:** Instill 1-2 drops to affected eye prn.
AMO Blink Tears Lubricating Eye Drops for Mild-Moderate Dry Eyes	Polyethylene Glycol 400 0.25%	**Adults:** Instill 1-2 drops to affected eye prn.
Bausch & Lomb Advanced Eye Relief Dry Eye Environmental Lubricant Eye Drops	Glycerin 1%	**Adults:** Instill 1 or 2 drops in the affected eye prn.
Bausch & Lomb Advanced Eye Relief Dry Eye Rejuvenation Lubricant Eye Drops	Glycerin/Propylene Glycol 0.3%-1%	**Adults:** Instill 1 or 2 drops in the affected eye prn.
Bausch & Lomb Advanced Eye Relief Night Time Lubricant Eye Ointment (Preservative Free)	Mineral Oil/White Petrolatum 20%-80%	**Adults:** Apply a small amount (¼ inch) of ointment to the inside of lower eyelid one or more times daily.
Bausch & Lomb Soothe Lubricant Eye Drops	Glycerin/Propylene Glycol 0.6%-0.6%	**Adults:** Instill 1 or 2 drops in the affected eye prn.
Bion Tears Lubricant Eye Drops	Dextran 70/Hydroxypropyl Methylcellulose 2910 0.1%-0.3%	**Adults:** Instill 1-2 drops to affected eye prn.
Clear Eyes Eye Drops for Dry Eyes	Carboxymethylcellulose Sodium/ Glycerine 1.0%-0.25%	**Adults:** Instill 1-2 drops to affected eye prn.
GenTeal Gel	Hypromellose 0.3%	**Adults:** Instill 1 or 2 drops in the affected eye prn.
GenTeal Mild Dry Eyes Drops	Hypromellose 0.2%	**Adults:** Instill 1-2 drops to affected eye prn.
GenTeal Moderate Dry Eyes Drops	Hypromellose 0.3%	**Adults:** Instill 1-2 drops to affected eye prn.
GenTeal PM Ointment	Mineral Oil/White Petrolatum 15%-85%	**Adults:** Apply a small amount (¼ inch) of oint to the inside of lower eyelid one or more times daily.
GenTeal Lubricant Eye Drops for Moderate to Severe Dry Eye Relief, Gel Drops	Carboxymethylcellulose Sodium/ Hypromellose 0.25%-0.3%	**Adults:** Instill 1-2 drops to affected eye prn.
Murine Tears Lubricant Eye Drops	Polyvinyl Alcohol/Povidone 0.5%-0.6%	**Adults:** Instill 1-2 drops to affected eye prn.
Optics Laboratory Minidrops Eye Therapy	Polyvinylpyrrolidone/ Polyvinyl Alcohol 6mg-14mg	**Adults:** Instill 1-2 drops to affected eye prn.
Rohto Zi For Eyes Lubricant Eye Drops	Povidone 1.8%	**Adults:** Instill 1-2 drops to affected eye prn.

(Continued)

TABLE 10. ARTIFICIAL TEAR PRODUCTS (cont.)

Brand Name	Ingredient/Strength	Dose
Soothe XP Emollient Lubricant Eye Drops	Light Mineral Oil/Mineral Oil 1%-4.5%	**Adults:** Instill 1-2 drops in the affected eye prn, or as directed by your doctor.
Systane Lubricant Eye Drops	Polyethylene Glycol 400/ Propylene Glycol 0.4%-0.3%	**Adults:** Instill 1-2 drops to affected eye prn.
Systane Nighttime Lubricant Eye Ointment	Mineral Oil/White Petrolatum 3%-94%	**Adults:** Place ¼ inch oint inside eyelid.
Systane Preservative Free Lubricant Eye Drops	Polyethylene Glycol 400/Propylene Glycol 0.4%-0.3%	**Adults:** Instill 1 or 2 drops in the affected eye prn.
Systane Ultra Lubricant Eye Drops	Polyethylene Glycol 400/Propylene Glycol 0.4%-0.3%	**Adults:** Instill 1 or 2 drops in the affected eye prn.
Tears Naturale Forte Lubricant Eye Drops	Dextran 70/Glycerin/Hydroxypropyl Methylcellulose 1%-0.2%-0.3%	**Adults:** Instill 1-2 drops to affected eye prn.
Tears Naturale Free Lubricant Eye Drops	Dextran 70/Hydroxypropyl Methylcellulose 2910 0.1%-0.3%	**Adults:** Instill 1-2 drops to affected eye prn.
Tears Naturale II Polyquad Lubricant Eye Drops	Dextran 70/Hydroxypropyl Methylcellulose 2910 0.1%-0.3%	**Adults:** Instill 1-2 drops to affected eye prn.
Tears Naturale P.M. Lubricant Eye Ointment	White Petrolatum/Mineral Oil 94%-3%	**Adults:** Place ¼ inch oint inside eyelid qd.
TheraTears Liquid Gel Lubricant Eye Gel	Sodium Carboxymethylcellulose 1%	**Adults:** Instill 1-2 drops to affected eye prn.
TheraTears Lubricant Eye Drops	Sodium Carboxymethylcellulose 0.25%	**Adults:** Instill 1-2 drops to affected eye prn.
Visine Pure Tears Lubricant Eye Drops	Glycerin/Hypromellose/Polyethylene Glycol 400 0.2%-0.2%-1%	**Adults and Peds >6 yrs:** Instill 1-2 drops to affected eye prn.
Viva-Drops Lubricant Eye Drops	Polysorbate 80	**Adults:** Instill 1-2 drops to affected eye prn.

TABLE 11. CANKER AND COLD SORE PRODUCTS

Brand Name	Ingredient/Strength	Dose
Abreva Cold Sore/Fever Blister Treatment	Docosanol 10%	**Adults & Peds ≥12 yrs:** Use 5 times a day until healed. **Max:** 10 days.
Abreva Pump Cold Sore/Fever Blister Treatment	Docosanol 10%	**Adults & Peds ≥12 yrs:** Use 5 times a day until healed. **Max:** 10 days.
Anbesol Cold Sore Therapy Ointment	Allantoin/Benzocaine/Camphor/White Petrolatum 1%-20%-3%-64.9%	**Adults & Peds ≥2 yrs:** Apply to affected area up to tid-qid.
Anbesol Jr. Gel	Benzocaine 10%	**Adults & Peds ≥2 yrs:** Apply to affected area up to qid.
Anbesol Maximum Strength Gel	Benzocaine 20%	**Adults & Peds ≥2 yrs:** Apply to affected area up to qid.
Anbesol Maximum Strength Liquid	Benzocaine 20%	**Adults & Peds ≥2 yrs:** Apply to affected area up to qid.
Anbesol Regular Strength Gel	Benzocaine 10%	**Adults & Peds ≥2 yrs:** Apply to affected area up to qid.
Anbesol Regular Strength Liquid	Benzocaine 10%	**Adults & Peds ≥2 yrs:** Apply to affected area up to qid.
Baby Anbesol	Benzocaine 7.5%	**Peds ≥4 months:** Apply to affected area up to qid.
Campho-Phenique Cold Sore Gel	Camphor/Phenol 10.8%-4.7%	**Adults & Peds ≥2 yrs:** Apply to affected area qd-tid.
ChapStick Cold Sore Therapy	Allantoin/Benzocaine/Camphor/White Petrolatum 1%-20%-3%-64.9%	**Adults & Peds ≥2 yrs:** Apply to affected area up to tid-qid.
Chloraseptic Max Sore Throat Relief	Phenol 1.5%/Glycerin 33%	**Peds ≥3 yrs:** Apply to affected area for 15 seconds, then spit. Use q2h.
Chloraseptic Pocket Pump Sore Throat Spray	Phenol 1.4%	**Adults & Peds ≥12 yrs:** Spray 5 times to affected area for 15 seconds, then spit. Use q2h. **Peds 3-12 yrs:** Spray 3 times to affected area for 15 seconds, then spit. Use q2h.
Dr. Snapz Swabplus Mouth Sore Relief Swabs	Benzocaine 20%	**Adults & Peds ≥2 yrs:** Apply to affected area up to qid.
Herpecin-L Lip Balm Stick, SPF 30	Dimethicone/Methyl Anthranilate/Octyl Methoxycinnamate/Octyl Salicylate/Oxybenzone 1%-5%-7.5%-5%-6%	**Adults & Peds ≥12 yrs:** Apply prn to cold sore.
Kank-A Soft Brush Tooth/Mouth Pain Gel	Benzocaine 20%	**Adults & Peds ≥2 yrs:** Apply to affected area up to qid.
Kanka-A Mouth Pain Liquid	Benzocaine 20%/Compound Benzoin Tincture	**Adults & Peds ≥2 yrs:** Apply to affected area up to qid. **Max:** q2h.
Novitra Cold Sore Maximum Strength Cream	Zincum Oxydatum 2X/HPUS	**Adults & Peds ≥2 yrs:** Apply to affected area q2-3h, 6 to 8 times daily.
Orabase with Benzocaine Paste	Benzocaine 20%	**Adults & Peds ≥2 yrs:** Apply to affected area up to qid.
Orajel Ultra Mouth Sore Medicine Film-Forming Gel	Benzocaine/Menthol 15%-2%	**Adults & Peds ≥2 yrs:** Apply to affected area up to qid.
Orajel Mouth Sore Medicine Gel	Benzocaine/Benzalkonium Chloride/Zinc Chloride 20%-0.02%-0.1%	**Adults & Peds ≥2 yrs:** Apply to affected area up to qid.
Orajel Antiseptic Mouth Sore Rinse	Hydrogen Peroxide 1.5%	**Adults & Peds ≥2 yrs:** Rinse with 2 tsp for 1 minute, then spit. Use up to qid.
Orajel Medicated Mouth Sore Swabs	Benzocaine 20%	**Adults & Peds ≥2 yrs:** Apply to affected area up to qid.

(Continued)

TABLE 11. CANKER AND COLD SORE PRODUCTS (cont.)

Brand Name	Ingredient/Strength	Dose
Orajel Medicated Cold Sore Brush	Allantoin/Benzocaine/Dimethicone/White Petrolatum 0.5%-20%-2%-65%	**Adults & Peds ≥2 yrs:** Apply to affected area up to tid-qid.
Orajel Protective Mouth Sore Discs	Benzocaine 15mg	**Adults & Peds ≥2 yrs:** Apply to affected area q2h prn.
Releev 1-Day Cold Sore Treatment	Benzalkonium Chloride 0.13%	**Adults & Peds ≥2 yrs:** Apply to clean dry affected area tid-qid.
Zilactin	Benzyl Alcohol 10%	**Adults & Peds ≥2 yrs:** Apply to affected area up to qid.
Zilactin B	Benzocaine 10%	**Adults & Peds ≥2 yrs:** Apply to affected area up to qid.
Zilactin L	Benzyl Alcohol 10%	**Adults & Peds ≥2 yrs:** Apply to affected area up to qid.
Zilactin Tooth & Gum	Benzocaine 20%	**Adults & Peds ≥2 yrs:** Apply to affected area up to qid.

TABLE 12. CONTACT DERMATITIS PRODUCTS

Brand Name	Ingredient/Strength	Dose
ANTIHISTAMINE		
Benadryl Itch Stopping Extra Strength Gel	Diphenhydramine HCl 2%	**Adults & Peds ≥2 yrs:** Apply to affected area tid-qid.
ANTIHISTAMINE COMBINATION		
Benadryl Extra Strength Itch-Stopping Cream	Diphenhydramine HCl/Zinc Acetate 2%-0.1%	**Adults & Peds ≥2 yrs:** Apply to affected area tid-qid.
Benadryl Extra Strength Spray	Diphenhydramine HCl/Zinc Acetate 2%-0.1%	**Adults & Peds ≥2 yrs:** Apply to affected area tid-qid.
Benadryl Extra Strength Itch Relief Stick	Diphenhydramine HCl/Zinc Acetate 2%-0.1%	**Adults & Peds ≥2 yrs:** Apply to affected area tid-qid.
Benadryl Original Strength Itch Stopping Cream	Diphenhydramine HCl/Zinc Acetate 1%-0.1%	**Adults & Peds ≥2 yrs:** Apply to affected area tid-qid.
CalaGel Anti-Itch Gel	Diphenhydramine HCl/Zinc Acetate/Benzenthonium Chloride 2%-0.215%-0.15%	**Adults & Peds ≥2 yrs:** Apply to affected area no more than tid.
Ivarest Double Relief Formula	Diphenhydramine HCl/Benzyl Alcohol/Calamine 2%-10.5%-14%	**Adults & Peds ≥2 yrs:** Apply to affected area tid-qid.
ASTRINGENT		
Domeboro Astringent Solution Powder Packets	Aluminum Acetate (combination of Calcium Acetate 893mg and Aluminum Sulfate 1191mg)	**Adults & Peds:** Dissolve 1-3 pkts and apply to affected area for 15-30 min tid.
Ivy-Dry Super with Zytrel	Zinc Acetate/Benzyl Alcohol/Camphor/Menthol 2%-10%-0.5%-0.25%	**Adults & Peds ≥6 yrs:** Apply to affected area tid.
Ivy-Dry Anti-Itch Cream with Zytrel	Zinc Acetate/Camphor/Menthol 2%-0.6%-0.4%	**Adults & Peds ≥6 yrs:** Apply to affected area tid.
Ivy-Dry Cream with Zytrel	Zinc Acetate/Camphor/Menthol 2%-0.6%-0.4%	**Adults & Peds ≥6 yrs:** Apply to affected area tid.
Ivy-Dry Kids with Zytrel	Zinc Acetate 2%	**Adults & Peds ≥2 yrs:** Apply to affected area tid.
ASTRINGENT COMBINATION		
Aveeno Calamine and Pramoxine HCl Anti-Itch Cream	Calamine/Camphor/Pramoxine HCl 3%-0.5%-1%	**Adults & Peds ≥2 yrs:** Apply to affected area tid-qid.
Aveeno Anti-Itch Concentrated Lotion	Calamine/Pramoxine HCl/Camphor 3%-1%-0.47%	**Adults & Peds ≥2 yrs:** Apply to affected area qid.
Caladryl Clear Anti-Itch Lotion	Zinc Acetate/Pramoxine HCl 0.1%-1%	**Adults & Peds ≥2 yrs:** Apply to affected area tid-qid.
Caladryl Anti-Itch Lotion	Calamine/Pramoxine HCl 8%-1%	**Adults & Peds ≥2 yrs:** Apply to affected area tid-qid.
Calamine Lotion (generic)	Calamine/Zinc Oxide 8%-8%	**Adults & Peds:** Apply to affected area prn.
Cortaid Poison Ivy Care Treatment Kit	(Scrub) Water, polyethylene, laureth-4, sodium lauryl sarcosinate, glycol distearate, acrylates/C10-30, alkyl acrylate crosspolymer, coco-glucoside, sodium hydroxide, microcrystalline wax, tetrasodium EDTA, glyceryl oleate, glyceryl stearate, quaternium-15, chromium hydroxide green, tocopherol (Spray) Zinc Acetate/Pramoxine 0.12%-1%	**Adults & Peds:** (Scrub) Apply quarter-sized amount into hand and rub onto affected area for 30 seconds. Rinse area thoroughly and pat dry. (Spray) Apply to affected area tid-qid.

(Continued)

TABLE 12. CONTACT DERMATITIS PRODUCTS (cont.)

BRAND NAME	INGREDIENT/STRENGTH	DOSE
CLEANSER		
Ivy-Dry Scrub with Zytrel	Polyethylene, sodium laureth sulfate, zinc lactate, panthenol, PEG-14M, nonoxynol-9, zinc gluconate, zinc acetate, glycerin, tocopheryl acetate, C12-15 pareth-9, *Aloe barbadensis* extract, carbomer, allantoin, sodium hydroxide	**Adults & Peds:** Gently rub into affected area for at least 30 seconds; rinse.
Cortaid Poison Ivy Care Toxin Removal Cloths	Water, laureth-4, sodium lauryl sarcosinate, glycerin, DMDM, hydantoin, methylparaben, tetrasodium EDTA, *Aloe barbadensis* leaf extract, citric acid	**Adults & Peds:** Wipe affected area at least 15 seconds. Rinse or wipe dry.
CORTICOSTEROID		
Aveeno 1% Hydrocortisone Anti-Itch Cream	Hydrocortisone 1%	**Adults & Peds ≥2 yrs:** Apply to affected area tid-qid.
Cortaid Advanced 12-Hour Anti-Itch Cream	Hydrocortisone 1%	**Adults & Peds ≥2 yrs:** Apply to affected area tid-qid.
Cortaid Intensive Therapy Cooling Spray	Hydrocortisone 1%	**Adults & Peds ≥2 yrs:** Apply to affected area tid-qid.
Cortaid Intensive Therapy Moisturizing Cream	Hydrocortisone 1%	**Adults & Peds ≥2 yrs:** Apply to affected area tid-qid.
Cortaid Maximum Strength Cream	Hydrocortisone 1%	**Adults & Peds ≥2 yrs:** Apply to affected area tid-qid.
Cortaid Maximum Strength Ointment	Hydrocortisone 1%	**Adults & Peds ≥2 yrs:** Apply to affected area tid-qid.
Cortizone-10 Easy Relief Applicator	Hydrocortisone 1%	**Adults & Peds ≥2 yrs:** Apply to affected area tid-qid.
Cortizone-10 Cooling Relief Gel	Hydrocortisone 1%	**Adults & Peds ≥2 yrs:** Apply to affected area tid-qid.
Cortizone-10 Creme	Hydrocortisone 1%	**Adults & Peds ≥2 yrs:** Apply to affected area tid-qid.
Cortizone-10 Ointment	Hydrocortisone 1%	**Adults & Peds ≥2 yrs:** Apply to affected area tid-qid.
Cortizone-10 Plus	Hydrocortisone 1%	**Adults & Peds ≥2 yrs:** Apply to affected area tid-qid.
Cortizone-10 Intensive Healing Formula	Hydrocortisone 1%	**Adults & Peds ≥2 yrs:** Apply to affected area tid-qid.
Corticool	Hydrocortisone 1%	**Adults & Peds ≥2 yrs:** Apply to affected area tid-qid.
Dermarest Eczema Medicated Lotion	Hydrocortisone 1%	**Adults & Peds ≥2 yrs:** Apply to affected area tid-qid.
COUNTERIRRITANT		
Gold Bond Quick Spray	Menthol/Benzethonium Chloride 1%-0.13%	**Adults & Peds ≥2 yrs:** Apply to affected area tid-qid.
Gold Bond Medicated Maximum Strength Anti-Itch Cream	Menthol/Pramoxine HCl 1%-1%	**Adults & Peds ≥2 yrs:** Apply to affected area tid-qid.
Ivy Block Lotion	Bentoquatam 5%	**Adults & Peds ≥6 yrs:** Apply 15 minutes before exposure risk and q4h for continued protection.
LOCAL ANESTHETIC		
Solarcaine Aloe Extra Burn Relief Gel	Lidocaine HCl 0.5%	**Adults & Peds ≥2 yrs:** Apply to affected area tid-qid.
Solarcaine Aloe Extra Burn Relief Spray	Lidocaine HCl 0.5%	**Adults & Peds ≥2 yrs:** Apply to affected area tid-qid.
Solarcaine First Aid Medicated Spray	Benzocaine/Triclosan 20%-0.13%	**Adults & Peds ≥2 yrs:** Apply to affected area qd-tid.

TABLE 12. CONTACT DERMATITIS PRODUCTS (cont.)

BRAND NAME	INGREDIENT/STRENGTH	DOSE
LOCAL ANESTHETIC COMBINATION		
Bactine Pain Relieving Cleansing Spray	Lidocaine/Benzalkonium Chloride 2.5%-0.13%	**Adults & Peds ≥2 yrs:** Apply to affected area qd-tid.
Bactine Original First Aid Liquid	Lidocaine HCl/Benzalkonium Chloride 2.5%-0.13%	**Adults & Peds ≥2 yrs:** Apply to affected area qd-tid.
Lanacane Maximum Strength Cream	Benzocaine/Benzethonium Chloride 20%-0.2%	**Adults & Peds ≥2 yrs:** Apply to affected area qd-tid.
Lanacane Antibacterial First Aid Spray	Benzocaine/Benzethonium Chloride 20%-0.2%	**Adults & Peds ≥2 yrs:** Apply to affected area qd-tid.
Lanacane Original Strength Cream	Benzocaine/Benzethonium Chloride 6%-0.2%	**Adults & Peds ≥2 yrs:** Apply to affected area qd-tid.
SKIN PROTECTANT		
Aveeno Skin Relief Moisturizing Cream	Dimethicone 2.5%	**Adults & Peds ≥2 yrs:** Apply to affected area tid-qid.
SKIN PROTECTANT COMBINATION		
Gold Bond Extra Strength Medicated Body Lotion	Dimethicone/Menthol 5%-0.5%	**Adults & Peds:** Apply to affected area tid-qid.
Gold Bond Medicated Body Lotion	Dimethicone/Menthol 5%-0.15%	**Adults & Peds:** Apply to affected area prn.
Gold Bond Medicated Powder	Zinc Oxide/Menthol 1%-0.15%	**Adults & Peds ≥2 yrs:** Apply to affected area tid-qid.
Gold Bond Medicated Extra Strength Powder	Zinc Oxide/Menthol 5%-0.8%	**Adults & Peds ≥2 yrs:** Apply to affected area tid-qid.
Vaseline Intensive Rescue Clinical Therapy Lotion	Dimethicone 1%	**Adults & Peds:** Apply to affected area prn.

TABLE 13. COUGH-COLD-FLU PRODUCTS

Brand Name	Analgesic	Antihistamine	Decongestant	Cough Suppressant	Expectorant	Dose
ANTIHISTAMINE + DECONGESTANT						
Actifed Cold & Allergy Tablets		Chlorpheniramine Maleate 4mg	Phenylephrine HCl 10mg			**Adults ≥12 yrs:** 1 tab q4h. **Max:** 6 tabs q24h.
Benadryl-D Allergy/Sinus Tablets		Diphenhydramine HCl 25mg	Phenylephrine HCl 10mg			**Adults & Peds ≥12 yrs:** 1 tab q4h. **Max:** 6 tabs q24h.
Children's Benadryl-D Allergy & Sinus Liquid		Diphenhydramine HCl 12.5mg/5mL	Phenylephrine HCl 5mg/5mL			**Adults ≥12 yrs:** 2 tsp (10mL) q4h. **Peds 6-<12 yrs:** 1 tsp (5mL) q4h. **Max:** 6 doses q24h.
Dimetapp Children's Cold & Allergy Elixir		Brompheniramine Maleate 1mg/5mL	Phenylephrine HCl 2.5mg/5mL			**Adults & Peds ≥12 yrs:** 4 tsp q4h. **Peds 6-<12 yrs:** 2 tsp q4h. **Max:** 6 doses q24h.
Dimetapp Nighttime Cold & Congestion Liquid		Diphenhydramine HCl 6.25mg/5mL	Phenylephrine HCl 2.5mg/5mL			**Adults & Peds ≥12 yrs:** 4 tsp q4h. **Peds 6-<12 yrs:** 2 tsp q4h. **Max:** 6 doses q24h.
Dimetapp Children's Cold & Allergy Chewable Tablets		Brompheniramine Maleate 1mg	Phenylephrine HCl 2.5mg			**Peds 6-<12 yrs:** 2 tabs q4h. **Max:** 6 doses q24h.
Pediacare Children's Allergy & Cold		Diphenhydramine HCl 12.5mg/5mL	Phenylephrine HCl 5mg/5mL			**Peds 6-11 yrs:** 1 tsp q4h. **Max:** 6 doses q24h.
Robitussin Night Time Cough & Cold Liquid		Diphenhydramine HCl 6.25mg/5mL	Phenylephrine HCl 2.5mg/5mL			**Adults & Peds ≥12 yrs:** 4 tsp q4h. **Max:** 6 doses q24h.
Sudafed PE Maximum Strength Sinus & Allergy Tablets		Chlorpheniramine Maleate 4mg	Phenylephrine HCl 10mg			**Adults & Peds ≥12 yrs:** 1 tab q4h. **Max:** 6 doses q24h.
Sudafed PE Nighttime Nasal Decongestant Tablets		Diphenhydramine HCl 25mg	Phenylephrine HCl 10mg			**Adults & Peds ≥12 yrs:** 1 tab q4h. **Max:** 6 tabs q24h.
Theraflu Nighttime Cold & Cough Thin Strips		Diphenhydramine HCl 25mg/strip	Phenylephrine HCl 10mg/strip			**Adults ≥12 yrs:** 1 strip q4h. **Max:** 6 strips q24h.
Triaminic Cold & Allergy Liquid		Chlorpheniramine Maleate 1mg/5mL	Phenylephrine HCl 2.5mg/5mL			**Peds 6-<12 yrs:** 2 tsp (10mL) q4h. **Max:** 6 doses q24h.
Triaminic Nighttime Cold & Cough Liquid		Diphenhydramine HCl 6.25mg/5mL	Phenylephrine HCl 2.5mg/5mL			**Peds 6-12 yrs:** 2 tsp (10mL) q4h. **Max:** 6 doses q24h.
Triaminic Nighttime Cold & Cough Thin Strips		Diphenhydramine HCl 12.5mg/strip	Phenylephrine HCl 5mg/strip			**Peds 6-12 yrs:** 1 strip q4h. **Max:** 6 strips q24h.
ANTIHISTAMINE + DECONGESTANT + ANALGESIC						
Advil Allergy Sinus Caplets	Ibuprofen 200mg	Chlorpheniramine Maleate 2mg	Pseudoephedrine HCl 30mg			**Adults & Peds ≥12 yrs:** 1 tab q4-6h. **Max:** 6 tabs q24h.
Alka-Seltzer Plus Cold Original Effervescent Tablets	Aspirin 325mg	Chlorpheniramine Maleate 2mg	Phenylephrine Bitartrate 7.8mg			**Adults & Peds ≥12 yrs:** 2 tabs q4h. **Max:** 8 tabs q24h.

TABLE 13. COUGH-COLD-FLU PRODUCTS (cont.)

Brand Name	Analgesic	Antihistamine	Cough Suppressant	Decongestant	Expectorant	Dose
Benadryl Allergy & Cold Kapgels	Acetaminophen 325mg	Diphenhydramine HCl 12.5mg		Phenylephrine HCl 5mg		**Adults & Peds ≥12 yrs:** 2 caps q4h. **Max:** 12 caps q24h.
Benadryl Allergy & Sinus Headache Kapgels	Acetaminophen 325mg	Diphenhydramine HCl 12.5mg		Phenylephrine HCl 5mg		**Adults & Peds ≥12 yrs:** 2 caps q4h. **Max:** 12 caps q24h.
Benadryl Severe Allergy & Sinus Headache Caplets	Acetaminophen 325mg	Diphenhydramine HCl 25mg		Phenylephrine HCl 5mg		**Adults & Peds ≥12 yrs:** 2 tabs q4h. **Max:** 12 tabs q24h.
Comtrex Day & Night Severe Cold & Sinus Caplets	Acetaminophen 325mg	Chlorpheniramine Maleate 2mg (nighttime dose only)		Phenylephrine HCl 5mg		**Adults & Peds ≥12 yrs:** *Daytime:* 2 daytime tabs q4h. **Max:** 8 daytime tabs q24h. *Nighttime:* 2 nighttime tabs q24h. **Max:** 4 nighttime tabs q24h.
Contac Cold & Flu Maximum Strength Caplets	Acetaminophen 500mg	Chlorpheniramine Maleate 2mg		Phenylephrine HCl 5mg		**Adults & Peds ≥12 yrs:** 2 tabs q4-6h. **Max:** 8 tabs q24h.
Dristan Cold Multi-Symptom Tablets	Acetaminophen 325mg	Chlorpheniramine Maleate 2mg		Phenylephrine HCl 5mg		**Adults & Peds ≥12 yrs:** 2 tabs q4h. **Max:** 12 tabs q24h.
Sudafed PE Nighttime Cold Caplets	Acetaminophen 325mg	Diphenhydramine HCl 25mg		Phenylephrine HCl 5mg		**Adults & Peds ≥12 yrs:** 2 tabs q4h. **Max:** 12 tabs q24h.
Sudafed PE Severe Cold Formula Caplets	Acetaminophen 325mg	Diphenhydramine HCl 12.5mg		Phenylephrine HCl 5mg		**Adults & Peds ≥12 yrs:** 2 tabs q4h. **Max:** 12 tabs q24h. **Peds 6–<12 yrs:** 1 tab q4h. **Max:** 5 tabs q24h.
Theraflu Cold & Sore Throat Hot Liquid	Acetaminophen 325mg/packet	Pheniramine Maleate 20mg/packet		Phenylephrine HCl 10mg/packet		**Adults & Peds ≥12 yrs:** 1 packet q4h. **Max:** 6 packets q24h.
Theraflu Nighttime Severe Cold & Cough Hot Liquid	Acetaminophen 650mg/packet	Diphenhydramine HCl 25mg/packet		Phenylephrine HCl 10mg/packet		**Adults & Peds ≥12 yrs:** 1 packet q4h. **Max:** 6 packets q24h.
Theraflu Sugar-Free Nighttime Severe Cold & Cough Hot Liquid	Acetaminophen 650mg/packet	Diphenhydramine HCl 25mg/packet		Phenylephrine HCl 10mg/packet		**Adults & Peds ≥12 yrs:** 1 packet q4h. **Max:** 6 packets q24h.
Theraflu Flu & Sore Throat Hot Liquid	Acetaminophen 650mg/packet	Pheniramine Maleate 20mg/packet		Phenylephrine HCl 10mg/packet		**Adults & Peds ≥12 yrs:** 1 packet q4h. **Max:** 6 packets q24h.
Theraflu Nighttime Warming Relief Syrup	Acetaminophen 325mg/15mL	Diphenhydramine HCl 12.5mg/15mL		Phenylephrine HCl 5mg/15mL		**Adults & Peds ≥12 yrs:** 2 tbl (30mL) q4h. **Max:** 6 doses (12 tbl or 180 mL) q24h.
Theraflu Flu & Sore Throat Relief Syrup	Acetaminophen 325mg/15mL	Diphenhydramine HCl 12.5mg/15mL		Phenylephrine HCl 5mg/15mL		**Adults & Peds ≥12 yrs:** 2 tbl (30mL) q4h. **Max:** 6 doses (12 tbl or 180mL) q24h.
Tylenol Children's Plus Cold Liquid	Acetaminophen 160mg/5mL	Chlorpheniramine Maleate 1mg/5mL		Phenylephrine HCl 2.5mg/5mL		**Peds 6-11 yrs (48-95 lbs):** 2 tsp (10mL) q4h. **Max:** 5 doses q24h.
Tylenol Children's Plus Cold and Allergy Liquid	Acetaminophen 160mg/5mL	Diphenhydramine HCl 12.5mg/5mL		Phenylephrine HCl 2.5mg/5mL		**Peds 6-11 yrs (48-95 lbs):** 2 tsp (10mL) q4h. **Max:** 5 doses q24h.
Tylenol Sinus Congestion & Pain Nighttime Caplets	Acetaminophen 325mg	Chlorpheniramine Maleate 2mg		Phenylephrine HCl 5mg		**Adults & Peds ≥12 yrs:** 2 tabs q4h. **Max:** 12 tabs q24h.

(Continued)

TABLE 13. COUGH-COLD-FLU PRODUCTS (cont.)

Brand Name	Analgesic	Antihistamine	Decongestant	Cough Suppressant	Expectorant	Dose
Tylenol Allergy Multi-Symptom Rapid-Release Gelcaps/ Coolburst Caplets	Acetaminophen 325mg	Chlorpheniramine Maleate 2mg	Phenylephrine HCl 5mg			**Adults & Peds ≥12 yrs:** 2 tabs q4h. **Max:** 12 tabs q24h.
Tylenol Allergy Multi-Symptom Nighttime Coolburst Caplets	Acetaminophen 325mg	Diphenhydramine HCl 25mg	Phenylephrine HCl 5mg			**Adults & Peds ≥12 yrs:** 2 tabs q4h. **Max:** 12 tabs q24h.
Vicks NyQuil Sinus Liquicaps	Acetaminophen 325mg	Doxylamine Succinate 6.25mg	Phenylephrine HCl 5mg			**Adults & Peds ≥12 yrs:** 2 caps q4h. **Max:** 6 doses q24h.
COUGH SUPPRESSANT						
Delsym 12 Hour Cough Relief Liquid				Dextromethorphan HBr 30mg/5mL		**Adults & Peds ≥12 yrs:** 2 tsp q12h. **Max:** 4 tsp q24h. **Peds 6-<12 yrs:** 1 tsp q12h. **Max:** 2 tsp q24h. **Peds 4-<6 yrs:** ½ tsp q12h. **Max:** 1 tsp q24h.
PediaCare Long-Acting Cough Liquid				Dextromethorphan HBr 7.5mg/5mL		**Peds 6-11 yrs:** 2 tsp q6-8h. **Peds 4-5 yrs:** 1 tsp q6-8h. **Max:** 4 doses q24h.
Robitussin Cough Long-Acting Liquid				Dextromethorphan HBr 15mg/5mL		**Adults & Peds ≥12 yrs:** 2 tsp (10mL) q6-8h. **Max:** 4 doses q24h.
Robitussin CoughGels Liqui-gels				Dextromethorphan HBr 15mg		**Adults & Peds ≥12 yrs:** 2 caps q6-8h. **Max:** 8 caps q24h.
Robitussin Children's Cough Long-Acting Liquid				Dextromethorphan HBr 7.5mg/5mL		**Adults & Peds ≥12 yrs:** 4 tsp q6-8h. **Peds 6-12 yrs:** 2 tsp q6-8h. **Peds 4-6 yrs:** 1 tsp q6-8h. **Max:** 4 doses q24h.
Triaminic Long-Acting Cough Liquid				Dextromethorphan HBr 7.5mg/5mL		**Peds 6-11 yrs:** 2 tsp (10mL) q6-8h. **Peds 4-<6 yrs:** 1 tsp (5mL) q6-8h. **Max:** 4 doses q24h.
Triaminic Thin Strips Long-Acting Cough				Dextromethorphan HBr 7.5mg/strip		**Peds 6-11 yrs:** 2 strips q6-8h. **Peds 4-<6 yrs:** 1 strip q6-8h. **Max:** 4 doses q24h.
Vicks DayQuil Cough Liquid				Dextromethorphan HBr 15mg/15mL		**Adults & Peds ≥12 yrs:** 2 tbl (30mL) q6-8h. **Peds 6-12 yrs:** 1 tbl (15mL) q6-8h. **Max:** 4 doses q24h.
Vicks Formula 44 Custom Care Dry Cough Suppressant				Dextromethorphan HBr 30mg		**Adults & Peds ≥12 yrs:** 1 tbl (15mL) q6-8h. **Peds 6-<12 yrs:** 1½ tsp (7.5mL) q6-8h. **Max:** 4 doses q24h.
Vicks BabyRub				Petrolatum, fragrance, aloe extract, eucalyptus oil, lavender oil, rosemary oil		**Peds:** Gently massage on the chest, neck, and back to help soothe and comfort.

TABLE 13. COUGH-COLD-FLU PRODUCTS (cont.)

Brand Name	Analgesic	Antihistamine	Decongestant	Cough Suppressant	Expectorant	Dose
Vicks Formula 44 Custom Care Sore Throat Lozenges				Menthol 10mg Benzocaine 10mg		**Adults & Peds >5 yrs:** 1 lozenge q2h.
Vicks VapoRub Cream				Camphor 5.2%, Menthol 2.8%, Eucalyptus 1.2%		**Adults & Peds ≥2 yrs:** Apply q8h. **Max:** tid per 24h.
Vicks VapoRub Ointment				Camphor 4.8%, Menthol 2.6%, Eucalyptus 1.2%		**Adults & Peds ≥2 yrs:** Apply q8h. **Max:** tid per 24h.
Vicks VapoSteam				Camphor 6.2%		**Adults & Peds ≥2 yrs:** 1 tbl/quart q8h or 1½ tsp/pint q8h. **Max:** tid per 24h.
COUGH SUPPRESSANT + ANTIHISTAMINE						
Coricidin HBP Cough & Cold Tablets		Chlorpheniramine Maleate 4mg		Dextromethorphan HBr 30mg		**Adults & Peds ≥12 yrs:** 1 tab q6h. **Max:** 4 tabs q24h.
Dimetapp Children's Long-Acting Cough Plus Cold Elixir		Chlorpheniramine Maleate 1mg/5mL		Dextromethorphan HBr 7.5mg/5mL		**Peds ≥12 yrs:** 4 tsp (20mL) q6h. **6-<12 yrs:** 2 tsp (10 mL) q6h. **Max:** 4 doses q24h.
Robitussin Cough & Cold Long-Acting Liquid		Chlorpheniramine Maleate 2mg/5mL		Dextromethorphan HBr 15mg/5mL		**Adults ≥12 yrs:** 2 tsp (10mL) q6h. **Max:** 4 doses q24h.
Robitussin Children's Cough & Cold Long-Acting Liquid		Chlorpheniramine Maleate 1mg/5mL		Dextromethorphan HBr 7.5mg/5mL		**Adults & Peds ≥12 yrs:** 4 tsp (20mL) q6h. **Peds 6-<12 yrs:** 2 tsp (10 mL) q6h. **Max:** 4 doses q24h.
Triaminic Softchews Cough and Runny Nose		Chlorpheniramine Maleate 1mg		Dextromethorphan HBr 5mg		**Peds 6-<12 yrs:** 2 tabs q4-6h. **Max:** 5 doses q24h.
Vicks Children's NyQuil Liquid		Chlorpheniramine Maleate 2mg/15mL		Dextromethorphan HBr 15mg/15mL		**Adults ≥12 yrs:** 2 tbl (30mL) q6h. **Peds 6-11 yrs:** 1 tbl (15mL) q6h. **Max:** 4 doses q24h.
Vicks NyQuil Cough Liquid		Doxylamine Succinate 6.25mg/15mL		Dextromethorphan HBr 15mg/15mL		**Adults & Peds ≥12 yrs:** 2 tbl (30mL) q6h. **Max:** 4 doses q24h.
COUGH SUPPRESSANT + ANALGESIC						
Triaminic Cough & Sore Throat Liquid	Acetaminophen 160mg/5mL			Dextromethorphan HBr 5mg/5mL		**Peds 6-<12 yrs:** 2 tsp (10mL) q4h. **Peds 4-<6 yrs:** 1 tsp (5mL) q4h. **Max:** 5 doses q24h.
Triaminic Softchews Cough & Sore Throat	Acetaminophen 160mg			Dextromethorphan HBr 5mg		**Peds 6-<12 yrs:** 2 tabs q4h. **Peds 4-<6 yrs:** 1 tab q4h. **Max:** 5 doses q24h.
Tylenol Children's Plus Cough and Sore Throat Liquid	Acetaminophen 160mg/5mL			Dextromethorphan HBr 5mg/5mL		**Peds (48-95 lbs) 6-11 yrs:** 2 tsp (10mL) q4h. **Peds (36-47 lbs) 4-5 yrs:** 1 tsp (5mL) q4h. **Max:** 5 doses q24h.
Tylenol Cough & Sore Throat Daytime Liquid	Acetaminophen 1000mg/30mL			Dextromethorphan HBr 30mg/30mL		**Adults & Peds ≥12 yrs:** 2 tbl (30mL) q6h. **Max:** 8 tbl q24h.

(Continued)

TABLE 13. COUGH-COLD-FLU PRODUCTS (cont.)

Brand Name	Analgesic	Antihistamine	Decongestant	Cough Suppressant	Expectorant	Dose
COUGH SUPPRESSANT + ANTIHISTAMINE + ANALGESIC						
Alka-Seltzer Plus Flu Effervescent Tablets	Aspirin 500mg	Chlorpheniramine Maleate 2mg		Dextromethorphan HBr 15mg		**Adults & Peds ≥12 yrs:** 2 tabs q6h. **Max:** 8 tabs q24h.
Tylenol Children's Plus Cough & Runny Nose Liquid	Acetaminophen 160mg/5mL	Chlorpheniramine Maleate 1mg/5mL		Dextromethorphan HBr 5mg/5mL		**Peds 6-11 yrs (48-95 lbs):** 2 tsp (10mL), q4h. **Max:** 5 doses q24h.
Coricidin HBP Maximum Strength Flu Tablets	Acetaminophen 500mg	Chlorpheniramine Maleate 2mg		Dextromethorphan HBr 15mg		**Adults & Peds ≥12 yrs:** 2 tabs q6h. **Max:** 8 tabs q24h.
Coricidin HBP Nighttime Multi-Symptom Cold Liquid	Acetaminophen 500mg/15mL	Doxylamine 6.25mg/15mL		Dextromethorphan HBr 15mg/15mL		**Adults & Peds ≥12 yrs:** 2 tbl q6h. **Max:** 4 doses q24h.
Triaminic Multisymptom Fever	Acetaminophen 160mg/5mL	Chlorpheniramine Maleate 1mg/5mL		Dextromethorphan HBr 7.5mg/5mL		**Peds 6-<12 yrs:** 2 tsp (10mL) q6h. **Max:** 4 doses (40mL) q24h.
Tylenol Cough & Sore Throat Nighttime Cool Burst/Honey Lemon Warming Liquid	Acetaminophen 500mg/15mL	Doxylamine 6.25mg/15mL		Dextromethorphan HBr 15mg/15mL		**Adults & Peds ≥12 yrs:** 2 tbl q6h. **Max:** 8 tbl q24h.
Vicks Formula 44 Custom Care Cough & Cold PM	Acetaminophen 650mg/15mL	Chlorpheniramine Maleate 4mg/15mL		Dextromethorphan HBr 30mg/15mL		**Adults & Peds ≥12 yrs:** 1 tbl q6h. **Max:** 4 doses q24h.
Vicks NyQuil Cold & Flu Relief Liquicaps	Acetaminophen 325mg	Doxylamine Succinate 6.25mg		Dextromethorphan HBr 15mg		**Adults & Peds ≥12 yrs:** 2 caps q6h. **Max:** 4 doses q24h.
Vicks NyQuil Cold & Flu Relief Liquid	Acetaminophen 500mg/15mL	Doxylamine Succinate 6.25mg/15mL		Dextromethorphan HBr 15mg/15mL		**Adults & Peds ≥12 yrs:** 2 tbl (30mL) q6h. **Max:** 8 tbl (120mL) q24h.
COUGH SUPPRESSANT + ANTIHISTAMINE + ANALGESIC + DECONGESTANT						
Alka-Seltzer Plus Cold & Cough Liquid Gels	Acetaminophen 325mg	Chlorpheniramine Maleate 2mg	Phenylephrine HCl 5mg	Dextromethorphan HBr 10mg		**Adults & Peds ≥12 yrs:** 2 caps q4h. **Max:** 12 caps q24h.
Alka-Seltzer Plus Cold & Cough Effervescent Tablets	Aspirin 325mg	Chlorpheniramine Maleate 2mg	Phenylephrine Bitartrate 7.8mg	Dextromethorphan HBr 10mg		**Adults & Peds ≥12 yrs:** 2 tabs q4h. **Max:** 8 tabs q24h.
Alka-Seltzer Plus Night Cold Formula Liquid Gels	Acetaminophen 325mg	Doxylamine 6.25mg	Phenylephrine HCl 5mg	Dextromethorphan HBr 10mg		**Adults & Peds ≥12 yrs:** 2 caps q4h. **Max:** 12 caps q24h.
Alka-Seltzer Plus Cold & Cough Liquid	Acetaminophen 162.5mg/5mL	Chlorpheniramine Maleate 1mg/5mL	Phenylephrine HCl 2.5mg/5mL	Dextromethorphan HBr 5mg/5mL		**Adults & Peds ≥12 yrs:** 4 tsp q4h. **Max:** 24 tsp q24h.
Alka-Seltzer Plus Night Cold Liquid	Acetaminophen 162.5mg/5mL	Doxylamine Succinate 3.125/5mL	Phenylephrine HCl 2.5mg/5mL	Dextromethorphan HBr 5mg/5mL		**Adults & Peds ≥12 yrs:** 4 tsp q4h. **Max:** 24 tsp q24h.
Alka-Seltzer Plus Night Cold Formula Effervescent Tablets	Aspirin 500mg	Doxylamine 6.25mg	Phenylephrine Bitartrate 7.8mg	Dextromethorphan HBr 10mg		**Adults & Peds ≥12 yrs:** 2 tabs q4-6h. **Max:** 8 tabs q24h.
Robitussin Night Time Cough, Cold & Flu Liquid	Acetaminophen 160mg/5mL	Chlorpheniramine Maleate 1mg/5mL	Phenylephrine HCl 2.5mg/5mL	Dextromethorphan HBr 5mg/5mL		**Adults & Peds ≥12 yrs:** 4 tsp q4h. **Max:** 5 doses q24h.
Theraflu Nighttime Severe Cold & Cough Caplets	Acetaminophen 325mg	Chlorpheniramine Maleate 2mg	Phenylephrine HCl 5mg	Dextromethorphan HBr 10mg		**Adults & Peds ≥12 yrs:** 2 tabs q4h. **Max:** 12 tabs q24h.

TABLE 13. COUGH-COLD-FLU PRODUCTS (cont.)

Brand Name	Analgesic	Antihistamine	Cough Suppressant	Decongestant	Expectorant	Dose
Tylenol Children's Plus Multisymptom Cold Liquid	Acetaminophen 160mg/5mL	Chlorpheniramine Maleate 1mg/5mL	Dextromethorphan HBr 5mg/5mL	Phenylephrine HCl 2.5mg/5mL		**Peds 6-11 yrs (48-95 lbs):** 2 tsp (10mL) q4h. **Max:** 5 doses q24h.
Tylenol Children's Plus Flu Liquid	Acetaminophen 160mg/5mL	Chlorpheniramine Maleate 1mg/5mL	Dextromethorphan HBr 5mg/5mL	Phenylephrine HCl 2.5mg/5mL		**Peds 6-11 yrs (48-95 lbs):** 2 tsp (10mL) q4h. **Max:** 5 doses q24h.
Tylenol Cold Head Congestion Nighttime Caplets	Acetaminophen 325mg	Chlorpheniramine Maleate 2mg	Dextromethorphan HBr 10mg	Phenylephrine HCl 5mg		**Adults & Peds ≥12 yrs:** 2 tabs q4h. **Max:** 12 tabs q24h.
Tylenol Cold Multi-Symptom Nighttime Coolburst Caplets	Acetaminophen 325mg	Chlorpheniramine Maleate 2mg	Dextromethorphan HBr 10mg	Phenylephrine HCl 5mg		**Adults & Peds ≥12 yrs:** 2 tabs q4h. **Max:** 12 tabs q24h.
Tylenol Cold Multi-Symptom Nighttime Coolburst Liquid	Acetaminophen 325mg/15mL	Doxylamine 6.25mg/30mL	Dextromethorphan HBr 10mg/15mL	Phenylephrine HCl 5mg/15mL		**Adults & Peds ≥12 yrs:** 2 tbl (30mL) q4h. **Max:** 12 tbl (180mL) q24h.
Vicks NyQuil D Liquid	Acetaminophen 500mg/15mL	Doxylamine 6.25mg/15mL	Dextromethorphan HBr 15mg/15mL	Pseudoephedrine HCl 30mg/15mL		**Adults & Peds ≥12 yrs:** 2 tbl (30mL) q6h. **Max:** 4 doses q24h.
COUGH SUPPRESSANT + ANTIHISTAMINE + DECONGESTANT						
Dimetapp Children's Cold & Cough		Brompheniramine Maleate 1mg/5mL	Dextromethorphan HBr 5mg/5mL	Phenylephrine HCl 2.5mg/5mL		**Adults & Peds ≥12 yrs:** 4 tsp (20mL) q4h. **Peds 6-<12 yrs:** 2 tsp (10mL) q4h. **Max:** 6 doses q24h.
Theraflu Cold & Cough Hot Liquid		Pheniramine Maleate 20mg/packet	Dextromethorphan HBr 20mg/packet	Phenylephrine HCl 10mg/packet		**Adults & Peds ≥12 yrs:** 1 packet q4h. **Max:** 6 packets q24h.
Triaminic-D Multi-Symptom Cold		Chlorpheniramine Maleate 1mg/5mL	Dextromethorphan HBr 7.5mg/5mL	Pseudoephedrine HCl 15mg/5mL		**Peds 6-<12 yrs:** 2 tsp q6h. **Max:** 4 doses q24h.
COUGH SUPPRESSANT + DECONGESTANT						
PediaCare Children's Multi-Symptom Cold Liquid			Dextromethorphan HBr 5mg/5mL	Phenylephrine HCl 2.5mg/5mL		**Peds 6-11 yrs:** 2 tsp (10mL) q4h. **Peds 4-5 yrs:** 1 tsp (5mL) q4h. **Max:** 6 doses q24h.
Sudafed PE Children's Cold & Cough Liquid			Dextromethorphan HBr 5mg/5mL	Phenylephrine HCl 2.5mg/5mL		**Peds 6-11 yrs:** 2 tsp (10mL) q4h. **Peds 4-5 yrs:** 1 tsp (5mL) q4h. **Max:** 6 doses q24h.
Triaminic Day Time Cold & Cough Liquid			Dextromethorphan HBr 5mg/5mL	Phenylephrine HCl 2.5mg/5mL		**Peds 6-<12 yrs:** 2 tsp (10mL) q4h. **Peds 4-<6 yrs:** 1 tsp (5mL) q4h. **Max:** 6 doses q24h.
Vicks Formula 44 Custom Care Congestion			Dextromethorphan HBr 20mg/15mL	Phenylephrine HCl 10mg/15mL		**Adults & Peds ≥12 yrs:** 1 tbl (15mL) q4h. **Peds 6-<12 yrs:** 1½ tsp (7.5mL) q4h. **Max:** 6 doses q24h.
COUGH SUPPRESSANT + DECONGESTANT + ANALGESIC						
Alka-Seltzer Plus Day Cold Liquid Gels	Acetaminophen 325mg		Dextromethorphan HBr 10mg	Phenylephrine HCl 5mg		**Adults & Peds ≥12 yrs:** 2 caps q4h. **Max:** 12 caps q24h.
Alka-Seltzer Plus Day & Night Liquid Gels	Acetaminophen 325mg	Doxylamine 6.25mg (nighttime dose only)	Dextromethorphan HBr 10mg	Phenylephrine HCl 5mg		**Adults & Peds ≥12 yrs:** 2 caps q4h. **Max:** 12 caps q24h.

(Continued)

TABLE 13. COUGH-COLD-FLU PRODUCTS (cont.)

Brand Name	Analgesic	Antihistamine	Decongestant	Cough Suppressant	Expectorant	Dose
Alka-Seltzer Plus Day & Night Cold Formula Effervescent Tablets	Aspirin 325mg	Doxylamine 6.25mg (nighttime dose only)	Phenylephrine Bitartrate 7.8mg	Dextromethorphan HBr 10mg		**Adults & Peds ≥12 yrs:** 2 tabs q4h. **Max:** 8 tabs q24h.
Comtrex Non-Drowsy Cold & Cough Caplets	Acetaminophen 325mg		Phenylephrine HCl 5mg	Dextromethorphan HBr 10mg		**Adults & Peds ≥12 yrs:** 2 tabs q4h. **Max:** 12 tabs q24h.
Theraflu Daytime Severe Cold & Cough Caplets	Acetaminophen 325mg		Phenylephrine HCl 5mg	Dextromethorphan HBr 10mg		**Adults & Peds ≥12 yrs:** 2 tabs q4h. **Max:** 12 tabs q24h.
Theraflu Daytime Severe Cold & Cough Hot Liquid	Acetaminophen 650mg/packet		Phenylephrine HCl 10mg/packet	Dextromethorphan HBr 20mg/packet		**Adults & Peds ≥12 yrs:** 1 pkt q4h. **Max:** 6 pkts q24h.
Tylenol Cold Head Congestion Daytime Capsules	Acetaminophen 325mg		Phenylephrine HCl 5mg	Dextromethorphan HBr 10mg		**Adults & Peds ≥12 yrs:** 2 caps q4h. **Max:** 12 caps q24h.
Tylenol Cold Head Congestion Day/Night Pack	Acetaminophen 325mg	Chlorpheniramine maleate 2mg	Phenylephrine HCl 5mg	Dextromethorphan HBr 10mg		**Adults & Peds ≥12 yrs:** 2 tabs q4h. **Max:** 12 tabs q24h.
Tylenol Cold Multi-Symptom Daytime Rapid-Release Gelcaps/ Cool Burst Caplets	Acetaminophen 325mg		Phenylephrine HCl 5mg	Dextromethorphan HBr 10mg		**Adults & Peds ≥12 yrs:** 2 caps q4h. **Max:** 12 caps q24h.
Tylenol Cold Multi-Symptom Daytime Citrus Burst Liquid	Acetaminophen 325mg/15mL		Phenylephrine HCl 5mg/15mL	Dextromethorphan HBr 10mg/15mL		**Adults & Peds ≥12 yrs:** 2 tbl (30mL) q4h. **Max:** 6 doses (12 tbl) q24h.
Tylenol Cold Multi-Symptom Day/Night Pack	Acetaminophen 325mg	Chlorpheniramine maleate 2mg	Phenylephrine HCl 5mg	Dextromethorphan HBr 10mg		**Adults & Peds ≥12 yrs:** 2 caps q4h. **Max:** 12 caps q24h.
Vicks DayQuil Cold & Flu Relief Liquicaps	Acetaminophen 325mg		Phenylephrine HCl 5mg	Dextromethorphan HBr 10mg		**Adults & Peds ≥12 yrs:** 2 caps q4h. **Max:** 6 caps q24h.
Vicks DayQuil Cold & Flu Relief Liquid	Acetaminophen 325mg/15mL		Phenylephrine HCl 5mg/15mL	Dextromethorphan HBr 10mg/15mL		**Adults & Peds ≥12 yrs:** 2 tbl (30 mL) q4h. **Max:** 6 doses q24h. **Peds 6–<12 yrs:** 1 tbl (15mL) q4h. **Max:** 5 doses q24h.

COUGH SUPPRESSANT + DECONGESTANT + EXPECTORANT

Brand Name	Analgesic	Antihistamine	Decongestant	Cough Suppressant	Expectorant	Dose
Robitussin Cough & Cold CF Liquid			Phenylephrine HCl 5mg/5mL	Dextromethorphan HBr 10mg/5mL	Guaifenesin 100mg/5mL	**Adults & Peds ≥12 yrs:** 2 tsp q4h. **Max:** 6 doses q24h.
Robitussin Cough & Cold D			Pseudoephedrine HCl 30mg/5mL	Dextromethorphan HBr 15mg/5mL	Guaifenesin 200mg/5mL	**Adults & Peds ≥12 yrs:** 2 tsp q4h. **Max:** 4 doses q24h.

COUGH SUPPRESSANT + DECONGESTANT + EXPECTORANT + ANALGESIC

Brand Name	Analgesic	Antihistamine	Decongestant	Cough Suppressant	Expectorant	Dose
Sudafed PE Cold & Cough Caplets	Acetaminophen 325mg		Phenylephrine HCl 5mg	Dextromethorphan HBr 10mg	Guaifenesin 100mg	**Adults & Peds ≥12 yrs:** 2 tabs q4h. **Max:** 12 tabs q24h.
Tylenol Cold Multi-Symptom Severe Coolburst Liquid	Acetaminophen 325mg/15mL		Phenylephrine HCl 5mg/15mL	Dextromethorphan HBr 10mg/15mL	Guaifenesin 200mg/15mL	**Adults & Peds ≥12 yrs:** 2 tbl q4h. **Max:** 12 tbl q24h.
Tylenol Cold Multi-Symptom Severe Coolburst Caplets	Acetaminophen 325mg		Phenylephrine HCl 5mg	Dextromethorphan HBr 10mg	Guaifenesin 200mg	**Adults & Peds ≥12 yrs:** 2 tabs q4h. **Max:** 12 tabs q24h.

TABLE 13. COUGH-COLD-FLU PRODUCTS (cont.)

Brand Name	Analgesic	Antihistamine	Decongestant	Cough Suppressant	Expectorant	Dose
Tylenol Cold Severe Head Congestion Caplets	Acetaminophen 325mg		Phenylephrine HCl 5mg	Dextromethorphan HBr 10mg	Guaifenesin 200mg	**Adults & Peds ≥12 yrs:** 2 tabs q4h. **Max:** 12 tabs q24h.
COUGH SUPPRESSANT & EXPECTORANT						
Alka-Seltzer Plus Mucus & Congestion Effervescent Tablets				Dextromethorphan HBr 10mg	Guaifenesin 200mg	**Adults & Peds ≥12 yrs:** 2 tabs q4h. **Max:** 8 tabs q24h.
Coricidin HBP Chest Congestion & Cough Softgels				Dextromethorphan HBr 10mg	Guaifenesin 200mg	**Adults & Peds ≥12 yrs:** 1-2 caps q4h. **Max:** 12 caps q24h.
Mucinex Cough Mini-Melts (Orange Crème)				Dextromethorphan HBr 5mg	Guaifenesin 100mg	**Adults & Peds ≥12 yrs:** 2-4 pkts q4h. **Peds 6-<12 yrs:** 1-2 pkts q4h. **Max:** 6 doses q24h. **Peds 4-<6yrs:** 1 pkt q4h. **Max:** 6 doses q24h.
Mucinex DM Extended-Release Tablets				Dextromethorphan HBr 30mg	Guaifenesin 600mg	**Adults & Peds ≥12 yrs:** 1-2 tabs q12h. **Max:** 4 tabs q24h.
Robitussin Cough & Chest Congestion DM Max Liquid				Dextromethorphan HBr 10mg/5mL	Guaifenesin 200mg/5mL	**Adults & Peds ≥12 yrs:** 2 tsp q4h. **Max:** 6 doses q24h.
Robitussin Cough & Chest Congestion DM Liquid				Dextromethorphan HBr 10mg/5mL	Guaifenesin 100mg/5mL	**Adults & Peds ≥12 yrs:** 2 tsp q4h. **Max:** 6 doses q24h.
Robitussin Cough & Chest Congestion Sugar-Free DM				Dextromethorphan HBr 10mg/5mL	Guaifenesin 100mg/5mL	**Adults & Peds ≥12 yrs:** 2 tsp q4h. **Max:** 6 doses q24h.
Vicks Formula 44 Custom Care Chesty Cough				Dextromethorphan HBr 20mg/15mL	Guaifenesin 200mg/15mL	**Adults & Peds ≥12 yrs:** 1 tbl (15mL) q4h. **Peds 6-<12 yrs:** 1½ tsp (7.5mL) q4h. **Max:** 6 doses q24h.
Vicks Formula 44e Pediatric Cough & Chest Congestion Relief Liquid				Dextromethorphan HBr 10mg/15mL	Guaifenesin 100mg/15mL	**Adults & Peds ≥12 yrs:** 2 tbl q4h. **Peds 6-<12 yrs:** 1 tbl q4h. **Peds 4-<6 yrs:** ½ tbl q4h. **Max:** 6 doses q24h.
DECONGESTANT						
PediaCare Children's Decongestant Liquid			Phenylephrine HCl 2.5mg/5mL			**Peds 6-11 yrs:** 2 tsp (10mL) q4h. **Peds 4-5 yrs:** 1 tsp (5mL) q4h. **Max:** 6 doses q24h.
Sudafed 12-Hour Tablets			Pseudoephedrine HCl 120mg			**Adults & Peds ≥12 yrs:** 1 tab q12h. **Max:** 2 tabs q24h.
Sudafed 24-Hour Tablets			Pseudoephedrine HCl 240mg			**Adults & Peds ≥12 yrs:** 1 tab q24h. **Max:** 1 tab q24h.
Sudafed Children's Nasal Decongestant Liquid			Pseudoephedrine HCl 15mg/5mL			**Peds 6-11 yrs:** 2 tsp q4-6h. **Peds 4-5 yrs:** 1 tsp q4-6h. **Max:** 4 doses q24h.
Sudafed OM Sinus Cold Nasal Spray			Oxymetazoline HCl 0.05%			**Adults & Peds ≥6 yrs:** 2-3 sprays q10-12h. **Max:** 2 doses q24h.
Sudafed OM Sinus Congestion Nasal Spray			Oxymetazoline HCl 0.05%			**Adults & Peds ≥6 yrs:** 2-3 sprays q10-12h. **Max:** 2 doses q24h.

(Continued)

TABLE 13. COUGH-COLD-FLU PRODUCTS (cont.)

Brand Name	Analgesic	Antihistamine	Decongestant	Cough Suppressant	Expectorant	Dose
Sudafed PE Nasal Decongestant Tablets			Phenylephrine HCl 10mg			**Adults & Peds ≥12 yrs:** 1 tab q4h. **Max:** 6 tabs q24h.
Sudafed PE Children's Nasal Decongestant Liquid			Phenylephrine HCl 2.5mg/5mL			**Peds 6-11 yrs:** 2 tsp q4-6h. **Peds 4-5 yrs:** 1 tsp q4-6h. **Max:** 4 doses q24h.
Sudafed Nasal Decongestant Tablets			Pseudoephedrine HCl 30mg			**Adults ≥12 yrs:** 2 tabs q4-6h. **Max:** 8 tabs q24h. **Peds 6-12 yrs:** 1 tab q4-6h. **Max:** 4 tab q24h.
Triaminic Thin Strips Cold with Stuffy Nose			Phenylephrine HCl 2.5mg/strip			**Peds 6-<12 yrs:** 2 strips q4h. **Peds 4-<6 yrs:** 1 strip q4h. **Max:** 6 doses q24h.
Triaminic Decongestant Spray Nasal & Sinus Congestion			Xylometazoline HCl 0.05%			**Peds 2-<12 yrs:** 1-2 sprays q8-10h. **Max:** 3 doses q24h.
Vicks Sinex 12-Hour Nasal Spray			Oxymetazoline HCl 0.05%			**Adults & Peds ≥6 yrs:** 2-3 sprays q10-12h. **Max:** 2 doses q24h.
Vicks Sinex Nasal Spray			Phenylephrine HCl 0.5%			**Adults & Peds ≥12 yrs:** 2-3 sprays q4h. **Max:** 18 sprays q24h.
Vicks Sinex UltraFine Mist			Phenylephrine HCl 0.5%			**Adults & Peds ≥12 yrs:** 2-3 sprays q4h. **Max:** 18 sprays q24h.
Vicks Vapor Inhaler			Levmetamfetamine 50mg			**Adults & Peds ≥12 yrs:** 2 inhalations q2h. **Max:** 24 inhalations q24h. **Peds 6-<12 yrs:** 1 inhalation q2h. **Max:** 12 inhalations q24h.
DECONGESTANT + ANALGESIC						
Advil Children's Cold Liquid	Ibuprofen 100mg/5mL		Pseudoephedrine HCl 15mg/5mL			**Peds 6-11 yrs (48-95 lbs):** 2 tsp (10mL) q6h. **2-5 yrs (24-47 lbs):** 1 tsp (5mL) q6h. **Max:** 4 doses q24h.
Advil Cold & Sinus Caplets/Liqui-gels	Ibuprofen 200mg		Pseudoephedrine HCl 30mg			**Adults & Peds ≥12 yrs:** 1-2 caps q4-6h. **Max:** 6 caps q24h.
Alka-Seltzer Plus Sinus Formula Effervescent Tablets	Aspirin 325mg		Phenylephrine Bitartrate 7.8mg			**Adults & Peds ≥12 yrs:** 2 tabs q4h. **Max:** 8 tabs q24h.
Contac Cold & Flu Day & Night Caplets	Acetaminophen 500mg	Chlorpheniramine Maleate 2mg	Phenylephrine HCl 5mg			**Adults & Peds ≥12 yrs:** 2 tabs q4-6h. **Max:** 8 tabs q24h.
Contac Cold & Flu Non-Drowsy Maximum Strength Caplets	Acetaminophen 500mg		Phenylephrine HCl 5mg			**Adults & Peds ≥12 yrs:** 2 tabs q4-6h. **Max:** 8 tabs q24h.
Motrin Children's Cold Suspension	Ibuprofen 100mg/5mL		Pseudoephedrine HCl 15mg/5mL			**Peds 6-11 yrs (48-95 lbs):** 2 tsp (10mL) q6h. **2-5 yrs (24-47 lbs):** 1 tsp (5mL) q6h. **Max:** 4 doses q24h.
Sinutab Sinus Caplets	Acetaminophen 325mg		Phenylephrine HCl 5mg			**Adults & Peds ≥12 yrs:** 2 tabs q4h. **Max:** 12 tabs q24h.
Sudafed PE Sinus Headache Caplets	Acetaminophen 325mg		Phenylephrine HCl 5mg			**Adults & Peds ≥12 yrs:** 2 tabs q4h. **Max:** 12 tabs q24h.

TABLE 13. COUGH-COLD-FLU PRODUCTS (cont.)

Brand Name	Analgesic	Antihistamine	Decongestant	Cough Suppressant	Expectorant	Dose
Tylenol Sinus Congestion & Pain Daytime Rapid-Release Gelcaps/ Gelcaps/Cool Burst Caplets	Acetaminophen 325mg		Phenylephrine HCl 5mg			**Adults & Peds ≥12 yrs:** 2 caps q4h. **Max:** 12 caps q24h.
Vicks DayQuil Sinus Liquicaps	Acetaminophen 325mg		Phenylephrine HCl 5mg			**Adults & Peds ≥12 yrs:** 2 caps q4h. **Max:** 12 caps q24h.
DECONGESTANT + EXPECTORANT						
Mucinex Cold Liquid (Mixed Berry)			Phenylephrine HCl 2.5mg/5mL		Guaifenesin 100mg/5mL	**Peds 6-12 yrs:** 2 tsp (10mL) q4h. **Peds 4-5 yrs:** 1 tsp (5mL) q4h. **Max:** 6 doses q24h.
Mucinex D Extended-Release Tablets			Pseudoephedrine HCl 60mg		Guaifenesin 600mg	**Adults & Peds ≥12 yrs:** 2 tabs q12h. **Max:** 4 tabs q24h.
Sudafed PE Non-Drying Sinus Caplets			Phenylephrine HCl 5mg		Guaifenesin 200mg	**Adults & Peds ≥12 yrs:** 2 tabs q4h. **Max:** 12 tabs q24h.
Triaminic Chest & Nasal Congestion Syrup			Phenylephrine HCl 2.5mg/5mL		Guaifenesin 50mg/5mL	**Peds 6-<12 yrs:** 2 tsp (10mL) q4h. **Peds 4-<6 yrs:** 1 tsp (5mL) q4h. **Max:** 6 doses q24h.
DECONGESTANT + EXPECTORANT + ANALGESIC						
Theraflu Cold & Chest Congestion Warming Relief	Acetaminophen 325mg/15mL		Phenylephrine HCl 5mg/15mL		Guaifenesin 200mg/15mL	**Adults & Peds ≥12 yrs:** 2 tbl (30mL) q4h. **Max:** 6 doses q24h.
Tylenol Sinus Congestion & Severe Pain Coolburst Caplets	Acetaminophen 325mg		Phenylephrine HCl 5mg		Guaifenesin 200mg	**Adults & Peds ≥12 yrs:** 2 tabs q4h. **Max:** 12 tabs q24h.
Tylenol Sinus Severe Congestion Daytime Coolburst Caplets	Acetaminophen 325mg		Pseudoephedrine HCl 30mg		Guaifenesin 200mg	**Adults & Peds ≥12 yrs:** 2 tabs q4-6h. **Max:** 8 tabs q24h.
EXPECTORANT						
Mucinex Tablets					Guaifenesin 600mg	**Adults & Peds ≥12 yrs:** 1-2 tabs q12h. **Max:** 4 tabs q24h.
Mucinex Kids Mini-Melts (Bubble Gum)					Guaifenesin 100mg	**Adults & Peds ≥12 yrs:** 2-4 packets q4h. **Peds 6-<12 yrs:** 1-2 packets q4h. **Peds 4-<6 yrs:** 1 packet q4h. **Max:** 6 doses q24h.
Mucinex Maximum Strength					Guaifenesin 1200mg	**Adults & Peds ≥12 yrs:** 1 tab q12h. **Max:** 6 tabs q24h.
Robitussin Chest Congestion					Guaifenesin 100mg/5mL	**Adults & Peds ≥12 yrs:** 2-4 tsp q4h. **Max:** 6 doses q24h.
EXPECTORANT + ANALGESIC						
Comtrex Deep Chest Cold Caplets	Acetaminophen 325mg				Guaifenesin 200mg	**Adults & Peds ≥12 yrs:** 2 tabs q4h. **Max:** 12 tabs q24h.

(Continued)

TABLE 13. COUGH-COLD-FLU PRODUCTS (cont.)

BRAND NAME	ANALGESIC	ANTIHISTAMINE	DECONGESTANT	COUGH SUPPRESSANT	EXPECTORANT	DOSE
Theraflu Flu & Chest Congestion Hot Liquid	Acetaminophen 1000mg/packet				Guaifenesin 400mg/packet	**Adults & Peds ≥12 yrs:** 1 packet q6h. **Max:** 4 packets q24h.
EXPECTORANT + DECONGESTANT + ANALGESIC						
Robitussin Cough & Cold D			Pseudoephedrine HCl 30mg/5mL	Dextromethorphan HBr 15mg/5mL	Guaifenesin 200mg/5mL	**Adults & Peds ≥12 yrs:** 2 tsp q4h. **Max:** 4 doses q24h.
Tylenol Sinus Congestion & Severe Pain Caplets	Acetaminophen 325mg		Phenylephrine HCl 5mg		Guaifenesin 200mg	**Adults & Peds ≥12 yrs:** 2 tabs q4h. **Max:** 12 tabs q24h.
ANTIHISTAMINE + ANALGESIC						
Coricidin HBP Cold & Flu Tablets	Acetaminophen 325mg	Chlorpheniramine Maleate 2mg				**Adults & Peds ≥12 yrs:** 2 tabs q4-6h. **Max:** 12 tabs q24h.
Tylenol Severe Allergy Caplets	Acetaminophen 500mg	Diphenhydramine HCl 12.5mg				**Adults & Peds ≥12 yrs:** 2 tabs q4-6h. **Max:** 8 tabs q24h.

TABLE 14. DANDRUFF PRODUCTS

BRAND NAME	INGREDIENT/STRENGTH	DOSE
COAL TAR		
Denorex Therapeutic Protection 2-in-1 Shampoo	Coal Tar 2.5%	**Adults & Peds:** Use biw.
DHS Tar Shampoo	Coal Tar 0.5%	**Adults & Peds:** Use biw.
DHS Tar Gel Shampoo	Coal Tar 0.5%	**Adults & Peds:** Use biw.
Ionil T Shampoo	Coal Tar 1%	**Adults & Peds:** Use biw.
Ionil T Plus Shampoo	Coal Tar 2%	**Adults & Peds:** Use biw.
Neutrogena T-Gel Shampoo Original Formula	Coal Tar 0.5%	**Adults & Peds:** Use biw.
Neutrogena T-Gel Shampoo, Extra Strength	Coal Tar 1%	**Adults & Peds:** Use biw.
Neutrogena T-Gel Stubborn Itch Control Shampoo	Coal Tar 0.5%	**Adults & Peds:** Use biw.
CORTICOSTEROID		
Maximum Strength Scalpicin Liquid	Hydrocortisone 1%	**Adults & Peds ≥2 yrs:** Apply to affected area qd-qid.
KETOCONAZOLE		
Nizoral Anti-Dandruff Shampoo	Ketoconazole 1%	**Adults & Peds ≥12 yrs:** Use q3-4d up to 8 wks.
PYRITHIONE ZINC		
DHS Zinc Shampoo	Pyrithione Zinc 2%	**Adults & Peds:** Use biw.
Head & Shoulders Dry Scalp Care Dandruff Shampoo Plus Conditioner; Shampoo; Conditioner	Pyrithione Zinc 1%	**Adults & Peds:** Use biw.
Head & Shoulders Smooth & Silky Dandruff Shampoo Plus Conditioner; Shampoo; Conditioner	Pyrithione Zinc 1%	**Adults & Peds:** Use biw.
Head & Shoulders Citrus Breeze Dandruff Shampoo Plus Conditioner; Shampoo	Pyrithione Zinc 1%	**Adults & Peds:** Use biw.
Head & Shoulders Classic Clean Dandruff Shampoo Plus Conditioner; Shampoo; Conditioner	Pyrithione Zinc 1%	**Adults & Peds:** Use biw.
Head & Shoulders Extra Volume Dandruff Shampoo	Pyrithione Zinc 1%	**Adults & Peds:** Use biw.
Head & Shoulders Ocean Lift Dandruff Shampoo Plus Conditioner; Shampoo	Pyrithione Zinc 1%	**Adults & Peds:** Use biw.
Head & Shoulders Dandruff Refresh Shampoo Plus Conditioner; Shampoo	Pyrithione Zinc 1%	**Adults & Peds:** Use biw.
Head & Shoulders Restoring Shine Dandruff Shampoo Plus Conditioner; Shampoo	Pyrithione Zinc 1%	**Adults & Peds:** Use biw.
Head & Shoulders Sensitive Care Dandruff Shampoo Plus Conditioner; Shampoo	Pyrithione Zinc 1%	**Adults & Peds:** Use biw.
L'Oreal VIVE Pro Anti-Dandruff 2-in-1 Shampoo & Conditioner for Men	Pyrithione Zinc 1%	**Adults & Peds:** Use biw.
Neutrogena T-Gel Daily Control Dandruff Shampoo	Pyrithione Zinc 1%	**Adults & Peds:** Use biw.

(Continued)

TABLE 14. DANDRUFF PRODUCTS (cont.)

BRAND NAME	INGREDIENT/STRENGTH	DOSE
Neutrogena T-Gel Daily Control 2-in-1 Dandruff Shampoo Plus Conditioner	Pyrithione Zinc 1%	**Adults & Peds:** Use biw.
Pantene Pro-V Shampoo + Conditioner, Anti-Dandruff	Pyrithione Zinc 1%	**Adults & Peds:** Use biw.
Pert Plus Shampoo Plus Conditioner, Dandruff Control	Pyrithione Zinc 1%	**Adults & Peds:** Use biw.
Pert Plus 2-in-1 Dandruff Dismissed Shampoo	Pyrithione Zinc 0.45%	**Adults & Peds:** Use biw.
Selsun Salon 2-in-1 Pyrithione Zinc Shampoo	Pyrithione Zinc 1%	**Adults & Peds:** Use biw.
Suave for Men 2 in 1 Shampoo/ Conditioner, Dandruff	Pyrithione Zinc 0.5%	**Adults & Peds:** Use biw.
SALICYLIC ACID		
Denorex Dandruff Shampoo, Extra Strength	Salicylic Acid 3%	**Adults & Peds:** Use biw.
DHS SAL Shampoo	Salicylic Acid 3%	**Adults & Peds:** Use biw.
Ionil Plus Conditioning Shampoo	Salicylic Acid 2%	**Adults & Peds:** Use biw.
Neutrogena T/Gel Therapeutic Conditioner	Salicylic Acid 2%	**Adults & Peds:** Use biw.
Neutrogena T/Sal Therapeutic Shampoo	Salicylic Acid 3%	**Adults & Peds:** Use biw.
Scalpicin Anti-Itch Liquid Scalp Treatment	Salicylic Acid 3%	**Adults & Peds:** Apply to affected area qd-qid.
Selsun Blue Naturals Dandruff Shampoo	Salicylic Acid 3%	**Adults & Peds:** Use biw.
SELENIUM SULFIDE		
Head & Shoulders Dandruff Shampoo, Intensive Treatment	Selenium Sulfide 1%	**Adults & Peds:** Use biw.
Selsun Blue Dandruff Shampoo, Medicated Formula	Selenium Sulfide 1%	**Adults & Peds:** Use biw.
Selsun Blue 2-in-1	Selenium Sulfide 1%	**Adults & Peds:** Use biw.
Selsun Blue Normal to Oily Formula	Selenium Sulfide 1%	**Adults & Peds:** Use biw.
Selsun Blue Dandruff Shampoo, Moisturizing Formula	Selenium Sulfide 1%	**Adults & Peds:** Use biw.
SULFUR/SALICYLIC ACID		
Sebulex Medicated Dandruff Shampoo	Sulfur/Salicylic Acid 2%-2%	**Adults & Peds ≥12 yrs:** Use qod-qd.

TABLE 15. DIAPER RASH PRODUCTS

BRAND NAME	INGREDIENT/STRENGTH	DOSE
WHITE PETROLATUM		
Balmex Multi-Purpose Healing Ointment	White Petrolatum 51.1%	**Peds:** Apply prn.
Vaseline Baby, Baby Fresh Scent	White Petrolatum 100%	**Peds:** Apply prn.
Vaseline Petroleum Jelly	White Petrolatum 100%	**Peds:** Apply prn.
ZINC OXIDE		
Aveeno Baby Soothing Relief Diaper Rash Cream	Zinc Oxide 13%	**Peds:** Apply prn.
Balmex Diaper Rash Cream with ActivGuard	Zinc Oxide 11.3%	**Peds:** Apply prn.
Boudreaux's Butt Paste, Diaper Rash Ointment	Zinc Oxide 16%	**Peds:** Apply prn.
California Baby Diaper Rash Cream	Zinc Oxide 12%	**Peds:** Apply prn.
Canus Li'l Goat's Milk Ointment	Zinc Oxide 40%	**Peds:** Apply prn.
Desitin Rapid Relief	Zinc Oxide 10%	**Peds:** Apply prn.
Desitin Maximum Strength Paste	Zinc Oxide 40%	**Peds:** Apply prn.
Huggies Gentle Care Creamy Diaper Rash Ointment	Zinc Oxide 10%	**Peds:** Apply prn.
Johnson's No-More Rash Diaper Rash Cream	Zinc Oxide 13%	**Peds:** Apply prn.
Mustela Bebe Vitamin Barrier Cream	Zinc Oxide 10%	**Peds:** Apply prn.
COMBINATION PRODUCTS		
A+D Original Ointment, Diaper Rash and All-Purpose Skincare Formula	Petrolatum/Lanolin 53.4%-15.5%	**Peds:** Apply prn.
A+D Zinc Oxide Diaper Rash Cream with Aloe	Dimethicone/Zinc Oxide 1%-10%	**Peds:** Apply prn.
Lansinoh Diaper Rash Ointment	Dimethicone/USP Modified Lanolin/ Zinc Oxide 5.0%-15.5%-5.5%	**Peds:** Apply prn.
Triple Paste Medicated Ointment	Beeswax/Lanolin/Zinc Oxide (12.8%)	**Peds:** Apply prn.

TABLE 16. DRY SKIN PRODUCTS

BRAND NAME	INGREDIENT/STRENGTH	DOSE
AmLactin Moisturizing Cream	Water, Lactic Acid, Ammonium Hydroxide, Light Mineral Oil, Glyceryl Stearate, PEG-100 Stearate, Glycerin, Propylene Glycol, Magnesium Aluminum Silicate, Laureth 4, Polyoxyl 40 Stearate, Cetyl Alcohol, Methylcellulose, Methylparaben, Propylparaben	**Adults & Peds:** Apply bid.
AmLactin Moisturizing Lotion	Water, Lactic Acid, Ammonium Hydroxide, Light Mineral Oil, Glyceryl Stearate, PEG-100 Stearate, Glycerin, Propylene Glycol, Magnesium Aluminum Silicate, Laureth 4, Polyoxyl 40 Stearate, Cetyl Alcohol, Methylcellulose, Methylparaben, Propylparaben	**Adults & Peds:** Apply bid.
AmLactin XL Moisturizing Lotion	Water, Ammonium Lactate, Potassium Lactate, Sodium Lactate, Emulsifying Wax, Light Mineral Oil, White Petrolatum, Glycerin, Propylene Glycol, Stearic Acid, Xanthum Gum, Methyl and Propylparabens	**Adults & Peds:** Apply bid.
Aquaphor Baby Healing Ointment	Petrolatum, Mineral Oil, Ceresin, Lanolin Alcohol, Panthenol, Glycerin, Bisabolol	**Adults & Peds:** Apply prn.
Aquaphor Healing Ointment	Petrolatum, Mineral Oil, Ceresin, Lanolin Alcohol, Panthenol, Glycerin, Bisabolol	**Adults & Peds:** Apply to affected area prn.
Aquaphor Original Ointment	Petrolatum, Mineral Oil, Ceresin, Lanolin Alcohol	**Adults & Peds:** Apply to affected area prn.
Aveeno Baby Calming Comfort Lotion	Dimethicone, Avèna Sativa (Oat) Kernel Flour, Benzyl Alcohol, Cetyl Alcohol, Distearyldimonium Chloride, Fragrance, Glycerin, Isopropyl Palmitate, Petrolatum, Sodium Chloride, Water	**Adults & Peds:** Apply prn.
Aveeno Baby Continuous Protection Lotion SPF 55	Avobenzone, Homosalate, Octisalate, Octocrylene, Oxybenzone, Avena Sativa (Oat) Kernel Flour, Behenyl Alcohol, BHT, Butyloctyl Salicylate, Caprylyl Methicone, Diethylhexyl 2,6-Naphthalate, Dimethicone, Disodium EDTA, Ethylhexyl Stearate, Ethylhexyl Glycerin, Ethylparaben, Glyceryl Stearate, Methylparaben, PEG 100 Stearate, Phenoxyethanol, Propylparaben, Silica, Sodium Polyacrylate, Styrene Acrylate Copolymer, Trideceth 6, Trimethylsiloxysilicate, VP/Hexadecene Copolymer, Water, Xanthan Gum	**Adults & Peds ≥6 mo:** Apply before sun exposure prn.
Aveeno Baby Moisture Soothing Relief Moisture Cream	Water, Glycerin, Petrolatum, Mineral Oil, Cetyl Alcohol, Dimethicone, Avena Sativa (Oat) Kernel Flour, Carbomer, Sodium Hydroxide, Ceteareth-6, Hydrolyzed Milk Protein, Hydrolyzed Oats, Hydrolyzed Soy Protein, PEG-25 Soy Sterol, Tetrasodium EDTA, Methylparaben, Citric Acid, Sodium Citrate, Benzalkonium Chloride, Benzaldehyde, Butylene Glycol, Butylparaben, Ethylparaben, Ethyl Alcohol, Isobutylparaben, Phenoxyethanol, Propylparaben, Stearyl Alcohol	**Adults & Peds:** Apply prn.
Aveeno Baby Soothing Bath Treatment Packets	Colloidal Oatmeal 43%, Calcium Silicilate, Laureth-4 Mineral Oil	**Adults & Peds:** Bathe in 1 packet for 15-20 min qd-bid.
Aveeno Baby Daily Moisture Lotion	Dimethicone 1.2%, Water, Glycerin, Distearyldimonium Chloride, Petrolatum, Isopropyl Palmitate, Cetyl Alcohol, Avena Sativa (Oat) Kernel Flour, Allontoin, Benzyl Alcohol, Sodium Chloride	**Peds:** Apply prn.
Aveeno Daily Moisturizer, Ultra-Calming SPF 15	Avobenzone/Octinoxate/Octisalate (3%-7.5%-2%), Arachidyl Alcohol, Arachidyl Glucoside, Behenyl Alcohol, Benzyl Alcohol, Butylparaben, C12 15 Alkyl Benzoate, C12 16 Alkyl Hydroxyethyl Ethylcellulose, C13 14 Isoparaffin, Cetearyl Alcohol, Cetearyl Glucoside, Chrysanthemum Parthenium Extract (Feverfew), Cyclohexasiloxane, Cyclopentasiloxane, Dimethicone, Disodium EDTA, Ethylene Acrylic Acid Copolymer, Ethylparaben, Fragrance, Glycerin, Iodopropynyl Butylcarbamate, Isobutylparaben, Laureth 7, Magnesium Aspartate, Methylparaben, Panthenol, Phenoxyethanol, Phenyl Trimethicone, Polyacrylamide, Potassium Aspartate, Propylparaben, Sarcosine, Sodium Cocoyl Amino Acids, Steareth 2, Steareth 12, Tetradibutyl Pentaerithrityl Hydroxyhydrocinnamate, Water	**Adults:** Apply qd.

(Continued)

TABLE 16. DRY SKIN PRODUCTS (cont.)

Brand Name	Ingredient/Strength	Dose
Aveeno Daily Moisturizing Lotion	Dimethicone 1.25%, Avena Sativa (Oat) Kernel Flour, Benzyl Alcohol, Cetyl Alcohol, Distearyldimonium Chloride, Glycerin, Isopropyl Palmitate, Petrolatum, Sodium Chloride, Water	**Adults:** Apply prn.
Aveeno Intense Relief Hand Cream	Water, Glycerin, Distearyldimonium Chloride, Petrolatum, Isopropyl Palmitate, Cetyl Alcohol, Aluminum Starch Octenyl Succinate, Dimethicone, Avena Sativa (Oat) Kernel Flour, Benzyl Alcohol, Sodium Chloride	**Adults & Peds:** Apply prn.
Aveeno Moisturizing Bar for Dry Skin	Avena Stativa (Oat) Flour, Water, Cetearyl Alcohol, Stearic Acid, Sodium Cocoyl Isethionate, Water, Disodium Lauryl Sulfosuccinate, Glycerin, Hydrogenated Vegetable Oil, Titanium Dioxide, Citric Acid, Sodium Trideceth Sulfate, Hydrogenated Castor Oil	**Adults & Peds:** Use qd.
Aveeno Moisturizing Lotion, Skin Relief	Dimethicone 1.25%, Allantoin, Avena Sativa Kernel Flour (Oat), Benzyl Alcohol, Cetyl Alcohol, Distearyldimonium Chloride, Glycerin, Isopropyl Palmitate, Menthol, Petrolatum, Sodium Chloride, Triticum Vulgare Germ Protein (Wheat), Water	**Adult & Peds ≥2 yrs:** Apply tid-qid.
Aveeno Positively Radiant Moisturizing Lotion	Water, Glycerin, Emulsifying Wax, Ethylhexyl Isononanoate, Glycine Soja (Soybean) Seed Extract, Propylene Glycol Isoceteth-3 Acetate, Dimethicone, Polyacrylamide, Cyclomethicone, Stearic Acid, Phenoxyethanol, C13-14 Isoparaffin, Dimethicone Copolyol, Benzyl Alcohol, Titanium Dioxide, Fragrance, Iodopropynyl Butylcarbamate, Tocopherol Acetate, Panthenol, Panthenyl Ethylether, Glyceryl Laurate, Laureth-7, Methylparaben, Silica, Mica, Polymethyl Methacrylate, Cetearyl Alcohol, Tetrasodium EDTA, Butylparaben, Ethylparaben, Isobutylparaben, Propylparaben, DMDM Hydantoin, BHT, Citric Acid	**Adults:** Apply prn.
Aveeno Positively Radiant Daily Moisturizer SPF 15	Avobenzone/Octinoxate/Octisalate (3%-7.5%-2%), Arachidyl Alcohol, Arachidyl Glucoside, Behenyl Alcohol, Benzalkonium Chloride, Benzyl Alcohol, BHT, Bisphenylpropyl Dimethicone, Butylparaben, C12-15 Alkyl Benzoate, C13-14 Isoparaffin, Cetearyl Alcohol, Cetearyl Glucoside, Dimethicone, Disodium EDTA, Ethylene/Acrylic Acid Co-polymer, Ethylparaben, Fragrance, Glycerin, Glycine Soja (Soybean) Seed Extract, Iodopropyl Butylcarbamate, Isobutylparaben, Laureth-7, Methylparaben, Mica, Panthenol, Phenoxyethanol, Polyacrylamide, Polymethyl Methacrylate, Propylparaben, Silica, Steareth-2, Steareth-21, Titanium Dioxide, Water, Sodium Hydroxide, Citric Acid	**Adults:** Use daily.
Aveeno Positively Smooth Moisturizing Lotion	Water, Glycerin, Emulsifying Wax, Ethylhexyl Isononanoate, Glycine Soja Seed Extracts (Soybean), Propylene Glycol Isoceteth 3 Acetate, Dimethicone, Cyclomethicone, Polyacrylamide, Stearic Acid, Phenoxyethanol, C13-14 Isoparaffin, Dimethicone Copolyol, Benzyl Alcohol, Fragrance, DMDM Hydantoin, Glyceryl Laurate, Laureth 7, Methylparaben, Cetearyl Alcohol, Tetrasodium EDTA, Butylparaben, Ethylparaben, BHT, Propylparaben, Isobutylparaben, Iodopropynyl Butylcarbamate, Panthenyl Ethyl Ether, Tocopheryl Acetate, Panthenol	**Adults:** Apply prn.
Aveeno Radiant Skin Daily Moisturizer with SPF 15	Octinoxate (Octyl Methoxycinnamate)/Avobenzone/Octisalate (Octyl Salicylate) 7.5%-3%-2%; Arachidyl Alcohol, Arachidyl Glucoside, Behenyl Alcohol, Benzalkonium Chloride, Benzyl Alcohol, BHT, Bisphenylpropyl Dimethicone, Butylparaben, C12-15 Alkyl-Benzoate, C13-14 Isoparaffin, Cetearyl Alcohol, Cetearyl Glucoside, Dimethicone, Disodium EDTA, Ethylene/Acrylic Acid Copolymer, Ethylparaben, Fragrance, Glycerin, Glycine Soja (Soybean) Seed Extract, Iodopropynyl Butylcarbamate, Isobutylparaben, Laureth-7, Methylparaben, Mica, Panthenol, Phenoxyethanol, Polyacrylamide, Polymethylmethacrylate, Propylparaben, Silica, Steareth-2, Steareth-21, Titanium Dioxide, Water, Sodium Hydroxide, Citric Acid	**Adults:** Apply prn.

TABLE 16. DRY SKIN PRODUCTS (cont.)

Brand Name	Ingredient/Strength	Dose
Aveeno Creamy Moisturizing Oil	Water, Sesamum Indicum Seed Oil (Sesame), Di PPG 3 Myristyl Ether Adipate, Glycerin, Hydrogenated Polydecene, Dimethicone, Cetyl Alcohol, Avena Sativa (Oat) Kernel Oil, Prunus Amygdalus Dulcis Oil (Sweet Almond), Avena Sativa (Oat) Kernel Flour, Glyceryl Stearate, PEG 100 Stearate, Magnesium Aluminum Silicate, Xanthan Gum, Diazolidinyl Urea, Acrylates/C10 30 Alkyl Acrylate Crosspolymer, Lauroyl Lysine, Methylparaben, Ethylparaben, Propylparaben, Sodium Hydroxide, BHT, Tetrasodium EDTA, Fragrance	**Adults:** Apply after shower/bath prn.
Aveeno Intense Relief Overnight Cream	Dimethicone (1.3%), Avena Sativa (Oat) Kernel Extract, Avena Sativa (Oat) Kernel Flour, Avena Sativa (Oat) Kernel Oil, Benzyl Alcohol, Butyrospermum Parkii (Shea Butter), Cetyl Alcohol, Chamomilla Recutita (Matricaria) Flower Extract, Distearyldimonium Chloride, Glycerin, Isopropyl Palmitate, Petrolatum, Propylene Glycol, Sodium Chloride, Steareth 20, Water	**Adults:** Apply prn.
Aveeno Skin Relief Moisturizing Cream	Dimethicone (2.5%), Water, Glycerin, Distearyldimonium Chloride, Petrolatum, Cetyl Alcohol, Theobroma Cacao (Cocoa) Seed Butter, Cetearyl Alcohol, Avena Sativa (Oat) Kernel Flour, Di PPG 3 Myristyl Ether Adipate, Benzyl Alcohol, Ceteareth 20, Avena Sativa (Oat) Kernel Oil, Hydroxyethyl Cellulose, Menthol, Sodium Chloride, Butyrospermum Parkii (Shea Butter) Extract	**Adults & Peds** ≥2 yrs: Apply tid-qid.
Aveeno Ultra-Calming Night Cream	Water, Glycerin, C12 15 Alkyl Benzoate, Cetearyl Alcohol, Dimethicone, Arachidyl Alcohol, Cetyl Alcohol, Chrysanthemum Parthenium (Feverfew) Extract, Phenoxyethanol, Phenyl Trimethicone, Behenyl Alcohol, Cetearyl Glucoside, Ethylene Acrylic Acid Copolymer, Panthenol, Polyacrylamide, Arachidyl Glucoside, Sodium Cocoyl Amino Acids, Fragrance, C13 14 Isoparaffin, Cetyl Hydroxyethylcellulose, Methylparaben, Disodium EDTA, Sodium Polyacrylate, Pentaerythrityl Tetra Di T Butyl Hydroxyhydrocinnamate, Sarcosine, Laureth 7, Propylparaben, Ethylparaben, Magnesium Aspartate, Potassium Aspartate	**Adults:** Apply prn.
Aveeno Skin Relief Body Wash, Fragrance Free	Water, Glycerin, Cocamidopropyl Betaine, Sodium Laureth Sulfate, Decyl Glucoside, Avena Sativa (Oat) Kernel Flour, Glycol Stearate, Sodium Lauroampho PG Acetate Phosphate, Guar Hydroxypropyl-trimonium Chloride, Hydroxypropyltrimonium Hydrolyzed Wheat Protein, PEG 20 Glycerides, Hydroxypropyltrimonium Hydrolyzed Wheat Starch, PEG 150 Pentaerythrityl Tetrastearate, PEG 120 Methyl Glucose Trioleate, Propylene Glycol, Tetrasodium EDTA, PEG 6 Caprylic/Capric Glycerides, Quaternium 15, Coriandrum Sativum Extract, Elettaria Cardamomum Seed Extract, Conmiphora Myrrha Extract, SD Alcohol 39C. May Contain: Sodium Hydroxide, Citric Acid	**Adults:** Apply prn.
Carmol-10 Lotion	Urea 10%, Carbomer 940, Cetyl Alcohol, Isopropyl Palmitate, PEG 8 Doleate, PEG 8 Distearate, Propylene Glycol, Propylene Glycol Dipelargonate, Sodium Laureth Sulfate, Stearic Acid, Trolamine, Xanthan Gum	**Adults & Peds:** Apply prn.
Carmol-20 Cream	Urea 20%, Water, Isopropyl Myristate, Isopropyl Palmitate, Stearic Acid, Propylene Glycol, Trolamine, Sodium Laureth, Carbomer, Xanthan Gum, Fragrance	**Adults & Peds:** Apply qd-bid.
Cetaphil Daily Facial Moisturizer SPF 15 with Parsol 1789	Avobenzone 3%, Octocrylene 10%, Water, Diisopropyl Adipate, Cyclomethicone, Glyceryl Stearate, PEG-100 Stearate, Glycerin, Polymethyl Methacrylate, Phenoxyethanol, Benzyl Alcohol, Acrylates/C10-30 Alkyl Acrylate Crosspolymer, Tocopheryl Acetate, Carbomer 940, Disodium EDTA, Triethanolamine	**Adults & Peds:** Apply prn.

(Continued)

TABLE 16. DRY SKIN PRODUCTS (cont.)

BRAND NAME	INGREDIENT/STRENGTH	DOSE
Cetaphil Daily Advance Ultra Hydrating Lotion	Water, Glycerin, Hydrogenated Polyisobutene, Cetearyl Alcohol, Macadamia Integrifolia Seed Oil (Macadamia Nut Oil), Butyrospermum Parkii (Shea Butter), Acrylates/C10-30 Alkyl Acrylate Crosspolymer, Sodium Polyacrylate, Phenoxyethanol, Tocopheryl Acetate, Ceteareth-20, Stearoxytrimethylsilane, Stearyl Alcohol, Benzyl Alcohol, Farnesol, Sodium PCA, Panthenol, Cyclopentasiloxane, Dimethiconol, Citric Acid, Sodium Hydroxide	**Adults & Peds:** Apply prn.
Cetaphil UVA/UVB Defense SPF 50	Octinoxate/Octisalate/Octocrylene/Oxybenzone/Titanium Dioxide (7.5%-5%-7%-6%-5.7%), Water, Propylene Glycol, Glycerin, Dimethicone, VP/Eicosene Copolymer, Cyclohexasiloxane, Stearic Acid, Potassium Cetyl Phosphate, Glyceryl Stearate, PEG-100 Stearate, Aluminum Hydroxide, Dimethiconol, Disodium EDTA, Tocopherol, Cyclopentasiloxane, Triethanolamine, Phenoxyethanol, Ethylparaben, Chlorphenesin, Cetyl Alcohol, Acrylates/C10-30 Alkyl Acrylate Crosspolymer, Methylparaben, Xanthan Gum	**Adults & Peds:** Apply prn.
Cetaphil Moisturizing Cream	Water, Petrolatum, Glyceryl Polymethacrylate, Dicaprylyl Ether, Glycerin, Dimethicone, Glyceryl Stearate, Cetyl Alcohol, Prunus Amygdalus Dulcis (Sweet Almond) Oil, PEG-30 Glyceryl Stearate, Tocopheryl Acetate, Benzyl Alcohol, Phenoxyethanol, Sodium Hydroxide, Acrylates/C10-30 Alkyl Acrylate Crosspolymer, Dimethiconol, Disodium EDTA, Propylene Glycol	**Adults & Peds:** Apply prn.
Cetaphil Moisturizing Lotion	Water, Glycerin, Hydrogenated Polyisobutene, Cetearyl Alcohol, Ceteareth-20, Macadamia Nut Oil, Dimethicone, Tocopheryl Acetate, Stearoxytrimethylsilane, Stearyl Alcohol, Panthenol, Farnesol, Benzyl Alcohol, Phenoxyethanol, Acrylates/C10-30 Alkyl Acrylate Crosspolymer, Sodium Hydroxide, Citric Acid	**Adults & Peds:** Apply prn.
Cetaphil Therapeutic Hand Cream	Water, Glycerin, Cetearyl Alcohol, Oleth-12, PEG-2 Stearate, Butyrospermum Parkii, Ethylhexyl Methoxycinnamate, Dimethicone, Stearyl Alcohol, Glyceryl Stearate, PEG-100 Stearate, Methylparaben, Tocopherol, Arginine PCA, Chlorhexidine Digluconate	**Adults & Peds:** Apply prn.
Corn Huskers Lotion	Water, Glycerin, SD Alcohol 40, Sodium Calcium Alginate, Oleyl Sarcosin, Methylparaben, Guar Gum, Triethanolamine, Calcium Sulfate, Calcium Chloride, Fumaric Acid, Boric Acid, Fragrance	**Adults & Peds:** Apply prn.
Curel Continuous Comfort Original Formula	Water, Glycerin, Distearyldimonium Chloride, Petrolatum, Isopropyl Palmitate, Cetyl Alcohol, Butyrospermum Parkii (Shea Butter), Acacia Senegal Gum, Dimethicone, Fragrance, Sodium Chloride, Gelatin, Methylparaben, Propylparaben	**Adults:** Apply to skin prn.
Curel Continuous Comfort Fragrance Free	Water, Glycerin, Distearyldimonium Chloride, Petrolatum, Isopropyl Palmitate, Cetyl Alcohol, Acacia Senegal Gum, Dimethicone, Sodium Chloride, Gelatin, Methylparaben, Propylparaben	**Adults:** Apply to skin prn.
Curel Natural Healing Soothing Lotion	Water, Glycerin, Distearyldimonium Chloride, Petrolatum, Isopropryl Palmitate, Cetyl Alcohol, Lavandula Angustifolia (Lavender) Flower Extract, Anthemis Nobilis (Chamomile) Flower Extract, Avena Sativa (Oat) Meal Extract, Propylene Glycol, Pentylene Glycol, Dimethicone, Fragrance, Sodium Chloride, Methylparaben, Propylparaben, Caramel	**Adults:** Apply to skin prn.
Curel Natural Healing Nourishing Lotion	Water, Glycerin, Distearyldimonium Chloride, Petrolatum, Isopropryl Palmitate, Cetyl Alcohol, Butyrospermum Parkii (Shea Butter), Vanilla Planifolia Fruit Extract, Honey (Mel), Propylene Glycol, Butylene Glycol, Dipropylene Glycol, Dimethicone, Fragrance, Sodium Chloride, Methylparaben, Propylparaben, Caramel	**Adults:** Apply to skin prn.
Curel Ultra Healing Intensive Moisture Lotion	Water, Glycerin, Petrolatum, Cetearyl Alcohol, Benhentrimonium Chloride, Cetyl-PG Hydroxyethyl Palmitamide, Isopropyl Palmitate, Butyrospermum Parkii (Shea Butter), Avena Sativa (Oat) Meal Extract, Eucalyptus Globulus Leaf Extract, Citrus Aurantium Dulcis (orange) Peel Oil, Cyclopentasiloxane, Dimethicone, Acacia Senegal Gum, Gelatin, DMDM Hydantoin	**Adults:** Apply to skin prn.

TABLE 16. DRY SKIN PRODUCTS (cont.)

BRAND NAME	INGREDIENT/STRENGTH	DOSE
Eucerin Creme Original	Water, Petrolatum, Mineral Oil, Ceresin, Lanolin Alcohol Methylchloroisothiazolinone, Methylisothiazolinone	**Adults & Peds:** Apply prn.
Eucerin Dry Skin Therapy Calming Cream	Water, Glycerin, Cetyl Palmitate, Mineral Oil, Caprylic/Capric Triglycerides, Octyldodecanol, Cetyl Alcohol, Glycerly Stearate, Colloidal Oatmeal, Dimethicone, PEG-40 Stearate, Phenoxyethanol, DMDM Hydantoin, Iodopropynyl Butylcarbamate	**Adults & Peds >2 yrs:** Apply prn.
Eucerin Plus Intensive Repair Lotion	Water, Mineral Oil, PEG-7 Hydrogenated Castor Oil, Isohexadecane, Sodium Lactate, Urea, Glycerin, Isopropyl Palmitate, Panthenol, Microcrystalline Wax, Magnesium Sulfate, Lanolin Alcohol, Bisabolol, Methylchloroisothiazolinone, Methylisothiazolinone	**Adults:** Apply prn.
Eucerin Sensitive Facial Skin Gentle Hydrating Cleanser	Water, Sodium Laureth Sulfate, Cocamidopropyl Betaine, Disodium Cocamphodiacetate, Glycol Distearate, PEG 7 Glyceryl Cocoate, Cocamide MEA, Laureth 10, Citric Acid, PEG 120 Methyl Glucose Dioleate, Lanolin Alcohol, Imidazolidinyl Urea	**Adults:** Use qd.
Eucerin Plus Intensive Repair Hand Creme	Water, Glycerin, Urea, Glyceryl Stearate, Stearyl Alcohol, Dicaprylyl Ether, Sodium Lactate, Dimethicone, PEG-40 Stearate, Cyclopenta-siloxane, Cyclohexasiloxane, Aluminum Starch Octenylsuccinate, Lactic Acid, Xanthan Gum, Phenoxyethanol, Methylparaben, Propylparaben	**Adults & Peds:** Apply qd.
Eucerin Lotion Daily Replenishing	Water, Sunflower Seed Oil, Petrolatum, Glycerin, Glyceryl Stearate SE, Octyldodecanol, Caprylic/Capric Triglycerides, Stearic Acid, Dimethicone, Cetearyl Alcohol, Lanolin Alcohol, Panthenol, Tocopheryl Acetate, Cholesterol, Carbomer, Disodium EDTA, Sodium Hydroxide, Phenoxyethanol, Methylparaben, Ethylparaben, Propylparaben, Butylparaben, Isobutylparaben, BHT	**Adults & Peds:** Apply qd.
Eucerin Lotion Original	Water, Mineral Oil, Isopropyl Myristate, PEG-40 Sorbitan Peroleate, Glyceryl Lanolate, Sorbitol, Propylene Glycol, Cetyl Palmitate, Magnesium Sulfate, Aluminum Stearate, Lanolin Alcohol, BHT, Methylchloroisothiazolinone, Methylisothiazolinone	**Adults & Peds:** Apply qd.
Eucerin Plus Smoothing Essentials	Water, Glycerin, Caprylic/Capric Triglyceride, Cetearyl Alcohol, Urea, Hydrogenated Coco Glycerides, Isopropyl Stearate, Octyldodecanol, Sodium Lactate, Dimethicone, Arginine HCl, Glyceryl Stearate SE, Myristyl Myristate, Carnitine, Chondrus Crispus (Carrageenan), Sodium Cetearyl Sulfate, Lactic Acid, Sodium Citrate, Citric Acid, Acrylates/C10 30 Alkyl Acrylate Crosspolymer, Phenoxyethanol, Methylparaben, Benzyl Alcohol, Propylparaben, Potassium Sorbate	**Adults:** Apply qd.
Eucerin Redness Relief Daily Perfecting Lotion SPF 15	Octinoxate, Octisalate, Titanium Dioxide, Water, Glycerine, Dimethicone, Polyglyceryl-3 Methylglucose Distearate, Butyrospermum Parkii (Shea Butter), Lauroyl Lysine, Squalane, Alcohol Denat., Sorbitan Stearate, Phenoxyethanol, Butylene Glycol, Magnesium Aluminum Silicate, Glycyrrhiza Inflata Root Extract, Xanthan Gum, Methylparaben, Propylparaben, Ethylparaben, Iodopropynyl Butylcarbamate, Trimethoxycaprylylsilane, Chromium Oxide Greens, Chromium Hydroxide Green, Ultramarines	**Adults & Peds:** Apply prn.
Eucerin Redness Relief Soothing Cleanser	Water, Glycerin, Sodium Laureth Sulfate, Carbomer, Phenoxyethanol, PEG-40 Hydrogenated Castor Oil, Sodium Methyl Cocoyl Taurate, PEG-7 Glyceryl Cocoate, Decyl Glucoside, Glycyrrhiza Inflata Root Extract, Xanthan Gum, Sodium Hydroxide, Methylparaben, Butylparaben, Ethylparaben, Isobutylparaben, Propylparaben, Benzophenone-4	**Adults & Peds:** Use qam and qpm.
Eucerin Redness Relief Soothing Moisture Lotion SPF 15	Water, Glycerin, Dimethicone, Polyglyceryl 3 Methylglucose Distearate, Butyrospermum Parkii (Shea SPF 15 Butter), Squalane, Alcohol Denat., Dicaprylyl Carbonate, Sorbitan Stearate, Lauroyl Lysine, Glycyrrhiza Inflata Root Extract, Phenoxyethanol, 1, 2 Hexanediol, Magnesium Aluminum Silicate, Xanthan Gum, Trimethoxycaprylylsilane, Methylparaben, Propylparaben, Ethylparaben	**Adults & Peds:** Apply qam and qpm.

(Continued)

TABLE 16. DRY SKIN PRODUCTS (cont.)

Brand Name	Ingredient/Strength	Dose
Eucerin Redness Relief Soothing Night Crème	Water, Glycerin, Panthenol, Caprylic/Capric Triglyceride, Dicaprylyl Carbonate, Octyldodecanol, C12-15 Alkyl Benzoate, Dimethicone, Squalane, Tapioca Starch, Cetearyl Alcohol, Glyceryl Stearate Citrate, Myristyl Myristate, Butylene Glycol, Benzyl Alcohol, Glycyrrhiza Inflata Root Extract, Carbomer, Phenoxyethanol, Ammonium Acryloydimethyltaurate/VP Copolymer, Sodium Hydroxide, Methylparaben, Propylparaben, Iodopropynyl Butylcarbamate	**Adults & Peds:** Apply qpm.
Gold Bond Ultimate Healing Lotion	Water, Glycerin, Dimethicone, Petrolatum, Jojoba Esters, Cetyl Alcohol, Aloe Barbadensis Leaf Juice, Stearyl Alcohol, Distearyldimonium Chloride, Cetearyl Alcohol, Steareth 21, Steareth 2, Propylene Glycol, Chamomilla Recutita Flower Extract (Matricaria), Polysorbate 60, Stearamidopropyl PG Dimonium Chloride Phosphate, Methyl Gluceth 20, Tocopheryl Acetate, Magnesium Ascorbyl Phosphate, Hydrolyzed Collagen, Hydrolyzed Elastin, Retinyl Palmitate, Hydrolyzed Jojoba Esters, Glyceryl Stearate, Dipotassium EDTA, Fragrance, Trietanolamine, Diazolidinyl Urea, Methylparaben, Propylparaben	**Adults & Peds:** Apply prn.
Gold Bond Ultimate Comfort Body Powder	Corn Starch, Sodium Bicarbonate, Silica, Fragrance, Ascrobyl Palmitate, Aloe Barbadensis Leaf Extract, Lavandula Angustifolia Extract, Chamomilla Recutita Flower Extract, Rosmarinus Officinalis Leaf Extract, Acacia Farnesiana Extract, Tocopheryl Acetate, Retinyl Palmitate, Polyoxymethylene Urea, Isopropyl Myristate, Benzethonium Chloride	**Adults & Peds:** Apply prn.
Keri Moisture Therapy Advance Extra Dry Skin Lotion	Water, Glycerin, Stearic Acid, Hydrogenated Polyisobutene, Petrolatum, Cetyl Alcohol, Aloe Barbadensis Leaf Juice, Tocopheryl Acetate, Cyclopentasiloxane, Dimethicone Copolyol, Glyceryl Stearate, PEG-100 Stearate, Dimethicone, Carbomer, Methylparaben, PEG-5 Soya Sterol, Magnesium Aluminum Silicate, Propylparaben, Phenoxyethanol, Disodium EDTA, Diazolidinyl Urea, Sodium Hydroxide, Fragrance	**Adults & Peds:** Apply prn.
Keri Lotion, Sensitive Skin	Water, Glycerin, Stearic Acid, Hydrogenated Polyisobutene, Petrolatum, Cetyl Alcohol, Aloe Barbadensis Leaf Juice, Tocopheryl Acetate (Vitamin E Acetate), Cyclopenta Siloxane, Dimethicone Copolyol, Glyceryl Stearate, PEG 100 Stearate, Dimethicone, Carbomer, Methylparaben, PEG 5 Soy Sterol, Magnesium Aluminum Silicate, Propylparaben, Phenoxyethanol, Disodium EDTA, Diazolidinyl Urea, Sodium Hydroxide	**Adults:** Apply prn.
Keri Original Formula Lotion	Water, Mineral Oil, Glycerin, Glycerol Stearate, PEG-40 Stearate, PEG-4 Dilaurate, Laureth-4, Carbomer, Methylparaben, Propylparaben, Fragrance, DMDM Hydantoin, Iodopropynyl Butylcarbamate, Aloe Barbadensis Leaf Juice, Helianthus Annuus (Sunflower) Seed Oil, Sodium Hydroxide, Disodium EDTA, Tocopheryl Acetate (Vitamin E Acetate)	**Adults & Peds:** Apply prn.
Keri Nourishing Shea Butter Lotion	Water, Mineral Oil, Glycerin, Butyrospermum Parkii (Shea Butter), PEG-40 Stearate, Glyceryl Stearate, PEG-4 Dilaurate, Laureth 4, Aloe Barbadensis Leaf Juice, Helianthus Annuus Seed Oil, Tocopheryl Acetate, Carbomer, Methylparaben, Propylparaben, DMDM Hydantoin, Iodopropynyl Butylcarbamate, Sodium Hydroxide, Disodium EDTA, Fragrance, PEG-100 Stearate	**Adults & Peds:** Apply prn.
Keri Age Defy & Protect Lotion	Octinoxate/Oxybenzone (7.5%-2%), Water, Ammonium Lactate, Cetearyl Alcohol, Glycerin, Ceteth-20, Galactoarabinan, Propylene Glycol Myristyl Ether Acetate, C12-15 Alkyl Benzoate, Sodium Hydroxypropyl Starch Phosphate, Octyldodecyl Neopentanoate, Dimethicone, Neopentyl Glycol Diethylhexanoate, Neopentyl Glycol Diisostearate, Xanthan Gum, Disodium EDTA, DMDM Hydantoin, Iodopropynyl Butylcarbamate, Tocopheryl Acetate (Vitamin E Acetate), Fragrance	**Adults & Peds:** Apply prn.

TABLE 16. DRY SKIN PRODUCTS (cont.)

Brand Name	Ingredient/Strength	Dose
Keri Long Lasting Hand Cream	Water, Cetearyl Alcohol and Polysorbate 60, Mineral Oil, Cetyl Alcohol, Caprylic/Capric Triglycerides, Propylene Glycol, Dimethicone, Methylparaben, Tocopheryl Acetate (Vitamin E Acetate), Propylparaben, Disodium EDTA	**Adults & Peds:** Apply prn.
Keri Overnight Deep Conditioning	Water, Butyrospermum Parkii (Shea Butter), Glycerin, Cetearyl Alcohol, Steareth-30, Ceteareth-10, Phenoxyethanol, Methylparaben, Ethylparaben, Butylparaben, Propylparaben, Dipentaerythrityl Tetrahydroxystearate/Tetraisostearate, Hydrogenated Polyisobutene, Cetyl Alcohol, Glycyrrhiza Glabra (Licorice) Root Extract, Butylene Glycol, Pyrus Malus (Apple) Fruit Extract, Dimethicone, Cyclopentasiloxane, Cyclohexasiloxane, Triethanolamine, Hydrogenated Castor Oil, Acrylates/C10-30 Alkyl Acrylate Crosspolymer, Disodium EDTA, Carbomer, Fragrance, Tocopheryl Acetate*, Caprylic/Capric Triglyceride, Hydrogenated Lecithin, Hydroxylated Lecithin, BHT, Lecithin, Ascorbyl Palmitate, Retinyl Palmitate, Helianthus Annuus (Sunflower) Seed Oil, Glyceryl Polymethacrylate, Propylene Glycol, Palmitoyl Oligopeptide, Panthenol, Niacinamide, Phytonadione	**Adults & Peds:** Apply prn.
Keri Renewal Milk Body Lotion	Water, Caprylic/Capric Triglyceride, Helianthus Annuus (Sunflower) Seed Oil, Glycerin, PEG-20 Methyl Glucose Sesquistearate, Methyl Glucose Sesquistearate, Sodium Pyruvate, Dimethicone, Beeswax, Phenoxyethanol, Polyacrylamide, Tocopheryl Acetate, Borago Officinalis Extract, Lactic Acid, Bifida Ferment Lysate, Methylparaben, C13-14 Isoparaffin, Carbomer, Sodium Hydroxide, Propylparaben, Propylene Glycol, Allantoin, Acrylates/C10-30 Alkyl Acrylate Crosspolymer, Disodium EDTA, Laureth-7, Ethylparaben, Butylparaben, BHT, Asorbyl Palmitate, Glyceryl Stearate, Glyceryl Oleate, Citric Acid, Hydrolyzed Fibronectin, Glycosphingolipids, Phospholipids, Cholesterol, Whey Protein	**Adults & Peds:** Apply prn.
Keri Renewal Serum for Dry Skin	Water, Urea, Propylene Glycol, Cyclopentasiloxane, Cyclomethicone, Lactobionic Acid, Gluconolactone, PEG/PPG-18/18 Dimethicone, Arginine, Butylene Glycol, Glycerin, Ammonium Hydroxide, Dimethiconol, Chlorphenesin, Methylparaben	**Adults & Peds:** Apply prn.
Lac-Hydrin Five Lotion	Water, Lactic Acid, Ammonium Hydroxide, Glycerin, Petrolatum, Squalane, Steareth-2, POE-21-Stearyl Ether, Propylene Glycol Dioctanoate, Cetyl Alcohol, Cetyl Palmitate, Magnesium Aluminum Silicate, Diazolidinyl Urea, Dimethicone, Methylchloroisothiazoline, Methylisothiazolinone	**Adults & Peds:** Apply bid.
Lubriderm Advanced Therapy Hand Cream	Water, Glycerin, Distearyldimonium Chloride, Petrolatum, Isopropyl Palmitate, Cetyl Alcohol, Aluminum Starch Octenylsuccinate, Dimethicone, Avena Sativa (Oat) Kernel Flour, Benzyl Alcohol, Methylparaben, Sodium Chloride, Tocopheryl Acetate, Lecithin, Retinyl Palmitate	**Adults & Peds:** Apply qd.
Lubriderm Advanced Therapy Moisturizing Lotion	Water, Mineral Oil, Glycerin, Cetyl Alcohol, Sorbitol, Caprylic/Capric Triglyceride, Cetearyl Alcohol, Stearic Acid, Dimethicone, Polysorbate 60, Tocopheryl Acetate, Panthenol, Phenoxyethanol, Lecithin, Carbomer, Sodium Hydroxide, Ceteareth-20, Diazolidinyl Urea, Sodium Citrate, Methylparaben, Titanium Dioxide, BHT, Sodium Pyruvate, Retinyl Palmitate, Propylparaben, Fragrance, Citric Acid, Ethylparaben, Tocopherol	**Adults & Peds:** Apply qd.
Lubriderm Advanced Therapy Triple Smoothing Lotion	Water, Glycerin, Glycolic Acid, Cetyl Alcohol, Dimethicone, Stearyl Alcohol, Isopropyl Palmitate, Caprylic/Capric Triglyceride, Potassium Hydroxide, Ethylhexyl Palmitate, Glyceryl Stearate, PEG-100 Stearate, Cetearyl Alcohol, Petrolatum, Cyclopentasiloxane, Ceteareth-20, Urea, Cyclohexasiloxane, DMDM Hydantoin, Methylparaben, Disodium EDTA, Xanthan Gum, Fragrance, Panthenol, Tocopheryl Acetate, Retinyl Palmitate	**Adults & Peds:** Apply qd.

(Continued)

TABLE 16. DRY SKIN PRODUCTS (cont.)

Brand Name	Ingredient/Strength	Dose
Lubriderm Daily Moisture Fragrance Free Lotion	Water, Mineral Oil, Glycerin, Caprylic/Capric Triglyceride, Cetyl Alcohol, Phenoxyethanol, Panthenol, Cetearyl Alcohol, Stearic Acid, Dimethicone, Carbomer, Ceteareth-20, Sodium Hydroxide, Sodium Citrate, Methylparaben, Propylparaben, Citric Acid, Ethylparaben	**Adults & Peds:** Apply qd.
Lubriderm Daily Moisture Lotion	Water, Mineral Oil, Glycerin, Caprylic/Capric Triglyceride, Stearic Acid, Cetyl Alcohol, Panthenol, Cetearyl Alcohol, Dimethicone, Carbomer, Ceteareth-20, Sodium Hydroxide, Sodium Citrate, Methylparaben, Phenoxyethanol, Propylparaben, Fragrance, Citric Acid, Ethylparaben	**Adults & Peds:** Apply qd.
Lubriderm Sensitive Skin Therapy Moisturizing Lotion	Water, Butylene Glycol, Mineral Oil, Petrolatum, Glycerin, Cetyl Alcohol, Propylene Glycol Dicaprylate/Dicaprate, PEG-40 Stearate, C11-13 Isoparaffin, Glyceryl Stearate, Tri-PPG-3 Myristyl Ether Citrate, Emulsifying Wax, Dimethicone, DMDM Hydantoin, Methylparaben, Carbomer, Ethylparaben, Propylparaben, Titanium Dioxide, Disodium EDTA, Sodium Hydroxide, Butylparaben, Xanthan Gum	**Adults & Peds:** Apply qd.
Lubriderm Daily Moisturizer Lotion, SPF 15	Octyl Methoxycinnamate/Octyl Salicylate/Oxybenzone (7.5%-4%-3%), Purified Water, C 12-15 Alkyl Benzoate, Cetearyl Alcohol, Ceteareth-20, Cetyl Alcohol, Glyceryl Monostearate, Propylene Glycol, White Petrolatum, Diazolidinyl Urea, Trolamine, Edetate Disodium, Xanthan Gum, Acrylates/C 10-30 Alkyl Acrylate Crosspolymer, Vitamin E, Iodopropynyl Butylcarbamate, Fragrance, Carbomer	**Adults & Peds >6 mo:** Apply prn.
Lubriderm Intense Skin Repair Body Cream	Water, Glycerin, Petrolatum, Mineral Oil, Cetyl Alcohol, Dimethicone, Avena Sativa (Oat) Kernel Flour, Carbomer, Ceteareth-6, Methylparaben, Sodium Citrate, Sodium Hydroxide, Tetrasodium EDTA, Stearyl Alcohol, Citric Acid, Benzalkonium Chloride, Ethylparaben, Propylparaben, Hydrolyzed Milk Protein, Benzaldehyde, Butyrospermum Parkii (Shea Butter), Hydrolyzed Soy Protein, Glyceryl Stearate, C12-15 Alkyl Benzoate, Polysorbate 80, Glycine Soja (Soybean) Sterols	**Adults & Peds:** Apply qd.
Lubriderm Intense Skin Repair Body Lotion	Water, Glycerin, Ethylhexyl Isononanoate, Mineral Oil, Petrolatum, Cetyl Alcohol, Sorbitan Monostearate, Hydrogenated Polydecene, Sodium Behenoyl Lactylate, Synthetic Wax, Trimethylpentanediol/Adipic Acid/Glycerin Crosspolymer, Butyrospermum Parkii (Shea Butter), Tri- PPG-3 Myristyl Ether Citrate, Propylene Glycol, Diazolidinyl Urea, Sorbityl Laurate, Glyceryl Stearate, Disodium EDTA, Triethanolamine, C12-15 Alkyl Benzoate, Fragrance, Polysorbate 80, Glycine Soja (Soybean) Sterols, Iodopropynyl Butylcarbamate	**Adults & Peds:** Apply qd.
Lubriderm Intense Skin Repair Body Lotion with Itch Relief	Water, Glycerin, Distearyldimonium Chloride, Petrolatum, Isopropyl Palmitate, Cetyl Alcohol, Dimethicone, Avena Sativa (Oat) Kernel Flour, Avena Sativa (Oat) Kernel Oil, Mineral Oil, Steareth-20, Methylparaben, Benzalkonium Chloride, Avena Sativa (Oat) Kernel Extract, Sodium Chloride, Panthenol, Butyrospermum Parkii (Shea Butter), Glyceryl Stearate C12-15 Alkyl Benzoate, Polysorbate 80, Glycine Soja (Soybean) Sterols, Titanium Dioxide	**Adults & Peds:** Apply qd or prn.
Lubriderm Skin Nourishing Moisturizing Lotion with Premium Oat Extract	Water, Glycerin, Caprylic/Capric Triglycerides, Glycerin, Glyceryl Stearate SE, Petrolatum, Camellia Oleifera Seed Oil, Castor Oil, Cocoa Butter, Cetyl Alcohol, Wax, Brassica Alba Seed Extract, Oat Kernel Extract, Cassia Angustifolia Seed Polysaccharide, Glyceryl Stearate, PEG 100 Stearate, Diazolidinyl Urea, Xanthan Gum Disodium EDTA, Fragrance, Iodopropynyl Butylcarbamate, Soybean Oil	**Adults:** Apply qd.
Lubriderm Skin Nourishing Moisturizing Lotion with Shea and Cocoa Butters	Water, Glycerin, Cetyl Alcohol, Glyceryl Stearate SE, Petrolatum, Emulsifying Wax, Caprylic/Capric Triglyceride, Castor Oil, Octyldodecanol, Shea Butter, Cocoa Butter, Dimethicone, Tocopheryl Acetate, Diazolidinyl Urea, Xanthan Gum, Disodium EDTA, Fragrance, Iodopropynyl Butylcarbamate	**Adults:** Apply qd.

TABLE 16. DRY SKIN PRODUCTS (cont.)

BRAND NAME	INGREDIENT/STRENGTH	DOSE
Lubriderm Skin Nourishing Moisturizing Lotion with Sea Kelp Extract	Water, Glycerin, Glyceryl Stearate SE, Cetyl Alcohol, Emulsifying Wax, Petrolatum, Caprylic/Capric Triglyceride, Castor Oil, Octyldodecanol, Dimethicone, Diazolidinyl Urea, Propylene Glycol, Xanthan Gum, Disodium EDTA, Fragrance, Giant Kelp Leaf Extract, Iodopropynyl Butylcarbamate	**Adults:** Apply qd.
Neutrogena Norwegian Formula Body Moisturizer	Water, Glycerin, Distearyldimonium Chloride, Petrolatum, Isopropyl Palmitate, Cetyl Alcohol, Dimethicone, Colloidal Oatmeal, Cetearyl Alcohol, Sodium Cetearyl Sulfate, Sodium Sulfate, Sodium Chloride, Benzyl Alcohol, Fragrance	**Adults & Peds:** Apply prn.
Neutrogena Norwegian Formula Hand Cream	Water Purified, Glycerin, Cetearyl Alcohol, Stearic Acid, Sodium Cetearyl Sulfate, Methylparaben, Propylparaben, Dilauryl Thiodipropionate, Sodium Sulfate, Fragrance	**Adults & Peds:** Apply prn.
Neutrogena Deep Moisture Body Cream	Water, Glycerin, Distearyldimonium Chloride, Petrolatum, Isopropyl Palmitate, Cetyl Alcohol, Dimethicone, Panthenol, Butyrospermum Parkii, Cocoa (Theobroma Cacao) Seed Butter, Mango (Mangifera Indica) Seed Butter, Benzyl Alcohol, BHT, Sodium Chloride, Yellow 5, Yellow 6, Fragrance	**Adults & Peds:** Apply qd.
Neutrogena Norwegian Formula Deep Moisture Hand Cream	Water, Glycerin, Distearyldimonium Chloride, Petrolatum, Isopropyl Palmitate, Cetyl Alcohol, Dimethicone, Panthenol, Butyrospermum Parkii, Cocoa Seed Butter (Theobroma Cacao), Mango Seed Butter (Mangifera Indica), Benzyl Alcohol, Phytantriol, BHT, Sodium Chloride, Yellow 5, Yellow 6, Fragrance	**Adults:** Apply prn.
Nivea Body Age Defying Moisturizer For Body	Water, Glycerin, Mineral Oil, Caprylic/Capric Triglycerides, Cetyl Alcohol, Dimethicone, Glyceryl Stearate, Cyclopentasiloxane, Cyclohexasiloxane, PEG-40 Stearate, Creatine, 1-Methylhydantoin-2-Imide, Ubiquinone, Fragrance, Carbomer, Sodium Hydroxide, Phenoxyethanol, Methylparaben, Propylparaben	**Adults:** Apply to damp skin prn.
Nivea Essentially Enriched Lotion	Water, Mineral Oil, C13-16 Isoparaffin, Glycerin, Isopropyl Palmitate, Petrolatum, PEG-40, Sorbitan Perisostearate, Polyglyceryl-3 Diisostearate, Prunus Amygdalus Dulcis (Sweet Almond) Oil, Tocopheryl Acetate, Taurine, Sea Salt, Magnesium Sulfate, Fragrance, Citric Acid, Sodium Citrate, Potassium Sorbate	**Adults & Peds >2 yrs:** Apply prn.
Nivea Body Original Moisture Daily Lotion, Dry Skin	Water, Mineral Oil, Glycerin, Isopropyl Palmitate, Glyceryl Stearate SE, Cetearyl Alcohol, Tocopheryl Acetate, Lanolin Alcohol, Isopropyl Myristate, Simethicone, Fragrance, Carbomer, Hydroxypropyl Methylcellulose, Sodium Hydroxide, Methylcellulose, Sodium Hydroxide, Methylchloroisothiazolinone, Methylisothiazolinone	**Adults:** Apply to damp skin prn.
Nivea Smooth Sensation Body Oil	Mineral Oil, Caprylic/Capric Triglycerides, Persea Gratissima Oil (Avocado), Fragrance	**Adults:** Apply to damp skin prn.
Nivea Smooth Sensation Daily Lotion, Dry Skin	Water, Glycerin, Mineral Oil, Caprylic/Capric Triglycerides, Cetyl Alcohol, Dimethicone, Glyceryl Stearate, Cyclopentasiloxane, Cyclohexasiloxane, PEG-40 Stearate, Ginkgo Biloba Leaf Extract, Tocopheryl Acetate, Butyrospermum Parkii (Shea Butter), Phenoxyethanol, Fragrance, Carbomer, Sodium Hydroxide, EDTA, Methylparaben, Propylparaben	**Adults:** Apply to damp skin prn.
Nivea Creme	Triple Purified Water, Mineral Oil, Petrolatum, Glycerin, Microcrystalline Wax, Lanolin Alcohol, Paraffin, Panthenol, Magnesium Sulfate, Decyl Oleate, Octyldodecanol, Aluminum Stearate, Methylchloroisothiazolinone, Methylisothiazolinone, Citric Acid, Magnesium Stearate, Fragrance	**Adults & Peds:** Apply prn.

(Continued)

TABLE 16. DRY SKIN PRODUCTS (cont.)

Brand Name	Ingredient/Strength	Dose
Vaseline Intensive Care Cocoa Butter Deep Conditioning Lotion	Water, Petrolatum, Glycerin, Stearic Acid, Isopropyl Palmitate, Glycol Stearate, Dimethicone, Theobroma Cacao Seed Butter (Cocoa), Butyrospermum Parkii (Shea Butter), Helianthus Annuus Seed Oil or Glycine Soja Oil (Sunflower, Soybean), Glycine Soja Sterol (Soybean), Tocopheryl Acetate (Vitamin E Acetate), Retinyl Palmitate (Vitamin A Palmitate), Sodium Stearoyl-2-Lactylate, Collagen Amino Acids, Urea, Glyceryl Stearate, Cetyl Alcohol, Magnesium Aluminum Silicate, Carbomer, Lecithin, Mineral Water, Sodium PCA, Potassium Lactate, Lactic Acid, Fragrance, Stearamide AMP, Triethanolamine, Methylparaben, DMDM Hydantoin, Disodium EDTA, Caramel, Titanium Dioxide	**Adults & Peds:** Apply prn.
Vaseline Intensive Care Healthy Hand & Nail Lotion	Water, Potassium Lactate, Sodium Hydroxypropyl Starch Phosphate, Glycerin, Stearic Acid, Mineral Oil, Dimethicone, Lactic Acid, Glycol Stearate, PEG 100 Stearate, Keratin, Glycine Soja Sterol (Soybean), Lecithin, Tocopheryl Acetate (Vitamin E Acetate), Retinyl Palmitate (Vitamin A Palmitate), Healianthus Annuus Seed Oil (Sunflower), Sodium PCA, Sodium Stearoyl Lactate, Urea, Collagen Amino Acids, Ethylhexyl Methoxycinnamate, Petrolatum, Mineral Water, Cetyl Alcohol, Stearamide AMP, Cyclomethicone, Magnesium Aluminum Silicate, Glyceryl Stearate, Fragrance, Xanthan Gum, Corn Oil, BHT, Disodium EDTA, Methylparaben, DMDM Hydantoin	**Adults & Peds:** Apply prn.
Vaseline Intensive Care Aloe Cool & Fresh Moisturizing Lotion	Water, Glycerin, Stearic Acid, Glycol Stearate, Aloe Barbadensis Leaf Juice (Aloe Vera), Cucumis Sativus Extract (Cucumber), Helianthus Annuus Seed Oil (Sunflower), Glycine Soja Oil (Soybean), Glycine Soja Sterol (Soybean), Sodium Stearoyl-2 Lactylate, Tocopheryl Acetate (Vitamin E Acetate), Retinyl Palmitate (Vitamin A Palmitate), Sodium Acrylate/Acryloyldimethyl Taurate Copolymer, Dimethicone, Glyceryl Stearate, Cetyl Alcohol, Lecithin, Mineral Water, Sodium PCA, Potassium Lactate, Lactic Acid, Collagen Amino Acids, Urea, Fragrance, Triethanolamine, DMDM Hydantoin, Iodopropynyl Butylcarbamate, Disodium EDTA, Titanium Dioxide	**Adults & Peds:** Apply prn.
Vaseline Intensive Care Lotion Total Moisture	Water, Glycerin, Stearic Acid, Glycol Stearate, Petrolatum, Isopropyl Palmitate, Glycine Soja Sterol (Soybean), Helianthus Annuus Seed Oil (Sunflower), Glycine Soja Oil (Soybean), Avena Sativa Kernel Protein (Oat), Sodium Stearoyl-2 Lactylate, Tocopheryl Acetate (Vitamin E Acetate), Retinyl Palmitate (Vitamin A Palmitate), Panthenol (Provitamin B5), Carbomer, Lecithin, Keratin, Dimethicone, Glyceryl Stearate, Cetyl Alcohol, Sodium PCA, Potassium Lactate, Lactic Acid, Collagen Amino Acids, Mineral Water, Fragrance, Triethanolamine, Magnesium Aluminum Silicate, Urea, Methylparaben, DMDM Hydantoin, Iodopropynyl Butylcarbamate, Disodium EDTA, Titanium Dioxide	**Adults & Peds:** Apply prn.
Vaseline Intensive Rescue Moisture Locking Lotion	Water, Glycerin, Petrolatum, Stearic Acid, Glycol Stearate, Dimethicone, Isopropyl Isostearate, Tapioca Starch, Cetyl Alcohol, Glyceryl Stearate, Magnesium Aluminum Silicate, Carbomer, Ethylene Brassylate, Triethanolamine, Disodium EDTA, Phenoxyethanol, Methylparaben, Propylparaben, Titanium Dioxide (CI 77891)	**Adults & Peds:** Apply prn.
Vaseline Jelly	White Petrolatum	**Adults & Peds:** Apply prn.
Vaseline Intensive Rescue Clinical Therapy Lotion	Dimethicone (1.0%), Water, Glycerin, Isopropyl Palmitate, Distearlydimonium Chloride, Cetyl Alcohol, Mineral Oil, Steareth-21, Borago Officinalis Seed Oil, Glycine Soja (Soybean) Sterol, Petrolatum, Tocopheryl Acetate, Fragrance (Lightly fragranced only), Stearic Acid, Lecithin, Tapioca Starch, Stearyl Stearate, Sodium Chloride, Linoleic Acid, Linolenic Acid, Ethylene Brassylate (Unfragranced only), Methylparaben, Propylparaben	**Adults & Peds:** Apply prn.

TABLE 16. DRY SKIN PRODUCTS (cont.)

Brand Name	Ingredient/Strength	Dose
Vaseline Intensive Rescue Heal & Repair Balm	Water, Petrolatum, Glycerin, Cyclopentasiloxane, Caprylic/Capric Triglyceride, Isopropyl Palmitate, Stearic Acid, Glycol Stearate, Sodium Hydroxypropyl Starch Phosphate, Peg-100 Stearate, Cetyl Alcohol, Glyceryl Stearate, Ethylene Brassylate, Disodium EDTA, Potassium Hydroxide, Phenoxyethanol, Methylparaben, Propylparaben	**Adults & Peds:** Apply prn.
Vaseline Intensive Rescue Moisture Locking Body Butter	Water, Petrolatum, Glycerin, Dimethicone, Cyclopentasiloxane, Stearic Acid, Hydrogenated Polyisobutene, Ethylhexyl Cocoate, Hydrogenated Didecene, Glycol Stearate, Paraffin, Theobroma Cacao (Cocoa) Seed Butter, Butyrospermum Parkii (Shea Butter), Potato Starch Modified, PEG-90 Diisostearate, Dimethiconol, Disteareth-75 IPDI, Glyceryl Stearate, Sodium Acrylate/Sodium Acryloyldimethyl Taurate Copolymer, Microcrystalline Wax, Xanthan Gum, Triethanolamine, Polysorbate 80, Dimethicone Copolyol, Cetyl Alcohol, Isohexadecane, Phenoxyethanol, Disodium EDTA, Ethylene Brassylate, Methylparaben, Propylparaben	**Adults & Peds:** Apply prn.
Vaseline Intensive Rescue Healing Hand Cream	Water, Glycerin, Isopropyl Palmitate, Distearlydimonium Chloride, Cetyl Alcohol, Mineral Oil, Steareth-21, Dimethicone, Petrolatum, Tocopheryl Acetate (Vitamin E Acetate), Borago Officinalis Seed Oil, Tapioca Starch, Stearic Acid, Glycine Soja (Soybean) Sterol, Lecithin, Linoleic Acid, Stearyl Stearate, Sodium Chloride, DMDM Hydantoin, Ethylene Brassylate, Methylparaben, Propylparaben, Titanium Dioxide	**Adults & Peds:** Apply prn.

TABLE 17. HEADACHE/MIGRAINE PRODUCTS

BRAND NAME	INGREDIENT/STRENGTH	DOSE
ACETAMINOPHEN		
Anacin Extra Strength Aspirin Free Tablets	Acetaminophen 500mg	**Adults & Peds ≥12 yrs:** 2 tabs q6h. **Max:** 8 tabs q24h.
Tylenol 8 Hour Caplets	Acetaminophen 650mg	**Adults & Peds ≥12 yrs:** 2 tabs q8h prn. **Max:** 6 tabs q24h.
Tylenol Arthritis Caplets	Acetaminophen 650mg	**Adults:** 2 tabs q8h prn. **Max:** 6 tabs q24h.
Tylenol Arthritis Geltabs	Acetaminophen 650mg	**Adults:** 2 tabs q8h prn. **Max:** 6 tabs q24h.
Tylenol Children's Meltaways Tablets	Acetaminophen 80mg	**Peds 2-3 yrs (24-35 lbs):** 2 tabs. **4-5 (36-47 lbs):** 3 tabs. **6-8 yrs (48-59 lbs):** 4 tabs. **9-10 yrs (60-71 lbs):** 5 tabs. **11 yrs (72-95 lbs):** 6 tabs. **Max:** 5 doses q24h.
Tylenol Children's Suspension	Acetaminophen 160mg/5mL	**Peds 2-3 yrs (24-35 lbs):** 1 tsp (5mL). **4-5 yrs (36-47 lbs):** 1.5 tsp (7.5mL). **6-8 yrs (48-59 lbs):** 2 tsp (10mL). **9-10 yrs (60-71 lbs):** 2.5 tsp (12.5mL). **11 yrs (72-95 lbs):** 3 tsp (15mL). May repeat q4h. **Max:** 5 doses q24h.
Tylenol Extra Strength Caplets	Acetaminophen 500mg	**Adults & Peds ≥12 yrs:** 2 tabs q4-6h prn. **Max:** 8 tabs q24h.
Tylenol Extra Strength Cool Caplets	Acetaminophen 500mg	**Adults & Peds ≥12 yrs:** 2 tabs q4-6h prn. **Max:** 8 tabs q24h.
Tylenol Extra Strength Rapid Release Gelcaps	Acetaminophen 500mg	**Adults & Peds ≥12 yrs:** 2 caps q4-6h prn. **Max:** 8 caps q24h.
Tylenol Extra Strength Rapid Blast Liquid	Acetaminophen 1000mg/30mL	**Adults & Peds ≥12 yrs:** 2 tbl (30mL) q4-6h prn. **Max:** 8 tbl (120mL) q24h.
Tylenol Extra Strength EZ Tabs	Acetaminophen 500mg	**Adults & Peds ≥12 yrs:** 2 tabs q4-6h prn. **Max:** 8 tabs q24h.
Tylenol Infants' Drops	Acetaminophen 80mg/0.8mL	**Peds 2-3 yrs (24-35 lbs):** 1.6 mL q4h prn. **Max:** 5 doses (8mL) q24h.
Tylenol Junior Meltaways Tablets	Acetaminophen 160mg	**Peds 6-8 yrs (48-59 lbs):** 2 tabs. **9-10 yrs (60-71 lbs):** 2.5 tabs. **11 yrs (72-95 lbs):** 3 tabs. **12 yrs (≥96 lbs):** 4 tabs. May repeat q4h. **Max:** 5 doses q24h.
Tylenol Regular Strength Tablets	Acetaminophen 325mg	**Adults & Peds ≥12 yrs:** 2 tabs q4-6h prn. **Max:** 12 tabs q24h. **Peds 6-11 yrs:** 1 tab q4-6h. **Max:** 5 tabs q24h.
ACETAMINOPHEN COMBINATIONS		
Anacin Advanced Headache Tablets	Acetaminophen/Aspirin/Caffeine 250mg-250mg-65mg	**Adults & Peds ≥12 yrs:** 2 tabs q6h. **Max:** 8 tabs q24h.
Excedrin Extra Strength Caplets	Acetaminophen/Aspirin/Caffeine 250mg-250mg-65mg	**Adults & Peds ≥12 yrs:** 2 tabs q6h. **Max:** 8 tabs q24h.
Excedrin Extra Strength Express Gels	Acetaminophen/Aspirin/Caffeine 250mg-250mg-65mg	**Adults & Peds ≥12 yrs:** 2 caps q6h. **Max:** 8 caps q24h.
Excedrin Extra Strength Geltabs	Acetaminophen/Aspirin/Caffeine 250mg-250mg-65mg	**Adults & Peds ≥12 yrs:** 2 tabs q6h. **Max:** 8 tabs q24h.
Excedrin Extra Strength Tablets	Acetaminophen/Aspirin/Caffeine 250mg-250mg-65mg	**Adults & Peds ≥12 yrs:** 2 tabs q6h. **Max:** 8 tabs q24h.
Excedrin Migraine Caplets	Acetaminophen/Aspirin/Caffeine 250mg-250mg-65mg	**Adults:** 2 tabs. **Max:** 2 tabs q24h.
Excedrin Migraine Geltabs	Acetaminophen/Aspirin/Caffeine 250mg-250mg-65mg	**Adults:** 2 tabs. **Max:** 2 tabs q24h.
Excedrin Migraine Tablets	Acetaminophen/Aspirin/Caffeine 250mg-250mg-65mg	**Adults:** 2 tabs. **Max:** 2 tabs q24h.
Excedrin Sinus Headache Caplets	Acetaminophen/Phenylephrine HCl 325mg-5mg	**Adults & Peds ≥12 yrs:** 2 tabs q4h. **Max:** 12 tabs q24h.

(Continued)

TABLE 17. HEADACHE/MIGRAINE PRODUCTS (cont.)

Brand Name	Ingredient/Strength	Dose
Excedrin Tension Headache Caplets	Acetaminophen/Caffeine 500mg-65mg	**Adults & Peds ≥12 yrs:** 2 tabs q6h. **Max:** 8 tabs q24h.
Excedrin Tension Headache Express Gels	Acetaminophen/Caffeine 500mg-65mg	**Adults & Peds ≥12 yrs:** 2 caps q6h. **Max:** 8 caps q24h.
Excedrin Tension Headache Geltabs	Acetaminophen/Caffeine 500mg-65mg	**Adults & Peds ≥12 yrs:** 2 tabs q6h. **Max:** 8 tabs q24h.
Goody's Body Pain Powder	Acetaminophen/Aspirin 325mg-500mg	**Adults & Peds ≥12 yrs:** 1 powder q4-6h. **Max:** 4 powders q24h.
Goody's Cool Orange	Acetaminophen/Aspirin/Caffeine 325mg-500mg-65mg	**Adults & Peds ≥12 yrs:** 1 powder q6h. **Max:** 4 powders q24h.
Goody's Extra Strength Headache Powders	Acetaminophen/Aspirin/Caffeine 260mg-520mg-32.5mg	**Adults & Peds ≥12 yrs:** 1 powder q4-6h. **Max:** 4 powders q24h.
Sudafed PE Sinus Headache	Acetaminophen/Phenylephrine HCl 325mg-5mg	**Adults & Peds ≥12 yrs:** 2 tabs q4h. **Max:** 12 tabs q24h.
Tylenol Sinus Congestion and Pain Daytime Cool Burst Caplet	Acetaminophen/Phenylephrine HCl 325mg-5mg	**Adults & Peds ≥12 yrs:** 2 tabs q4h. **Max:** 12 tabs q24h.
Tylenol Sinus Congestion & Pain Daytime Rapid Release Gelcaps	Acetaminophen/Phenylephrine HCl 325mg-5mg	**Adults & Peds ≥12 yrs:** 2 caps q4h. **Max:** 12 caps q24h.
Vanquish Caplets	Acetaminophen/Aspirin/Caffeine 194mg-227mg-33mg	**Adults & Peds ≥12 yrs:** 2 tabs q6h. **Max:** 8 tabs q24h.
ACETAMINOPHEN/SLEEP AIDS		
Excedrin PM Caplets	Acetaminophen/Diphenhydramine 500mg-38mg	**Adults & Peds ≥12 yrs:** 2 tabs qhs. **Max:** 2 tabs q24h.
Excedrin PM Tablets	Acetaminophen/Diphenhydramine Citrate 500mg-38mg	**Adults & Peds ≥12 yrs:** 2 tabs qhs. **Max:** 2 tabs q24h.
Goody's PM Powder	Acetaminophen/Diphenhydramine 1000mg-76mg/dose	**Adults & Peds ≥12 yrs:** 1 packet (2 powders) qhs.
Tylenol PM Caplets	Acetaminophen/Diphenhydramine 500mg-25mg	**Adults & Peds ≥12 yrs:** 2 tabs qhs. **Max:** 2 tabs q24h.
Tylenol PM Geltabs	Acetaminophen/Diphenhydramine 500mg-25mg	**Adults & Peds ≥12 yrs:** 2 tabs qhs. **Max:** 2 tabs q24h.
Tylenol PM Rapid Release Gels	Acetaminophen/Diphenhydramine 500mg-25mg	**Adults & Peds ≥12 yrs:** 2 caps qhs. **Max:** 2 caps q24h.
Tylenol PM Vanilla Liquid	Acetaminophen/Diphenhydramine 1000mg-50mg/30mL	**Adults & Peds ≥12 yrs:** 2 tbl (30mL) qhs. **Max:** 2 tbl (30mL) q24h.
Tylenol Sinus Congestion and Pain Nighttime	Acetaminophen/Chlorpheniramine/ Phenylephrine HCl 325mg-2mg-5mg	**Adults & Peds ≥12 yrs:** 2 caps q4h. **Max:** 12 caps q24h.
NONSTEROIDAL ANTI-INFLAMMATORY DRUGS (NSAIDs)		
Advil Caplets	Ibuprofen 200mg	**Adults & Peds ≥12 yrs:** 1-2 tabs q4-6h. **Max:** 6 tabs q24h.
Advil Children's Suspension	Ibuprofen 100mg/5mL	**Peds 2-3 yrs (24-35 lbs):** 1 tsp (5mL). **4-5 yrs (36-47 lbs):** 1.5 tsp (7.5mL). **6-8 yrs (48-59 lbs):** 2 tsp (10mL). **9-10 yrs (60-71 lbs):** 2.5 tsp (12.5mL). **11 yrs (72-95 lbs):** 3 tsp (15mL). May repeat q6-8h. **Max:** 4 doses q24h.
Advil Gel Caplets	Ibuprofen 200mg	**Adults & Peds ≥12 yrs:** 1-2 tabs q4-6h. **Max:** 6 tabs q24h.
Advil Infants' Concentrated Drops	Ibuprofen 50mg/1.25mL	**Peds 6-11 months (12-17 lbs):** 1.25mL. **12-23 months (18-23 lbs):** 1.875mL. May repeat q6-8h. **Max:** 4 doses q24h.
Advil Liqui-Gels	Ibuprofen 200mg	**Adults & Peds ≥12 yrs:** 1-2 caps q4-6h. **Max:** 6 caps q24h.

TABLE 17. HEADACHE/MIGRAINE PRODUCTS (cont.)

BRAND NAME	INGREDIENT/STRENGTH	DOSE
Advil Migraine Capsules	Ibuprofen 200mg	**Adults:** 2 caps prn. **Max:** 2 caps q24h.
Advil Tablets	Ibuprofen 200mg	**Adults & Peds ≥12 yrs:** 1-2 tabs q4-6h. **Max:** 6 tabs q24h.
Aleve Caplets	Naproxen Sodium 220mg	**Adults & Peds ≥12 yrs:** 1 tab q8-12h. May take 1 additional tab within 1 hour of first dose. **Max:** 2 tabs q8-12h or 3 tabs q24h.
Aleve Liquid Gels	Naproxen Sodium 220mg	**Adults & Peds ≥12 yrs:** 1 cap q8-12h. May take 1 additional cap within 1 hr of first dose. **Max:** 2 caps q8-12hr or 3 caps q24h.
Aleve Smooth Gels	Naproxen Sodium 220mg	**Adults & Peds ≥12 yrs:** 1 cap q8-12h. May take 1 additional cap within 1 hour of first dose. **Max:** 2 caps q8-12h or 3 caps q24h.
Aleve Tablets	Naproxen Sodium 220mg	**Adults & Peds ≥12 yrs:** 1 tab q8-12h. May take 1 additional tab within 1 hour of first dose. **Max:** 2 tabs q8-12h or 3 tabs q24h.
Motrin Children's Suspension	Ibuprofen 100mg/5mL	**Peds 2-5 yrs (24-47 lbs):** 1 tsp (5mL). **6-11 yrs (48-95 lbs):** 2 tsp (10mL). May repeat q6h. **Max:** 4 doses q24h.
Motrin IB Caplets	Ibuprofen 200mg	**Adults & Peds ≥12 yrs:** 1-2 tabs q4-6h. **Max:** 6 tabs q24h.
Motrin IB Tablets	Ibuprofen 200mg	**Adults & Peds ≥12 yrs:** 1-2 tabs q4-6h. **Max:** 6 tabs q24h.
Motrin Infants' Drops	Ibuprofen 50mg/1.25mL	**Peds 6-11 months (12-17 lbs):** 1.25mL. **12-23 months (18-23 lbs):** 1.875mL. May repeat q6-8h. **Max:** 4 doses q24h.
Motrin Junior Strength Caplets	Ibuprofen 100mg	**Peds 6-8 yrs (48-59 lbs):** 2 tabs. **9-10 yrs (60-71 lbs):** 2.5 tabs. **11 yrs (72-95 lbs):** 3 tabs. May repeat q6-8h. **Max:** 4 doses q24h.
Motrin Junior Strength Chewable Tablets	Ibuprofen 100mg	**Peds 2-3 yrs (24-35 lbs):** 1 tab. **4-5 yrs (36-47 lbs):** 1.5 tabs. **6-8 yrs (48-59 lbs):** 2 tabs. **9-10 yrs (60-71 lbs):** 2.5 tabs. **11 yrs (72-95 lbs):** 3 tabs. May repeat q6-8h. **Max:** 4 doses q24h.
NSAID COMBINATIONS		
Advil Allergy Sinus Caplets	Ibuprofen/Chlorpheniramine/ Pseudoephedrine HCl 200mg-2mg-30mg	**Adults & Peds ≥12 yrs:** 1 tab q4-6h. **Max:** 6 tabs q24h.
Advil Cold & Sinus Caplets	Ibuprofen/Pseudoephedrine HCl 200mg-30mg	**Adults & Peds ≥12 yrs:** 1-2 tabs q4-6h. **Max:** 6 tabs q24h.
Advil Cold & Sinus Liqui-Gels	Ibuprofen/Pseudoephedrine HCl 200mg-30mg	**Adults & Peds ≥12 yrs:** 1-2 caps q4-6h. **Max:** 6 caps q24h.
Aleve-D Sinus & Cold	Naproxen Sodium/Pseudoephedrine HCl 220mg-120mg	**Adults & Peds ≥12 yrs:** 1 tab q12h. **Max:** 2 tabs q24h.
NSAID SLEEP AIDS		
Advil PM Caplets	Ibuprofen/Diphenhydramine Citrate 200mg-38mg	**Adults & Peds ≥12 yrs:** 2 tabs qhs. **Max:** 2 tabs q24hrs.
Advil PM Liqui-Gels	Ibuprofen/Diphenhydramine HCl 200mg-25mg	**Adults & Peds ≥12 yrs:** 2 caps qhs. **Max:** 2 caps q24hrs.
SALICYLATES		
Anacin 81 Tablets	Aspirin 81mg	**Adults & Peds ≥12 yrs:** 2 tabs q6h. **Max:** 8 tabs q24h.
Bayer Aspirin Extra Strength Caplets	Aspirin 500mg	**Adults & Peds ≥12 yrs:** 1-2 tabs q4-6h. **Max:** 8 tabs q24h.

(Continued)

TABLE 17. HEADACHE/MIGRAINE PRODUCTS (cont.)

BRAND NAME	INGREDIENT/STRENGTH	DOSE
Bayer Aspirin Safety Coated Caplets	Aspirin 325mg	**Adults & Peds ≥12 yrs:** 1-2 tabs q4h. **Max:** 12 tabs q24h.
Bayer Genuine Aspirin Tablets	Aspirin 325mg	**Adults & Peds ≥12 yrs:** 1-2 tabs q4h or 3 tabs q6h. **Max:** 12 tabs q24h.
Bayer Low-Dose Aspirin Chewable Tablets	Aspirin 81mg	**Adults & Peds ≥12 yrs:** 4-8 tabs q4h. **Max:** 48 tabs q24h.
Bayer Low-Dose Aspirin Safety Coated Tablets	Aspirin 81mg	**Adults & Peds ≥12 yrs:** 4-8 tabs q4h. **Max:** 48 tabs q24h.
Doan's Extra Strength Caplets	Magnesium Salicylate Tetrahydrate 580mg	**Adults & Peds ≥12 yrs:** 2 tabs q6h. **Max:** 8 tabs q24h.
Ecotrin Low Strength Tablets	Aspirin 81mg	**Adults:** 4-8 tabs q4h. **Max:** 48 tabs q24h.
Ecotrin Regular Strength Tablets	Aspirin 325mg	**Adults & Peds ≥12 yrs:** 1-2 tabs q4h. **Max:** 12 tabs q24h.
Halfprin 162mg Tablets	Aspirin 162mg	**Adults & Peds ≥12 yrs:** 2-4 tabs q4h. **Max:** 24 tabs q24h.
Halfprin 81mg Tablets	Aspirin 81mg	**Adults & Peds ≥12 yrs:** 4-8 tabs q4h. **Max:** 48 tabs q24h.
St. Joseph Aspirin Chewable Tablets	Aspirin 81mg	**Adults & Peds ≥12 yrs:** 4-8 tabs q4h. **Max:** 48 tabs q24h.
St. Joseph Enteric Safety-Coated Tablets	Aspirin 81mg	**Adults & Peds ≥12 yrs:** 4-8 tabs q4h. **Max:** 48 tabs q24h.
SALICYLATES, BUFFERED		
Alka-Seltzer Extra Strength Effervescent Tablets	Aspirin/Citric Acid/Sodium Bicarbonate 500mg-1000mg-1985mg	**Adults & Peds ≥12 yrs:** 2 tabs q6h. **Max:** 7 tabs q24h. **≥60 yrs: Max:** 3 tabs q24h.
Alka-Seltzer Original Effervescent Tablets	Aspirin/Citric Acid/Sodium Bicarbonate 325mg-1000mg-1916mg	**Adults & Peds ≥12 yrs:** 2 tabs q4h. **Max:** 8 tabs q24h. **≥60 yrs: Max:** 4 tabs q24h.
Ascriptin Maximum Strength Tablets	Aspirin Buffered with Maalox/Calcium Carbonate 500mg	**Adults & Peds ≥12 yrs:** 2 tabs q4h. **Max:** 8 tabs q24h.
Ascriptin Regular Strength Tablets	Aspirin 325mg Buffered with Maalox/Calcium Carbonate	**Adults & Peds ≥12 yrs:** 2 tabs q4h. **Max:** 12 tabs q24h.
Bayer Extra Strength Plus Caplets	Aspirin 500mg Buffered with Calcium Carbonate	**Adults & Peds ≥12 yrs:** 1-2 tabs q4-6h. **Max:** 8 tabs q24h.
Bayer Women's Low Dose Aspirin Caplets	Aspirin 81mg Buffered with Calcium Carbonate 777mg	**Adults & Peds ≥12 yrs:** 4-8 tabs q4h. **Max:** 10 tabs q24h.
Bufferin Extra Strength Tablets	Aspirin 500mg Buffered with Calcium Carbonate/Magnesium Oxide/Magnesium Carbonate	**Adults & Peds ≥12 yrs:** 2 tabs q6h. **Max:** 8 tabs q24h.
Bufferin Tablets	Aspirin 325mg Buffered with Benzoic Acid/Citric Acid	**Adults & Peds ≥12 yrs:** 2 tabs q4h. **Max:** 12 tabs q24h.
SALICYLATE COMBINATIONS		
Alka-Seltzer Wake-Up Call!	Aspirin/Caffeine 500mg-65mg	**Adults & Peds ≥12 yrs:** 2 tabs q6h. **Max:** 8 tabs q24h. **≥60 yrs: Max:** 4 tabs q24h.
Anacin Max Strength Tablets	Aspirin/Caffeine 500mg-32mg	**Adults & Peds ≥12 yrs:** 2 tabs q6h. **Max:** 8 tabs q24h.
Anacin Tablets	Aspirin/Caffeine 400mg-32mg	**Adults & Peds ≥12 yrs:** 2 tabs q6h. **Max:** 8 tabs q24h.
Bayer Back & Body Pain Caplets	Aspirin/Caffeine 500mg-32.5mg	**Adults & Peds ≥12 yrs:** 2 tabs q6h. **Max:** 8 tabs q24h.
BC Arthritis Strength Powders	Aspirin/Caffeine/Salicylamide 742mg-38mg-222mg	**Adults & Peds ≥12 yrs:** 1 powder q3-4h. **Max:** 4 powders q24h.
BC Original Formula Powders	Aspirin/Caffeine/Salicylamide 650mg-33.3mg-195mg	**Adults & Peds ≥12 yrs:** 1 powder q3-4h. **Max:** 4 powders q24h.

TABLE 17. HEADACHE/MIGRAINE PRODUCTS (cont.)

Brand Name	Ingredient/Strength	Dose
SALICYLATES/SLEEP AIDS		
Alka-Seltzer PM	Aspirin/Diphenhydramine Citrate 325mg-38mg	**Adults & Peds ≥12 yrs:** 2 tabs qhs. **Max:** 2 tabs q24h.
Bayer PM Caplets	Aspirin/Diphenhydramine 500mg-38.3mg	**Adults & Peds ≥12 yrs:** 2 tabs qhs.
Doan's Extra Strength PM Caplets	Magnesium Salicylate Tetrahydrate/Diphenhydramine 580mg-25mg	**Adults & Peds ≥12 yrs:** 2 tabs qhs.

TABLE 18. HEMORRHOIDAL PRODUCTS

BRAND NAME	INGREDIENT/STRENGTH	DOSE
ANESTHETICS/ANESTHETIC COMBINATIONS		
Tucks Hemorrhoidal Ointment	Pramoxine HCl/Zinc Oxide/Mineral Oil 1%-12.5%-46.6%	**Adults ≥12 yrs:** Apply to affected area prn. **Max:** 5 times q24h.
Nupercainal Ointment	Dibucaine 1%	**Adults & Peds ≥12 yrs:** Apply to affected area tid-qid.
Preparation H Hemorrhoidal Cream, Maximum Strength Pain Relief	Glycerin/Phenylephrine HCl/ Pramoxine HCl/White Petrolatum 14.4%-0.25%-1%-15%	**Adults ≥12 yrs:** Apply to affected area prn. **Max:** 4 times q24h.
Tronolane Anesthetic Hemorrhoid Cream	Pramoxine HCl/Zinc Oxide 1%-5%	**Adults:** Apply to affected area prn. **Max:** 5 times q24h.
BULK-FORMING LAXATIVES		
Citrucel Caplets	Methylcellulose 500mg	**Adults ≥12 yrs:** 2 tabs qd prn. **Max:** 12 tabs q24h. **Peds 6-12 yrs:** 1 tab qd prn. **Max:** 6 tabs q24h.
Citrucel Powder	Methylcellulose 2g/tbl	**Adults ≥12 yrs:** 1 tbl (11.5g) qd-tid. **Peds 6-12 yrs:** ½ tbl (5.75g) qd.
Equalactin Chewable Tablet	Calcium Polycarbophil 625mg	**Adults & Peds ≥12 yrs:** 2 tabs qd. **Max:** 8 tabs qd. **Peds 6-12 yrs:** 1 tab qd. **Max:** 4 tabs qd. **Peds 2 to <6 yrs:** 1 tab qd. **Max:** 2 tabs qd.
Fibercon Caplets	Calcium Polycarbophil 625mg	**Adults & Peds ≥12 yrs:** 2 tabs qd. **Max:** 8 tabs qd. **Peds 6-<12 yrs:** 1 tab qd. **Max:** 4 tabs qd.
Konsyl Easy Mix Powder	Psyllium 4.3g/tsp	**Adults ≥12 yrs:** 1 tsp qd-qid. **Peds 6-12 yrs:** ½ tsp qd-tid.
Konsyl Fiber Caplets	Calcium Polycarbophil 625mg	**Adults ≥12 yrs:** 2 tabs qd-qid. **Max:** 8 tabs q24h. **Peds 6-12 yrs:** 1 tab qd-tid. **Max:** 3 tabs q24h.
Konsyl Orange Powder	Psyllium 3.4g/tbl	**Adults & Peds ≥12 yrs:** 1 tbl qd-tid. **Peds 6-12 yrs:** ½ tbl qd-tid.
Konsyl Original Powder	Psyllium 6g/tsp	**Adults ≥12 yrs:** 1 tsp qd-tid. **Peds 6-12 yrs:** ½ tsp qd-tid.
Konsyl-D Powder	Psyllium 3.4g/tsp	**Adults ≥12 yrs:** 1 tsp qd-tid. **Peds 6-12 yrs:** ½ tsp qd-tid.
Metamucil Capsules	Psyllium 0.52g	**Adults & Peds ≥12 yrs:** 5 caps qd-tid.
Metamucil Original Texture Powder	Psyllium 3.4g/tbl	**Adults & Peds ≥12 yrs:** 1 tbl up to tid. **Peds 6-11 yrs:** ½ tbl up to tid.
Metamucil Smooth Texture Powder (Orange)	Psyllium 3.4g/tbl	**Adults & Peds ≥12 yrs:** 1 tbl up to tid. **Peds 6-11 yrs:** ½ tbl up to tid.
Metamucil Wafers	Psyllium 3.4g/dose	**Adults ≥12 yrs:** 2 wafers qd-tid. **Peds 6-12 yrs:** 1 wafer qd-tid.
HYDROCORTISONE		
Tucks Anti-Itch Ointment	Hydrocortisone Acetate 1.12%	**Adults & Peds ≥12 yrs:** Apply to affected area ud. **Max:** Apply to affected area tid-qid q24h.
Preparation H Anti-Itch Cream	Hydrocortisone 1.0%	**Adults & Peds ≥12 yrs:** Apply to affected area tid-qid.
STOOL SOFTENER		
Colace Capsules	Docusate Sodium 100mg	**Adults ≥12 yrs:** 1-3 caps qd. **Peds 2-12 yrs:** 1 cap qd.
Colace Capsules	Docusate Sodium 50mg	**Adults ≥12 yrs:** 1-6 caps qd. **Peds 2-12 yrs:** 1-3 caps qd.
Colace Liquid	Docusate Sodium 10mg/mL	**Adults ≥12 yrs:** 5-15mL qd-bid. **Peds 2-12 yrs:** 5-15mL qd.
Colace Syrup	Docusate Sodium 60mg/15mL	**Adults ≥12 yrs:** 1-6 tbl qd. **Peds 2-12 yrs:** 1-2.5 tbl qd.

(Continued)

TABLE 18. HEMORRHOIDAL PRODUCTS (cont.)

Brand Name	Ingredient/Strength	Dose
Docusol Constipation Relief, Mini Enemas	Docusate Sodium 283mg	**Adults ≥12 yrs:** Take 1-3 units qd. **Peds 6-12 yrs:** Take 1 unit qd.
Dulcolax Stool Softener Capsules	Docusate Sodium 100mg	**Adults ≥12 yrs:** 1-3 caps qd. **Peds 2-12 yrs:** 1 cap qd.
Fleet Pedia-Lax Liquid Stool Softener	Docusate 50mg/tbl	**Peds 2-12 yrs:** 1-3 tbl qd. **Max:** 3 tbl.
Fleet Sof-Lax	Docusate 100mg	**Adults & Peds ≥12 yrs:** 1-3 softgels qd. **Peds 2-12 yrs:** 1 softgel qd.
Kaopectate Liqui-Gels	Docusate Calcium 240mg	**Adults & Peds ≥12 yrs:** 1 cap qd until normal bowel movement.
Phillips Stool Softener Capsules	Docusate Sodium 100mg	**Adults ≥12 yrs:** 1-3 caps qd. **Peds 6-12 yrs:** 1 cap qd.
WITCH HAZEL/WITCH HAZEL COMBINATIONS		
Hemspray Hemorrhoid Relief Spray	Witch Hazel/Glycerin/ Phenylephrine HCl/Camphor 50%-20%-0.25%-0.15%	**Adults & Peds ≥12 yrs:** Apply to affected area prn. **Max:** 5 times q24h.
Preparation H Hemorrhoidal Cooling Gel	Phenylephrine HCl/Witch Hazel 0.25%-50.0%	**Adults ≥12 yrs:** Apply to affected area prn. **Max:** 4 times q24h.
Preparation H Medicated Wipes	Witch Hazel 50%	**Adults & Peds ≥12 yrs:** Apply to affected area prn. **Max:** 6 times q24h.
T.N. Dickinson's Witch Hazel Hemorrhoidal Pads	Witch Hazel 50%	**Adults & Peds ≥12 yrs:** Apply to affected area prn. **Max:** 6 times q24h.
Tucks Medicated Pads	Witch Hazel 50%	**Adults & Peds ≥12 yrs:** Apply to affected area prn. **Max:** 6 times q24h.
Tucks Take Alongs Medicated Towelettes	Witch Hazel 50%	**Adults & Peds ≥12 yrs:** Apply to affected area prn. **Max:** 6 times q24h.
MISCELLANEOUS		
Preparation H Hemorrhoidal Ointment	Mineral Oil/Petrolatum/ Phenylephrine HCl/Shark Liver Oil 14%-71.9%-0.25%-3.0%	**Adults ≥12 yrs:** Apply to affected area prn. **Max:** 4 times q24h.
Preparation H Hemorrhoidal Suppositories	Cocoa Butter/Phenylephrine HCl/ Shark Liver Oil 85.5%-0.25%-3.0%	**Adults & Peds ≥12 yrs:** Insert 1 supp prn. **Max:** 4 times q24h.
Tronolane Suppositories	Hard Fat/Phenylephrine HCl 88.7%-0.25%	**Adults & Peds ≥12 yrs:** Insert 1 supp prn. **Max:** 4 times q24h.
Tucks Topical Starch Hemorrhoidal Suppositories	Topical Starch 51%	**Adults & Peds ≥12 yrs:** Insert 1 supp prn. **Max:** 6 times q24h.

TABLE 19. INSOMNIA PRODUCTS

BRAND NAME	INGREDIENT/STRENGTH	DOSE
DIPHENHYDRAMINE		
Nytol Quick Caps Caplets	Diphenhydramine 25mg	**Adults & Peds** ≥**12 yrs:** 2 tabs qhs.
Nytol Quick Gels Capsules	Diphenhydramine 50mg	**Adults & Peds** ≥**12 yrs:** 1 cap qhs.
Simply Sleep Nighttime Sleep Aid Caplets	Diphenhydramine 25mg	**Adults & Peds** ≥**12 yrs:** 2 tabs qhs.
Sominex Original Formula	Diphenhydramine 25mg	**Adults & Peds** ≥**12 yrs:** 2 tabs qhs.
Sominex Maximum Strength Formula	Diphenhydramine 50mg	**Adults & Peds** ≥**12 yrs:** 1 tab qhs.
Unisom Nighttime Sleep-Aid Sleep Gels	Diphenhydramine 50mg	**Adults & Peds** ≥**12 yrs:** 1 cap qhs.
Unisom Sleepmelt	Diphenhydramine 25mg	**Adults & Peds** ≥**12 yrs:** 2 tabs qhs.
DIPHENHYDRAMINE COMBINATION		
Alka-Seltzer PM	Aspirin/Diphenhydramine Citrate 325mg-38mg	**Adults & Peds** ≥**12 yrs:** 2 tabs qhs.
Bayer PM Relief Caplets	Aspirin/Diphenhydramine Citrate 500mg-38.3mg	**Adults & Peds** ≥**12 yrs:** 2 tabs qhs.
Doan's Extra Strength PM Caplets	Magnesium Salicylate Tetrahydrate/ Diphenhydramine 580mg-25mg	**Adults & Peds** ≥**12 yrs:** 2 tabs qhs.
Excedrin PM Caplets	Acetaminophen/Diphenhydramine Citrate 500mg-38mg	**Adults & Peds** ≥**12 yrs:** 2 tabs qhs.
Excedrin PM Tablets	Acetaminophen/Diphenhydramine Citrate 500mg-38mg	**Adults & Peds** ≥**12 yrs:** 2 tabs qhs.
Goody's PM Powders	Acetaminophen/Diphenhydramine Citrate 1000mg-76mg/dose	**Adults & Peds** ≥**12 yrs:** 1 packet (2 powders) qhs.
Tylenol PM Caplets	Acetaminophen/Diphenhydramine HCl 500mg-25mg	**Adults & Peds** ≥**12 yrs:** 2 tabs qhs.
Tylenol PM Rapid Release Gelcaps	Acetaminophen/Diphenhydramine HCl 500mg-25mg	**Adults & Peds** ≥**12 yrs:** 2 caps qhs.
Tylenol PM Geltabs	Acetaminophen/Diphenhydramine HCl 500mg-25mg	**Adults & Peds** ≥**12 yrs:** 2 tabs qhs.
Tylenol PM Liquid	Acetaminophen/Diphenhydramine HCl 1000mg-50mg/30mL	**Adults & Peds** ≥**12 yrs:** 2 tbl (30mL) qhs. **Max:** 2 tbl (30mL) q24h.
DOXYLAMINE		
Unisom Nighttime Sleep-Aid Sleep Tabs	Doxylamine Succinate 25mg	**Adults & Peds** ≥**12 yrs:** 1 tab 30 min before hs.

TABLE 20. IS IT A COLD, THE FLU, OR AN ALLERGY?

	COLD	FLU	AIRBORNE ALLERGY
SYMPTOMS			
Chest discomfort	Mild to moderate	Common; can become severe	Sometimes
Cough	Common (hacking cough)	Sometimes	Sometimes
Duration	3-14 days	Days to weeks	Weeks (eg, 6 weeks for ragweed or grass pollen seasons)
Extreme exhaustion	Never	Early and prominent	Never
Fatigue, weakness	Sometimes	Can last up to 2-3 weeks	Sometimes
Fever	Rare	Characteristic, high (100-102°F); lasts 3-4 days	Never
General aches, pains	Slight	Usual; often severe	Never
Headache	Rare	Common	Sometimes
Itchy eyes	Rare or never	Rare or never	Common
Runny nose	Common		Common
Sneezing	Usual	Sometimes	Usual
Sore throat	Common	Sometimes	Sometimes
Stuffy nose	Common	Sometimes	Common
TREATMENT*			
	Antihistamines	Amantadine	Antihistamines
	Decongestants	Rimantadine	Nasal steroids
	Nonsteroidal anti-inflammatories	Oseltamivir	Decongestants
		Zanamivir	
PREVENTION			
	Wash your hands often; avoid close contact with anyone with a cold	Annual vaccination Amantadine Rimantadine Oseltamivir	Avoid allergens such as pollen, house flies, dust mites, mold, pet dander, cockroaches
COMPLICATIONS			
	Sinus infection	Bronchitis	Sinus infections
	Middle ear infection	Pneumonia	Asthma
	Asthma	Can be life-threatening	

Adapted from the National Institute of Allergy and Infectious Diseases, November 2008.

*Used only for temporary relief of cold symptoms.

TABLE 21. LAXATIVE PRODUCTS

Brand Name	Ingredient/Strength	Dose
BULK-FORMING		
Citrucel Caplets	Methylcellulose 500mg	**Adults & Peds ≥12 yrs:** 2 tabs qd prn. **Max:** 12 tabs q24h. **Peds 6-<12yrs:** 1 tab qd prn. **Max:** 6 tabs q24h.
Citrucel Powder	Methylcellulose 2g/tbl	**Adults & Peds ≥12 yrs:** 1 tbl (11.5g) qd-tid. **Peds 6-<12 yrs:** ½ tbl (5.75g) qd.
Equalactin Chewable Tablet	Calcium Polycarbophil 625mg	**Adults & Peds ≥12 yrs:** 2 tabs qd. **Max:** 8 tabs q24h. **Peds 6-11 yrs:** 1 tab qd. **Max:** 4 tabs q24h. **Peds 2-5 yrs:** 1 tab qd. **Max:** 2 tabs q24h.
Fibercon Caplets	Calcium Polycarbophil 625mg	**Adults & Peds ≥12 yrs:** 2 tabs qd. **Max:** 8 tabs qd.
Konsyl Easy Mix Powder	Psyllium 4.3g/tsp	**Adults & Peds ≥12 yrs:** 1 tsp qd-tid. **Peds 6-<12 yrs:** ½ tsp qd-tid.
Konsyl Fiber Caplets	Calcium Polycarbophil 625mg	**Adults:** 2 tabs qd-qid. **Max:** 8 tabs q24h. **Peds 6-12 yrs:** 1 tab qd-tid. **Max:** 3 tabs q24h.
Konsyl Orange Powder	Psyllium 3.4g/tbl	**Adults & Peds ≥12 yrs:** 1 tbl qd-tid. **Peds 7-11 yrs:** ½ tbl qd-tid.
Konsyl Original Powder	Psyllium 6g/tsp	**Adults & Peds ≥12 yrs:** 1 tsp qd-tid. **Peds 7-11 yrs:** ½ tsp qd-tid.
Konsyl-D Powder	Psyllium 3.4g/tsp	**Adults & Peds ≥12 yrs:** 1 tsp qd-tid. **Peds 7-11 yrs:** ½ tsp qd-tid.
Metamucil Capsules	Psyllium 0.52g	**Adults & Peds ≥12 yrs:** 5 caps qd-tid.
Metamucil Original Texture Powder (orange)	Psyllium 3.4g/tbl	**Adults & Peds ≥12 yrs:** 1 tbl up to tid. **Peds 6-11 yrs:** ½ tbl up to tid.
Metamucil Smooth Texture Powder (orange)	Psyllium 3.4g/tbl	**Adults & Peds ≥12 yrs:** 1 tbl up to tid. **Peds 6-11 yrs:** ½ tbl up to tid.
Metamucil Wafers	Psyllium 3.4g/dose	**Adults & Peds ≥12 yrs:** 2 wafers qd-tid. **Peds 6-11 yrs:** 1 wafer qd-tid.
HYPEROSMOTICS		
Colace Glycerin Suppositories for Adults and Children	Glycerin 2.1g	**Adults & Peds ≥6 yrs:** 1 supp. **Max:** 1 supp q24h.
Colace Glycerin Suppositories for Infants and Children	Glycerin 1.2g	**Peds 2-5 yrs:** 1 supp. **Max:** 1 supp q24h.
Fleet Mineral Oil Enema	Mineral Oil 118mL	**Adults & Peds ≥12 yrs:** 1 bottle (118mL). **Peds 2-<12 yrs:** ½ bottle (59mL).
Fleet Pedia-Lax Glycerin Suppositories	Glycerin 1g	**Peds 2-6 yrs:** 1 supp. ud.
Fleet Pedia-Lax Liquid Glycerin Suppositories	Glycerin 2.3g	**Peds 2-6 yrs:** 1 supp. ud.
SALINES		
Fleet Enema	Monobasic Sodium Phosphate/Dibasic Sodium Phosphate 19g-7g/118mL	**Adults & Peds ≥12 yrs:** 1 bottle (118mL).
Fleet Enema Extra	Monobasic Sodium Phosphate/Dibasic Sodium Phosphate 19g-7g/197mL	**Adults & Peds ≥12 yrs:** 1 bottle (197mL).
Fleet Pedia-Lax Chewable Tablets	Magnesium Hydroxide 400mg	**Peds 6-<12 yrs:** 3-6 tabs qd. **Max:** 6 tabs q24h. **Peds 2-<6 yrs:** 1-3 tabs qd. **Max:** 3 tabs q24h.
Fleet Pedia-Lax Enema	Monobasic Sodium Phosphate/Dibasic Sodium Phosphate 9.5g-3.5g/59mL	**Peds 5-11 yrs:** 1 bottle (59mL). **Peds 2-<5 yrs:** ½ bottle (29.5mL).

(Continued)

TABLE 21. LAXATIVE PRODUCTS (cont.)

BRAND NAME	INGREDIENT/STRENGTH	DOSE
Magnesium Citrate Solution	Magnesium Citrate 1.75g/30mL	**Adults & Peds ≥12 yrs:** 300mL. **Peds 6-<12 yrs:** 90-210mL. **Peds 2-<6 yrs:** 60mL.
Phillips Antacid/Laxative Chewable Tablets	Magnesium Hydroxide 311mg	**Adults & Peds ≥12 yrs:** 8 tabs qd. **Peds 6-11 yrs:** 4 tabs qd. **Peds 3-5 yrs:** 2 tabs qd.
Phillips Cramp-Free Laxative Caplets	Magnesium 500mg	**Adults & Peds ≥12 yrs:** Take 2-4 tabs qd. **Max:** 4 tabs q24h.
Phillips Milk of Magnesia Concentrated Liquid	Magnesium Hydroxide 800mg/5mL	**Adults & Peds ≥12 yrs:** 1-2 tbl qd. **Peds 6-11 yrs:** ½-1 tbl qd.
Phillips Milk of Magnesia Liquid	Magnesium Hydroxide 400mg/5mL	**Adults & Peds ≥12 yrs:** 2-4 tbl qd. **Peds 6-11 yrs:** 1-2 tbl qd.
SALINE COMBINATION		
Phillips M-O Liquid	Magnesium Hydroxide/Mineral Oil 300mg-1.25mL/5mL	**Adults & Peds ≥12 yrs:** 3-4 tbl qd. **Peds 6-11 yrs:** 4-6 tsp qd.
STIMULANTS		
Alophen Enteric Coated Stimulant Laxative Pills	Bisacodyl 5mg	**Adults & Peds ≥12 yrs:** Take 1-3 tabs qd. **Peds 6-12 yrs:** Take 1 tab qd.
Carter's Laxative, Sodium Free Pills	Bisacodyl 5mg	**Adults & Peds ≥12 yrs:** Take 1-3 tabs (usually 2 tabs) qd. **Peds 6-<12 yrs:** Take 1 tab qd.
Castor Oil	Castor Oil	**Adults & Peds ≥12 yrs:** 15-60mL. **Peds 2-<12 yrs:** 5-15mL.
Doxidan Tablets	Bisacodyl 5mg	**Adults & Peds ≥12 yrs:** 1-3 tabs (usually 2) qd. **Peds 6-12 yrs:** 1 tab qd.
Dulcolax Suppository	Bisacodyl 10mg	**Adults & Peds ≥12 yrs:** 1 supp qd. **Peds 6-12 yrs:** ½ supp qd.
Dulcolax Tablets	Bisacodyl 5mg	**Adults & Peds ≥12 yrs:** 1-3 tabs (usually 2) qd. **Peds 6-<12 yrs:** 1 tab qd.
Ex-Lax Maximum Strength Tablets	Sennosides 25mg	**Adults & Peds ≥12 yrs:** 2 tabs qd-bid. **Peds 6-<12 yrs:** 1 tab qd-bid.
Ex-Lax Tablets	Sennosides 15mg	**Adults & Peds ≥12 yrs:** 2 tabs qd-bid. **Peds 6-<12 yrs:** 1 tab qd-bid.
Ex-Lax Ultra Stimulant Laxative Tablets	Bisacodyl 5mg	**Adults & Peds ≥12 yrs:** 1-3 tabs qd. **Peds 6-<12 yrs:** 1 tab qd-bid.
Fleet Bisacodyl Enema	Bisacodyl 10mg/30mL	**Adults & Peds ≥12 yrs:** 1 bottle (30mL).
Fleet Bisacodyl Suppositories	Bisacodyl 10mg	**Adults & Peds ≥12 yrs:** 1 supp qd. **Peds 6-<12 yrs:** ½ supp qd.
Fleet Pedia-Lax Quick Dissolve Strips	Sennosides 8.6mg	**Peds 6-<12 yrs:** 2 strips. **Max:** 4 strips q24h. **Peds 2-<6 yrs:** 1 strip. **Max:** 2 strips q24h.
Fleet Stimulant Laxative Tablets	Bisacodyl 5mg	**Adults & Peds ≥12 yrs:** 1-3 tabs (usually 2) qd. **Peds 6-<12 yrs:** 1 tab qd.
Perdiem Overnight Relief Tablets	Sennosides 15mg	**Adults & Peds ≥12 yrs:** 2 tabs qd-bid. **Peds 6-<12 yrs:** 1 tab qd-bid.
Senokot Tablets	Sennosides 8.6mg	**Adults & Peds ≥12 yrs:** 2 tabs qd. **Max:** 4 tabs bid. **Peds 6-<12 yrs:** 1 tab qd. **Max:** 2 tabs bid. **Peds 2-<6 yrs:** ½ tab qd. **Max:** 1 tab bid.
SenokotXTRA Tablets	Sennosides 17.2mg	**Adults & Peds ≥6 yrs:** Starting dose 1 tab qd. **Max:** 2 tabs bid. **Peds 2-<6 yrs:** ½ tab qd. **Max:** 1 tab bid.

TABLE 21. LAXATIVE PRODUCTS (cont.)

BRAND NAME	INGREDIENT/STRENGTH	DOSE
STIMULANT COMBINATIONS		
Konsyl Senna Prompt	Psyllium/Sennosides 500mg-9mg	**Adults & Peds ≥12 yrs:** 1-5 caps qd-bid.
Peri-Colace Tablets	Sennosides/Docusate 8.6mg-50mg	**Adults & Peds ≥12 yrs:** 2-4 tabs qd. **Peds 6-<12 yrs:** 1-2 tabs qd. **Peds 2-5 yrs:** 1 tab qd.
Senokot S Tablets	Sennosides/Docusate 8.6mg-50mg	**Adults ≥12 yrs:** 2 tabs qd. **Max:** 4 tabs bid. **Peds 6-<12 yrs:** 1 tab qd. **Max:** 2 tabs bid. **Peds 2-<6 yrs:** ½ tab qd. **Max:** 1 tab bid.
SURFACTANTS (STOOL SOFTENERS)		
Colace Capsules	Docusate Sodium 100mg	**Adults & Peds ≥12 yrs:** 1-3 caps qd. **Peds 2-<12 yrs:** 1 cap qd.
Colace Capsules	Docusate Sodium 50mg	**Adults & Peds ≥12 yrs:** 1-6 caps qd. **Peds 2-<12 yrs:** 1-3 caps qd.
Colace Liquid	Docusate Sodium 10mg/mL	**Adults & Peds ≥12 yrs:** 5-15mL qd-bid. **Peds 2-<12 yrs:** 5-15mL qd.
Colace Syrup	Docusate Sodium 60mg/15mL	**Adults & Peds ≥12 yrs:** 1-6 tbl qd. **Peds 2-<12 yrs:** 1-2½ tbl qd.
Docusol Constipation Relief, Mini Enemas	Docusate Sodium 283mg	**Adults & Peds ≥12 yrs:** Take 1-3 units qd. **Peds 6-12 yrs:** Take 1 unit qd.
Dulcolax Stool Softener Capsules	Docusate Sodium 100mg	**Adults & Peds ≥12 yrs:** 1-3 caps qd. **Peds 2-<12 yrs:** 1 cap qd.
Fleet Pedia-Lax Liquid Stool Softener	Docusate 50mg/tbl	**Peds 2-12 yrs:** 1-3 tbl qd. **Max:** 3 tbl.
Fleet Sof-Lax	Docusate 100mg	**Adults & Peds ≥12 yrs:** 1-3 softgels qd. **Peds 2-<12 yrs:** 1 softgel qd.
Kaopectate Liqui-Gels	Docusate Calcium 240mg	**Adults & Peds ≥12 yrs:** 1 cap qd until normal bowel movement.
Phillips Stool Softener Capsules	Docusate Sodium 100mg	**Adults & Peds ≥12 yrs:** 1-3 caps qd. **Peds 6-<12 yrs:** 1 cap qd.

TABLE 22. NASAL DECONGESTANT/MOISTURIZING PRODUCTS

Brand Name	Ingredient/Strength	Dose
PSEUDOEPHEDRINE		
Sudafed 12 Hour Tablets	Pseudoephedrine HCl 120mg	**Adults & Peds ≥12 yrs:** 1 tab q12h. **Max:** 2 tabs/day.
Sudafed 24 Hour Tablets	Pseudoephedrine HCl 240mg	**Adults & Peds ≥12 yrs:** 1 tab q24h. **Max:** 1 tab/day.
Sudafed Children's Nasal Decongestant Liquid	Pseudoephedrine HCl 15mg/5mL	**Peds 6-11 yrs:** 2 tsp q4-6h. **Peds 4-5 yrs:** 1 tsp q4-6h. **Max:** 4 doses q24h.
Sudafed Nasal Decongestant Tablets	Pseudoephedrine HCl 30mg	**Adults ≥12 yrs:** 2 tabs q4-6h. **Max:** 8 tabs/day. **Peds 6-12 yrs:** 1 tab q4-6h. **Max:** 4 tabs/day.
PHENYLEPHRINE		
Pediacare Children's Decongestant Liquid	Phenylephrine 2.5/5mL	**Peds 6-11 yrs:** 2 tsp q4h. **Peds 4-5 yrs:** 1 tsp q4h. **Max:** 6 doses q24h.
Sudafed PE	Phenylephrine 10mg	**Adults & Peds ≥12 yrs:** 1 tab q4h. **Max:** 6 tabs/day.
TOPICAL NASAL DECONGESTANTS		
4-Way Fast Acting Nasal Decongestant Spray	Phenylephrine HCl 1%	**Adults & Peds ≥12 yrs:** Instill 2-3 sprays per nostril q4h.
4-Way Mentholated Nasal Decongestant Spray	Phenylephrine HCl 1%	**Adults & Peds ≥12 yrs:** Instill 2-3 sprays per nostril q4h.
Afrin No Drip Extra Moisturizing Nasal Spray	Oxymetazoline HCl 0.05%	**Adults & Peds ≥6 yrs:** Instill 2-3 sprays per nostril q10-12h. **Max:** 2 doses q24h.
Afrin No Drip Sinus Nasal Spray	Oxymetazoline HCl 0.05%	**Adults & Peds ≥6 yrs:** Instill 2-3 sprays per nostril q10-12h. **Max:** 2 doses q24h.
Afrin No-Drip Original Pump Mist Nasal Spray	Oxymetazoline HCl 0.05%	**Adults & Peds ≥6 yrs:** Instill 2-3 sprays per nostril q10-12h. **Max:** 2 doses q24h.
Afrin No Drip Severe Congestion Nasal Spray	Oxymetazoline HCl 0.05%	**Adults & Peds ≥6 yrs:** Instill 2-3 sprays per nostril q10-12h. **Max:** 2 doses q24h.
Afrin No Drip All Night 12 Hour Pump Mist	Oxymetazoline HCl 0.05%	**Adults & Peds ≥6 yrs:** Instill 2-3 sprays per nostril q10-12h. **Max:** 2 doses q24h.
Benzedrex Inhaler	Propylhexedrine 250mg	**Adults & Peds ≥6 yrs:** Inhale 2 sprays per nostril q2h.
Dristan 12 Hour Nasal Spray	Oxymetazoline HCl 0.05%	**Adults & Peds ≥12 yrs:** Instill 2-3 sprays per nostril q10-12h. **Max:** 2 doses q24h.
Mucinex Full Force Nasal Spray	Oxymetazoline HCl 0.05%	**Adults & Peds ≥6 yrs:** Instill 2-3 sprays per nostril q10-12h. **Max:** 2 doses q24h.
Neo-Synephrine Nighttime Nasal Spray	Oxymetazoline HCl 0.05%	**Adults & Peds ≥6 yrs:** Instill 2-3 sprays per nostril q10-12h. **Max:** 2 doses q24h.
Neo-Synephrine Extra Strength Nasal Spray	Phenylephrine HCl 1%	**Adults & Peds ≥12 yrs:** Instill 2-3 sprays per nostril q4h.
Neo-Synephrine Mild Formula Nasal Spray	Phenylephrine HCl 0.25%	**Adults & Peds ≥6 yrs:** Instill 2-3 sprays per nostril q4h.
Neo-Synephrine Regular Strength Nasal Decongestant Spray	Phenylephrine HCl 0.5%	**Adults & Peds ≥12 yrs:** Instill 2-3 sprays per nostril q4h.
Nostrilla Complete Congestion Relief	Oxymetazoline HCl 0.05%	**Adults & Peds ≥6 yrs:** Instill 2-3 sprays per nostril q10-12h. **Max:** 2 doses q24h.
Nostrilla Original Fast Relief	Oxymetazoline HCl 0.05%	**Adults & Peds ≥6 yrs:** Instill 2-3 sprays per nostril q10-12h. **Max:** 2 doses q24h.
Sudafed Sinus Congestion 12 Hour Nasal Spray	Oxymetazoline HCl 0.05%	**Adults & Peds ≥6 yrs:** Spray 2-3 sprays per nostril q10-12h. **Max:** 2 doses q24h.
Sudafed Sinus Cold 12 Hour Nasal Spray	Oxymetazoline HCl 0.05%	**Adults & Peds ≥6 yrs:** Spray 2-3 sprays per nostril q10-12h. **Max:** 2 doses q24h.
Vicks Sinex 12 Hour Ultra Fine Mist For Sinus Relief	Oxymetazoline HCl 0.05%	**Adults & Peds ≥6 yrs:** Spray 2-3 sprays per nostril q10-12h. **Max:** 2 doses q24h.

(Continued)

TABLE 22. NASAL DECONGESTANT/MOISTURIZING PRODUCTS (cont.)

BRAND NAME	INGREDIENT/STRENGTH	DOSE
Vicks Sinex 12 Hour Nasal Spray	Oxymetazoline HCl 0.05%	**Adults & Peds ≥6 yrs:** Instill 2-3 sprays per nostril q10-12h. **Max:** 2 doses q24h.
Vicks Sinex Nasal Spray For Sinus Relief	Phenylephrine HCl 0.5%	**Adults & Peds ≥12 yrs:** Instill 2-3 sprays per nostril q4h.
Zicam Extreme Congestion Relief	Oxymetazoline HCl 0.05%	**Adults & Peds ≥6 yrs:** Instill 2-3 sprays per nostril q10-12h. **Max:** 2 doses q24h.
Zicam Intense Sinus Relief	Oxymetazoline HCl 0.05%	**Adults & Peds ≥6 yrs:** Instill 2-3 sprays per nostril q10-12h. **Max:** 2 doses q24h.
TOPICAL NASAL MOISTURIZERS		
4-Way Saline Moisturizing Mist	Water, Boric Acid, Glycerin, Sodium Chloride, Sodium Borate, Eucalyptol, Menthol, Polysorbate 80, Benzalkonium Chloride	**Adults & Peds ≥2 yrs:** Instill 2-3 sprays per nostril prn.
Ayr Allergy & Sinus Nasal Mist	Sodium Chloride 2.65%	**Adults & Peds:** Spray bid-tid prn.
Ayr Baby's Saline Nose Spray/Drops	Sodium Chloride 0.65%	**Peds:** Instill 2 to 6 drops in each nostril.
Ayr Saline Nasal Gel With Soothing Aloe	Water, Methyl Gluceth 10, Propylene Glycol, Glycerin, Glyceryl Polymethacrylate, Triethanolamine, Aloe Barbadensis Leaf Juice (Aloe Vera Gel), PEG/PPG 18/18 Dimethicone, Carbomer, Poloxamer 184, Sodium Chloride, Xanthan Gum, Diazolidinyl Urea, Methyl-paraben, Propylparaben, Glycine Soja Oil (Soybean), Geranium Maculatum Oil, Tocopheryl Acetate, Blue 1	**Adults & Peds:** Apply to nostril prn.
Ayr Saline Nasal Gel, No-Drip Sinus Spray	Water, Sodium Carbomethyl Starch, Propylene Glycol, Glycerin, Aloe Barbadensis Leaf Juice (Aloe Vera Gel), Sodium Chloride, Cetyl Pyridinium Chloride, Citric Acid, Disodium EDTA, Glycine Soja (Soybean Oil), Tocopheryl Acetate, Benzyl Alcohol, Benzalkonium Chloride, Geranium Maculatum Oil	**Adults & Peds:** Instill 1 spray in each nostril prn.
Ayr Saline Nasal Mist	Sodium Chloride 0.65%	**Adults & Peds:** Instill 2 sprays per nostril prn.
ENTSOL Mist, Buffered Hypertonic Nasal Irrigation Mist	Purified Water, Sodium Chloride, Sodium Phosphate Dibasic Edetate Disodium, Potassium Phosphate Monobasic, Benzalkonium Chloride	**Adults & Peds:** Instill 1-2 sprays per nostril prn.
ENTSOL Spray, Buffered Hypertonic Saline Nasal Spray	Purified Water, Sodium Chloride Phosphate Dibasic, Potassium Phosphate Monobasic	**Adults & Peds:** Instill 1 spray per nostril 2–6 times daily.
ENTSOL Nasal Gel with Aloe and Vitamin E	Water (Purified), Propylene Glycol, Aloe, Glycerin, Dimethicone Copolyol, Poloxamer 184, Methyl Gluceth 10, Triethanolamine, Carbomer, Sodium Chloride, Vitamin E, Disodium EDTA, Xanthan Gum, Benzalkonium Chloride	**Adults & Peds:** Use prn.
Little Noses Saline Spray/Drops, Non-Medicated	Sodium Chloride 0.65%	**Peds:** 2-6 drops per nostril as directed.
Nostrilla Conditioning Double Moisture	Benzalkonium Chloride Solution, Carboxy-methylcellulose Sodium, Eucalyptol, Glycine, Hyaluronic Acid Sodium, Polyethylene Glycol, Povidone, Propylene Glycol, Sodium Chloride (as 1.9% saline solution), Spearmint Oil, Wintergreen Oil, Water	**Adults & Peds:** Spray once per nostril prn.

TABLE 22. NASAL DECONGESTANT/MOISTURIZING PRODUCTS (cont.)

Brand Name	Ingredient/Strength	Dose
Ocean Premium Saline Nasal Spray	Sodium Chloride 0.65%	**Adults & Peds:** Instill 2 sprays per nostril prn.
Simply Saline Sterile Saline Nasal Mist	Sodium Chloride 0.9%	**Adults & Peds:** Use prn as directed.
SinoFresh Nasal & Sinus Care	Eucalyptus Globules 20x, Kalium Bichromicum 30x, Benzalkonium Chloride, Cetylpyridium Chloride, Dibasic Sodium Phosphate, Essential Oil Blend (wintergreen, spearmint, peppermint, and eucalyptus oils), Monobasic Sodium Phosphate, Polysorbate 80, Propylene Glycol, Purified Water, Sodium Chloride, Sorbitol Solution	**Adults & Peds:** 1-2 sprays per nostril bid.

TABLE 23. OPHTHALMIC DECONGESTANT/ANTIHISTAMINE PRODUCTS

BRAND NAME	INGREDIENT/STRENGTH	DOSE
KETOTIFEN		
Zaditor	Ketotifen 0.025%	**Adults & Peds >3 yrs:** Instill 1 drop in affected eye(s) bid every 8-12 hrs. **Max:** 2 doses qd.
Alaway	Ketotifen 0.025%	**Adults & Peds >3 yrs:** Instill 1 drop in affected eye(s) bid every 8-12 hrs. **Max:** 2 doses qd.
NAPHAZOLINE		
Bausch & Lomb Advanced Eye Relief Redness Maximum Relief	Naphazoline HCl/Hypromellose 0.03%-0.5%	**Adults:** Instill 1-2 drops to affected eye(s) qid.
Clear Eyes ACR Seasonal Relief	Naphazoline HCl/Glycerin/Zinc Sulfate 0.012%-0.2%-0.25%	**Adults:** Instill 1-2 drops to affected eye(s) qid.
Clear Eyes Redness Relief	Naphazoline HCl/Glycerin 0.012%-0.2%	**Adults:** Instill 1-2 drops to affected eye(s) qid.
Opcon-A Allergy Relief Drops	Naphazoline HCl/Pheniramine Maleate 0.03%-0.32%	**Adults & Peds ≥6 yrs:** Instill 1-2 drops to affected eye(s) qid.
Visine-A Allergy Relief Drops	Naphazoline HCl/ Pheniramine Maleate 0.025%-0.3%	**Adults & Peds ≥6 yrs:** Instill 1-2 drops to affected eye(s) qid.
Rohto V Cool Redness Relief Drops	Naphazoline HCl/ Polysorbate 80 0.012%-0.2%	**Adults:** Instill 1-2 drops to affected eye(s) qid.
OXYMETAZOLINE		
Visine L.R. Redness Reliever Drops	Oxymetazoline HCl 0.025%	**Adults & Peds ≥6 yrs:** Instill 1-2 drops to affected eye(s) q6h prn.
PHENYLEPHRINE		
Allergan Relief Redness Reliever & Lubricant Eye Drops	Phenylephrine HCl/ Polyvinyl Alcohol 0.12%-1.4%	**Adults:** Instill 1-2 drops to affected eye(s) qid.
TETRAHYDROZOLINE		
Visine Original Drops	Tetrahydrozoline HCl 0.05%	**Adults & Peds ≥6 yrs:** Instill 1-2 drops to affected eye(s) qid.
Visine Advanced Redness Reliever Drops	Tetrahydrozoline HCl/Polyethylene Glycol 400/ Povidone/Dextran 70 0.05%-1%-1%-0.1%	**Adults & Peds ≥6 yrs:** Instill 1-2 drops to affected eye(s) qid.
Murine Tears Plus Eye Drops	Tetrahydrozoline HCl/Polyvinyl Alcohol/ Povidone 0.05%-0.5%-0.6%	**Adults:** Instill 1-2 drops to affected eye(s) qid.
Rohto V. Arctic Eye Drops	Tetrahydrozoline HCl/Hypromellose 0.05%-0.35%	**Adults:** Instill 1-2 drops to affected eye(s) qid.
Rohto V. Ice Eye Drops	Tetrahydrozoline HCl/Hypromellose/Zinc Sulfate 0.05%-0.2%-0.25%	**Adults:** Instill 1-2 drops to affected eye(s) qid.
Visine A.C. Astringent Redness Reliever Drops	Tetrahydrozoline HCl/ Zinc Sulfate 0.05%-0.25%	**Adults & Peds ≥6 yrs:** Instill 1-2 drops to affected eye(s) qid.

TABLE 24. PSORIASIS PRODUCTS

Brand Name	Ingredient/Strength	Dose
COAL TAR		
Denorex Therapeutic Protection 2-in-1 Shampoo	Coal Tar 2.5%	**Adults & Peds:** Use at least biw.
DHS Tar Shampoo	Coal Tar 0.5%	**Adults & Peds:** Use tiw.
DHS Tar Gel Shampoo	Coal Tar 0.5%	**Adults & Peds:** Use tiw.
Ionil-T Plus Shampoo	Coal Tar 2%	**Adults & Peds:** Use at least biw.
Ionil-T Shampoo	Coal Tar 2%	**Adults & Peds:** Use at least biw.
MG217 Medicated Tar Lotion	Coal Tar 1%	**Adults & Peds:** Apply to affected area qd-qid.
MG217 Ointment	Coal Tar 2%	**Adults & Peds:** Apply to affected area qd-qid.
MG217 Tar Shampoo	Coal Tar 3%	**Adults & Peds:** Use at least biw.
Neutrogena T/Gel Shampoo Extra Strength	Coal Tar 1%	**Adults & Peds:** Use qod. **Max:** 4 times qweek.
Neutrogena T/Gel Shampoo Original Formula	Coal Tar 0.5%	**Adults & Peds:** Use at least biw.
Neutrogena T/Gel Stubborn Itch Shampoo	Coal Tar 0.5%	**Adults & Peds:** Use at least biw.
Psoriasin Gel	Coal Tar 1.25%	**Adults & Peds:** Apply to affected area qd-qid.
Psoriasin Liquid	Coal Tar 0.66%	**Adults & Peds:** Apply to affected area qd-qid.
Psoriasin Ointment	Coal Tar 2%	**Adults & Peds:** Apply to affected area qd-qid.
CORTICOSTEROID		
Aveeno Hydrocortisone 1% Anti-Itch Cream	Hydrocortisone 1%	**Adults & Peds ≥2 yrs:** Apply to affected area tid-qid.
Cortaid Advanced 12-Hour Anti-Itch Cream	Hydrocortisone 1%	**Adults & Peds ≥2 yrs:** Apply to affected area tid-qid.
Cortaid Intensive Therapy Cooling Spray	Hydrocortisone 1%	**Adults & Peds ≥2 yrs:** Apply to affected area tid-qid.
Cortaid Intensive Therapy Moisturizing Cream	Hydrocortisone 1%	**Adults & Peds ≥2 yrs:** Apply to affected area tid-qid.
Cortaid Maximum Strength Cream	Hydrocortisone 1%	**Adults & Peds ≥2 yrs:** Apply to affected area tid-qid.
Cortaid Maximum Strength Ointment	Hydrocortisone 1%	**Adults & Peds ≥2 yrs:** Apply to affected area tid-qid.
Cortizone-10 Creme	Hydrocortisone 1%	**Adults & Peds ≥2 yrs:** Apply to affected area tid-qid.
Cortizone-10 Creme Plus	Hydrocortisone 1%	**Adults & Peds ≥2 yrs:** Apply to affected area tid-qid.
Cortizone-10 Ointment	Hydrocortisone 1%	**Adults & Peds ≥2 yrs:** Apply to affected area tid-qid.
Cortizone-10 Intensive Healing Formula	Hydrocortisone 1%	**Adults & Peds ≥2 yrs:** Apply to affected area tid-qid.
Cortizone-10 Easy Relief Applicator	Hydrocortisone 1%	**Adults & Peds ≥2 yrs:** Apply to affected area tid-qid.
Cortizone-10 Cool Relief Gel	Hydrocortisone 1%	**Adults & Peds ≥2 yrs:** Apply to affected area tid-qid.
SALICYLIC ACID		
Dermarest Psoriasis Medicated Overnight Treatment	Salicylic Acid 3%	**Adults & Peds:** Apply to affected area qhs. **Max:** qid.
Dermarest Psoriasis Medicated Moisturizer	Salicylic Acid 2%	**Adults & Peds:** Apply to affected area qd-qid.
Dermarest Psoriasis Medicated Scalp Treatment	Salicylic Acid 3%	**Adults & Peds:** Apply to affected area qd-qid.
Dermarest Psoriasis Medicated Shampoo/Conditioner	Salicylic Acid 3%	**Adults & Peds:** Apply to affected area at least biw.

(Continued)

TABLE 24. PSORIASIS PRODUCTS (cont.)

Brand Name	Ingredient/Strength	Dose
Dermarest Psoriasis Medicated Skin Treatment	Salicylic Acid 3%	**Adults & Peds:** Apply to affected area qd-qid.
Neutrogena T/Gel Conditioner	Salicylic Acid 2%	**Adults & Peds:** Use at least biw.
Neutrogena T/Sal Shampoo	Salicylic Acid 3%	**Adults & Peds:** Use at least tiw.
Psoriasin Therapeutic Shampoo and Body Wash	Salicylic Acid 3%	**Adults & Peds:** Use biw.

TABLE 25. SMOKING CESSATION PRODUCTS

Brand Name	Ingredient/Strength	Dose
Commit Stop Smoking 2mg Lozenges	Nicotine Polacrilex 2mg	**Adults:** If smoking first cigarette >30 minutes after waking up use 2mg lozenge. **Weeks 1 to 6:** 1 lozenge q1-2h. **Weeks 7 to 9:** 1 lozenge q2-4h. **Weeks 10 to 12:** 1 lozenge q4-8h. **Max:** 5 lozenges/6 hours; 20 lozenges/day. Stop using at the end of 12 weeks.
Commit Stop Smoking 4mg Lozenges	Nicotine Polacrilex 4mg	**Adults:** If smoking first cigarette within 30 minutes after waking up use 4mg lozenge. **Weeks 1 to 6:** 1 lozenge q1-2h. **Weeks 7 to 9:** 1 lozenge q2-4h. **Weeks 10 to 12:** 1 lozenge q4-8h. **Max:** 5 lozenges/ 6 hours; 20 lozenges/day. Stop using at the end of 12 weeks.
NicoDerm CQ Step 1 Clear Patch	Nicotine 21mg	**Adults:** If smoking >10 cigarettes/day. **Weeks 1 to 6:** Apply one 21mg patch/day. **Weeks 7 to 8:** Apply one 14mg patch/day. **Weeks 9 to 10:** Apply one 7mg patch/day.
NicoDerm CQ Step 2 Clear Patch	Nicotine 14mg	**Adults:** If smoking <10 cigarettes/day. **Weeks 1 to 6:** Apply one 14mg patch/day. **Weeks 7 to 8:** Apply one 7mg patch/day.
NicoDerm CQ Step 3 Clear Patch	Nicotine 7mg	**Adults:** Apply 1 patch qd Weeks 9 to 10 if smoking >10 cigarettes/day or Weeks 7 to 8 if smoking ≤10 cigarettes/day.
Nicorette 2mg	Nicotine Polacrilex 2mg	**Adults:** If smoking <25 cigarettes/day use 2mg gum. **Weeks 1 to 6:** 1 piece q1-2h. **Weeks 7 to 9:** 1 piece q2-4h. **Weeks 10 to 12:** 1 piece q4-8h. **Max:** 24 pieces/day.
Nicorette 4mg	Nicotine Polacrilex 4mg	**Adults:** If smoking ≥25 cigarettes/day use 4mg gum. **Weeks 1 to 6:** 1 piece q1-2h. **Weeks 7 to 9:** 1 piece q2-4h. **Weeks 10 to 12:** 1 piece q4-8h. **Max:** 24 pieces/day.
Habitrol Nicotine Transdermal System Patch Step 1	Nicotine 21mg/24hr	**Adults:** If smoking >10 cigarettes/day. **Weeks 1 to 4:** Apply one 21mg patch/day. **Weeks 5 to 6:** Apply one 14mg patch/day. **Weeks 7 to 8:** Apply one 7mg patch/day.
Habitrol Nicotine Transdermal System Patch Step 2	Nicotine 14mg/24hr	**Adults:** If smoking >10 cigarettes/day. **Weeks 1 to 4:** Apply one 21mg patch/day. **Weeks 5 to 6:** Apply one 14mg patch/day. **Weeks 7 to 8:** Apply one 7mg patch/day. If smoking <10 cigarettes/day. **Weeks 1 to 6:** Apply one 14 mg patch/day. **Weeks 7 to 8:** Apply one 7mg patch/day.
Habitrol Nicotine Transdermal System Patch Step 3	Nicotine 7mg/24hr	**Adults:** If smoking >10 cigarettes/day. **Weeks 1 to 4:** Apply one 21mg patch/day. **Weeks 5 to 6:** Apply one 14mg patch/day. **Weeks 7 to 8:** Apply one 7mg patch/day. If smoking <10 cigarettes/day. **Weeks 1 to 6:** Apply one 14mg patch/day. **Weeks 7 to 8:** Apply one 7mg patch/day.

TABLE 26. WEIGHT MANAGEMENT PRODUCTS

Brand Name	Ingredient/Strength	Dose
Alli Weight-Loss Aid	Orlistat 60 mg	**Adults:** 1 cap with each fat-containing meal. **Max:** 3 caps per day.
Applied Nutrition Carb Blocker	Common Bean Extract, IsoPhase 2200, Soy Bean Oil, Bioperine Black Pepper Extract (95% Piperine) (Fruit), Conjugated Linoleic Acid (CLA), White Tea Extract (30% Polyphenols, 10% Caffeine) (Leaf)	**Adults:** Take 2 caps with meals bid.
Applied Nutrition Green Tea Fat Burner	Chromium (From Chromium Picolinate), Green Tea Extract (Leaf, 50% EGCG), Natural Caffeine, Xenedrol Blend [(Bitter Orange Extract) (Fruit, 6% Synephrine), Betaine HCl, Bladderwrack Powder, Cayenne Powder (Fruit), Eleuthero Powder (Root), Ginger Powder (Root), Gotu Kola Powder (Aerial), Licorice *(Glycyrrhiza glabra)* Powder (Root, rhizome), Maté (Yerba Maté) Powder (Leaf)]	**Adults:** Take 2 caps with meals bid.
Applied Nutrition Green Tea Triple Fat Burner	Vitamin C (as Ascorbic Acid), Vitamin E (as d-Alpha Tocopheryl Acetate), Niacin (as Niacinamide), Vitamin B6 (as Pyridoxine Hydrochloride), Folic Acid, Vitamin B12 (as Cyanocobalamin), Green Tea Extract (50% EGCG) (Leaf), White Tea Extract (50% EGCG) (Leaf), Orange Pekoe (Black) Tea Extract (50% EGCG) (Leaf), Natural Caffeine, Citrus *(Citrus spp.)* Bioflavonoids (10% Bioflavonoids) (Fruit)	**Adults:** Take 2 caps with meals bid.
Applied Nutrition 10-Day Hoodia Diet Capsules	Green Tea Extract (Leaf, 20% Caffeine), *Hoodia gordonii* (Aerial, 20:1), Natural Caffeine, Garcinia Extract (Fruit, 50% Hydroxycitric Acid), Choline (as Choline Bitartrate), Inositol, L-Methionine	**Adults:** Take 2 caps with meals bid.
Applied Nutrition Natural Fat Burner Capsules	Vitamin C (as Ascorbic Acid), Vitamin E (as d-Alpha Tocopheryl Acetate), Niacin (as Niacinamide), Vitamin B6 (as Pyridoxine Hydrochloride), Folic Acid, Vitamin B12 (as Cyanocobalamin), Green Tea Extract (leaf, 50% EGCG), Natural Caffeine, Red Leaf Lettuce-powder, Cassia Extract (6:1 bark), Cranberry *(Vaccinium macrocarpon)* Extract (fruit), Grapefruit Extract (40:1 fruit), Noni Extract (4:1 fruit), Blueberry *(Vaccinium angustifolium)* Extract (fruit), Pomegranate Extract (5:1 fruit), Apple Cider Vinegar Powder, Citrus *(Citrus spp.)* Bioflavonoids (fruit)	**Adults:** Take 2 caps with meals bid.
Aqua-Ban Maximum Strength Diuretic Tablets	Pamabrom 50mg	**Adults:** Take 1 tab qid. **Max:** 4 tabs q24h.
BioMD Nutraceuticals Metabolism T3 Capsules	Calcium Phosphate, Gum Guggul Extract, L-Tyrosine, *Garcinia Cambogia*, Dipotassium Phosphate, Sodium Phosphate, Disodium Phosphate, Phosphatidyl Choline	**Adults:** Take 2 caps with meals bid-tid. **Max:** 6 caps q24h.
Biotest Hot-Rox Capsules	A7-E Super-Thermogenic Gel XXX500 [Lauroyl Macrogol-32 Glycerides, P-Methylcarbonyl-ethylphenol, 3,17-Dihydroxy-Delta-5-Etiocholane-7-One Diethylcarbonate, Carbolin 19 (Forskolin 1,9-Carbonate), Piperine, Yohimbine HCl], Caffeine	**Adults:** Take 1-2 caps bid. **Max:** 4 caps q24h.

(Continued)

TABLE 26. WEIGHT MANAGEMENT PRODUCTS (cont.)

Brand Name	Ingredient/Strength	Dose
Carb Cutter Original Formula Tablets	Vitamin C (as Ascorbic Acid), Chromium (as Chromium Dinicotinate Glycinate), Absorptive Vegetable Fiber, Banaba Leaf Extract (Lagerstroemia speciosa), Gymnema Sylvestre Leaf and Gymnema Sylvestre Leaf Extract (25% Gymnemic Acids), Fenugreek Seed Extract, Super Hydroxycitric Extract of Garcinia cambogia Fruit], Vanadium (as BMOV), Guarana Seed Extract (Supplying 60mg Caffeine), Korean Ginseng Root Extract (5% Ginsenosides), Eleuthero Root Extract (0.8% Eleutherosides), Green Tea Leaf Extract (36% Total Polyphenols)	**Adults:** Take 1-2 tabs with meals bid.
Carb Cutter Phase 2 Starch Neutralizer Tablets	Phase 2 Starch Neutralizer (Phaseolus vulgaris from White Kidney Bean Extract), Gymnema sylvestre Leaf, Fenugreek Seed, Garcina cambogia Fruit Extract 50.0%, Hydroxycitric Acid, Vanadium (as Vanadyl Sulfate)	**Adults:** Take 1-2 tabs with meals bid.
Dexatrim Max	Thiamin, Riboflavin, Niacin, Vitamin B6, Vitamin B12, Pantothenic Acid, Chromium, Proprietary Herbal Blend (Green Tea and Oolong Tea Standardized Leaf Extracts), Epigalocatechin Gallate (EGCG), Caffeine, Asian Ginseng Root Extract	**Adults:** Take 1-2 caps with water, one in AM and one in afternoon. **Max:** 2 caps q24h.
Dexatrim Max₂O	Thiamin (B1), Riboflavin (B2), Niacin (B3), Vitamin B6, Vitamin B12, Pantothenic Acid, Chromium, Potassium, EGCG (Green Tea Extract), Panax Ginseng Extract, Folic Acid, Caffeine, Sodium	**Adults:** Dissolve 2 tabs in 16.9 ounces of water. **Max:** 6 tabs q24h.
Dexatrim Natural Extra Energy Formula Caplets	Calcium, Chromium, Green Tea Leaf Standardized Extract with Epigallocatechin Gallate (EGCG) and Caffeine, Asian (Panax) Ginseng Root	**Adults:** Take 1 tab with meals tid. **Max:** 3 tabs q24h.
Dexatrim Natural Green Tea Formula Caplets	Calcium, Chromium, Green Tea Leaf Standardized Extract, Asian (Panax) Ginseng Root	**Adults:** Take 1 tab with meal tid. **Max:** 3 tabs q24h.
Dexatrim Max Complex 7	Thiamine (B1), Riboflavin (B2), Niacin (B3), Vitamin B6, Vitamin B12, Pantothenic Acid, Chromium, Complex 7 Proprietary Herbal Blend (Green Tea and Oolong Tea Standardized Leaf Extracts (Camellia sinensis), Epigallocatechin Gallate (EGCG), Caffeine, Asian (Panax) Ginseng Root (4% Ginsenosides), 7-Keto [3-acetyl-7Oxo Dehydroepiandrosterone]	**Adults:** Take 2 caps qam. Second serving mid-afternoon. **Max:** 4 caps q24h.
EAS CLA Capsules	CLA (Conjugated Linoleic Acid 1.5g)	**Adults:** Take 2 caps with meals tid.
Estrin-D Capsules	Vitamin B6, Magnesium, Estrin-D Proprietary Blend (Yerbe Mate Leaf, Caffeine, Guarana Seed, Damiana Leaf and Stem, Green Tea, Ginger Root, Kola Nut, DHEA, Schisandra Fruit, Scutellaria Root, Coca Nut, Jujube Fruit, Thea Sinensis Complex Leaf)	**Adults:** Take 2 caps 30 min before meals. **Max:** 6 caps q24h.
Isatori Lean System 7 Advanced Metabolic Support Formula	Yerba Mate, Guarana Extract, Green Tea Leaf Extract, Dandelion Leaf, Advantra, 7-Keto, Bioperine, Fucus Nodosus, Pomegranate Extract	**Adults:** Take 3 caps with meals bid. **Max:** 6 caps q24h.
Metab-O-Fx Extreme	Guarana Seed, Yerba Maté Leaf, Kola Nut Seed, Bitter Orange Extract, Green Tea Extract, Cocoa Nut, Black Tea Extract, Korean Ginseng Root, Rhodiola rodsea Extract, Niacin (B3)	**Adults:** Take 1 tab with meal bid-tid. **Max:** 3 tabs q24h.

TABLE 26. WEIGHT MANAGEMENT PRODUCTS (cont.)

BRAND NAME	INGREDIENT/STRENGTH	DOSE
Metabolife Break Through	Proprietary Blend of Green Tea (Leaf) Extract, L-Tyrosine, Cayenne (Fruit), Caffeine	**Adults:** Take 2 tabs 1 hr before meals tid, at least 3-4 hrs apart. **Max:** 6 tabs q24h.
Metabolife Extreme Energy	Niacin, Pantothenic Acid (as D-Calcium Pantothenate), Magnesium (as Oxide/Amino Acid Chelate), Guarana Extract (Seed), Asian Ginseng Extract (Root), Green Tea Extract (Leaf), Yerba Mate Extract (Leaf), Eleuthero Extract (Root), *Rhodiola* Extract (Root), Theaine	**Adults:** Take 1-2 caps tid at least 3-4 hrs apart. **Max:** 4 caps q8h.
Metabolife Ultra Caplets	Calcium (as Hydroxycitrate), Chromium (as Chromium Picolinate), Sodium, Potassium, SuperCitriMax Garcinia Extract (Fruit) (Standardized for Hydroxycitric Acid), Caffeine, Co-Enzyme Q10	**Adults:** Take 2 tabs tid 30-60 min before meals, at least 3-4 hrs apart. **Max:** 6 tabs q24h.
Metabolife Caffeine Free Caplets	Thiamin (B1), Riboflavin (B2), Niacin (B3), Vitamin B6, Pantothenic Acid, Calcium, Chromium, Potassium, Garcinia Extract (Fruit), Sodium	**Adults:** Take 2 tabs tid 30-60 min before meals, at least 3-4 hrs apart. **Max:** 6 tabs q24h.
MHP TakeOff, Hi-Energy Fat Burner Capsules	*Citrus aurantium* Extract, Guarana Seed Extract and Green Tea Leaf Extract, L-Tyrosine, *Ginkgo biloba* Leaf Extract, Triple-Ginseng Concentrate (Contains: Panax Ginseng Root Extract, American Ginseng Root Extract and Eleuthro Root Extract. Adrenal Support Blend: Licorice Root Extract, Astragalus Root Extract and Schizandra Berry Extract.)	**Adults:** Take 2 caps qd or bid.
Natrol Carb Intercept with Phase 2 Starch Neutralizer Capsules	White Kidney Bean Extract	**Adults:** Take 2 caps before carbohydrate-containing meals.
Natrol CitriMax Plus	Calcium (from (-) Hydoxycitric Acid), Chromium (as Chromium Polynicotinate), (10(-) HydroxyCitric Acid (HCA) (from Garcinia Cambogia (Fruit), Uva Ursi (Leaf), Cascara Sagrada (bark)	**Adults:** Take 1 cap ½ hr before meals tid.
Natrol Green Tea 500mg Capsules	Green Tea Extract, Polyphenols, Catechins, Caffeine	**Adults:** Take 1 cap with meals qd.
Natural Balance Fat Magnet Capsules	Chitosan, Psyllium Husk, Malic Acid, Vegetarian Lipase, Aloe Vera	**Adults:** Take 2 caps with meals bid.
Nature Made Chromium Picolinate, Extra Strength	Chromium 350mg	**Adults:** Take 1 tab qd.
Nature's Bounty Super Green Tea Diet Capsules	Green Tea *(Camellia sinensis)* (Leaf), Caffeine, Guarana *(Paullinia cupana)* (Seed), Ginger *(Zingiber officinale)* (Root), Bladderwrack Extract *(Fucus vesiculosus)* (Whole Plant), Uva Ursi *(Arctistaohylos uva-ursi)* (Leaf), Vitamin B-6 (as Pyridoxine Hydrochloride), Chromium (as Chromium Polynicotinate)	**Adults:** Take 1 cap bid. **Max:** 2 caps q24h.
Nature's Bounty Xtreme Lean Zn-3 Ephedra Free Capsules	Methylxanthines (Caffeine), Green Tea Extract *(Camellia Sinensis)* (Leaf) (Standardized for Epigallocatechin gallate, Caffeine, Polyphenols), Metabromine Cocoa Extract (Standardized for Theobromine, Caffeine), Bitter Orange Extract *(Citrus Aurantium)* (Fruit) (Standardized for Synepherine, N-Methyltyramine, Hordenine, Octopamine and Tyramine), Tyrosine Complex (L-Tyrosine and Acetyl L-Tyrosine), L-Methionine, Ginger Extract *(Zingiber Officinale)* (Root), Grape Seed Extract (seed), Flavone Complex (Proprietary Blend of 3, 3', 4', 5-7-Tetrahydroxyflavone), DMAE (Dimethyl-aminoethanol), Vitamin C as Ascorbic Acid, Vitamin B6 as Pyridoxine Hydrochloride, Pantothenic Acid as d-Calcium Pantothenate, Magnesium as Magnesium Oxide	**Adults:** Take 2 caps bid. **Max:** 4 caps q24h.

(Continued)

TABLE 26. WEIGHT MANAGEMENT PRODUCTS (cont.)

Brand Name	Ingredient/Strength	Dose
Nunaturals LevelRight for Blood Sugar Management Capsules	*Gymenema sylvestre* Extract, Fenugreek Extract, Bitter Melon Extract, Siberian Ginseng Extract, Alpha Lipoic Acid, Cinnamon Bark Extract, Banaba Leaf Extract, Biotin, Chromium Polynicotinate, Chromium Picolinate, Vanadium	**Adults:** Take 1 cap with meals tid.
One-A-Day Weight Smart Dietary Supplement Tablets	Vitamin A (30% as Beta-Carotene), Vitamin C, Vitamin D, Vitamin E, Vitamin K, Thiamin (B1), Riboflavin (B2), Niacin, Vitamin B6, Folic Acid, Vitamin B12, Pantothenic Acid, Calcium (Elemental), Iron, Magnesium, Zinc, Selenium, Copper, Manganese, Chromium, Guarana Seed (Powder & Extract), Caffeine, Green Tea Powder (Leaf), Cayenne Pepper Powder (Fruit)	**Adults:** Take 1 tab with meals qd.
Prolab Enhanced CLA	CLA (Conjugated Linoleic Acid), Flax Seed Oil, Alpha Linoleic Acid, Linoleic Acid, Sunflower or Safflower Oil	**Adults:** Take 3 caps with meals qd.
Stacker 2 Ephedra Free Capsules	Kola Nut (Seeds), Yerba Mate (Leaves), Cassia Mimosoides Extract (Leaves/Stems/Pids), White Willow Bark, Caffeine (Anhydrous), Green Tea (Leaves), Guggulsterone (Whole Plant), Gymnema (Leaves), Tri-guggLyptoid3 complex	**Adults:** Take 1 cap after meals. **Max:** 3 caps q24h.
Tetrazene ES-50 Ultra High-Energy Weight Loss Catalyst Capsules	Vitamin B6 (as Pyridoxine HCl), Biotin, Tetrazene Proprietary Blend: KGM-90 (Super-Class) Pharmaceutical Grade Glucomannan, Glutamine, Olive Leaf Extract. ES-50 Thermogenic Complex: L-Tyrosine, *Camellia Sinensis* (Green Tea Leaf Extract, Standardized for EGCG and Caffeine), Pharmaceutical Grade Caffeine, Vinpocetine	**Adults:** Take 2 caps with meals tid. **Max:** 6 caps q24h.
Tetrazene KGM-90 Rapid Weight Loss Catalyst Capsules	Vitamin B6, Biotin, Propiatary Blend as Follows: KGM-90 (SuperClass Pharmaceutical Grade Glucomannan), Glutamine, Olive Leaf Extract	**Adults:** Take 2 caps with meals tid. **Max:** 6 caps q24h.
Twinlab GTF Chromium	Calcium from Dicalcium Phosphate Dehydrate, 200mcg Tablets Chromium from Chromium Yeast, Brewers Yeast	**Adults:** Take 1 tab qd.
Twinlab Mega L-Carnitine	L-Carnitine 500mg	**Adults:** Take 1 tab daily on an empty stomach.
Twinlab Metabolift, Ephedra Free Formula Capsules	Guarana Seed Extract, Citrus Aurantium Fruit Extract, Proprietary Thermogenic and Metabolic Blend, St. John's Wort Extract, L-Phenylalanine, Green Tea Leaf Extract, Quercetin Dihydrate, Citrus Bioflavonoid Complex, Ginger Root, Cayenne Fruit	**Adults:** Take 2 caps before each meal. **Max:** 6 caps q24h.
Ultra Diet Pep Tablets	Vitamin B12 (Cyanocobalamin), Vitamin B6 (as Pyridoxine HCl), Pantothenic Acid (as d-Calcium Pantothenate), Iodine DynaChrome Chromium (as Arginate/Chelidamate), Potassium (as Potassium Chloride), Green Tea Leaf Extract, Dandelion (Leaf), Ginger (Root), Passion Flower (Aerial Portion Extract), Kelp (Leaf), L-Tyrosine	**Adults:** Take 1 tab with meals bid.

TABLE 26. WEIGHT MANAGEMENT PRODUCTS (cont.)

Brand Name	Ingredient/Strength	Dose
XtremeLean Advanced Formula, Ephedra Free Capsules	Vitamin C (as Ascorbic Acid), Vitamin B-6 (as Pyridoxine Hydrochloride), Pantothenic Acid (as d-Calcium Pantothenate), Magnesium (as Magnesium Oxide), Proprietary XtremeLean, Thermo Complex (Yerba Maté Extract [Leaf])-(standardized for Methylxanthines [Caffeine])), Green Tea Extract *(Camellia sinensis)* (Leaf) (standardized for Epigallocatechin Gallate, Caffeine, Polyphenols), Metabromine Cocoa Extract (standardized for Theobromine, Caffeine), Bitter Orange Extract *(Citrus aurantium)* (Fruit) (standardized for Synepherine, N-Methyltyramine, Hordenine, Octopamine, Tyramine), Tyrosine Complex (L-Tyrosine, Acetyl L-Tyrosine), L-Methionine, Ginger Extract *(Zingiber officinale)* (Root), Grape Seed Extract (Seed), Flavone Complex (Proprietary Blend of: 3, 3', 4', 5-7- Pentahydroxyflavone, 3, 3', 4', 7 Tetrahydroxyflavone), DMAE (Dimethylaminoethanol)	**Adults:** Take 2 caps before meals bid.
Zantrex 3, Ephedrine Free	Rice Flour, Zantrex-3 Proprietary Blend Containing: Yerba Maté (Leaf), Caffeine, Guarana (Seed), Damiana (Leaf, Stem), Green Tea (Leaf), Kola Nut, *Schizonepeta* (Spica), *Piper nigrum* (Fruit), Tibetan Ginseng (Root), Panax Ginseng (Root), Maca Root, Cocoa Nut, Thea Sinensis Complex (Leaf), Niacin (B3)	**Adults:** Take 2 caps with meals qd. **Max:** 6 cap q24h.

TABLE 27. WOUND CARE PRODUCTS

BRAND NAME	INGREDIENT/STRENGTH	DOSE
NEOMYCIN/POLYMYXIN B/BACITRACIN COMBINATIONS		
Bacitracin Ointment	Bacitracin 500 U	**Adults & Peds:** Apply to affected area qd-tid.
Neosporin Ointment	Neomycin/polymyxin B/bacitracin 3.5mg-5,000 U-400 U	**Adults & Peds:** Apply to affected area qd-tid.
Neosporin Plus Pain Relief Cream	Neomycin/polymyxin B/pramoxine 3.5mg-10,000 U-10mg	**Adults & Peds:** Apply to affected area qd-tid.
Neosporin Plus Pain Relief Ointment	Neomycin/polymyxin B/bacitracin/pramoxine 3.5mg-10,000 U-500 U-10mg	**Adults & Peds:** Apply to affected area qd-tid.
Neosporin To Go Ointment	Neomycin/polymyxin B/bacitracin 3.5mg-5,000 U-400 U	**Adults & Peds:** Apply to affected area qd-tid.
Polysporin Ointment	Polymyxin B/bacitracin 10,000 U-500 U	**Adults & Peds:** Apply to affected area qd-tid.
Polysporin First Aid Antibiotic Powder	Polymyxin B/bacitracin 10,000 U-500 U	**Adults & Peds:** Apply to affected area qd-tid.
BENZALKONIUM CHLORIDE COMBINATIONS		
Bactine First Aid Liquid	Lidocaine HCl/benzalkonium chloride 2.5%-0.13%	**Adults & Peds ≥2 yrs:** Apply to affected area qd-tid.
Bactine Pain Relieving Cleansing Spray	Lidocaine HCl/benzalkonium chloride 2.5%-0.13%	**Adults & Peds ≥2 yrs:** Apply to affected area qd-tid.
Neosporin Neo To Go	Benzalkonium Cl/pramoxine HCl 0.13%-1%	**Adults & Peds ≥2 yrs:** Apply to affected area qd-tid.
BENZETHONIUM CHLORIDE COMBINATIONS		
Gold Bond First Aid Quick Spray	Menthol/benzethonium chloride 1%-0.13%	**Adults & Peds ≥2 yrs:** Apply to affected area tid-qid.
Lanacane Maximum Strength Cream Anti-Itch	Benzocaine/benzethonium chloride 20%-0.1%	**Adults & Peds ≥2 yrs:** Apply to affected area qd-tid.
Lanacane Anti-Itch Crème Medication	Benzocaine/benzethonium chloride 6%-0.2%	**Adults & Peds ≥2 yrs:** Apply to affected area qd-tid.
Lanacane Maximum Strength First Aid Spray	Benzocaine/benzethonium chloride 20%-0.2%	**Adults & Peds ≥2 yrs:** Apply to affected area qd-tid.
CHLORHEXIDINE GLUCONATE		
Hibiclens	Chlorhexidine gluconate 4%	**Adults & Peds:** Apply sparingly to affected area prn.
Hibistat Hand Antiseptic	Chlorhexidine gluconate/isopropyl alcohol 0.5%-70%	**Adults:** Wipe until dry.
IODINE		
Betadine Skin Cleanser	Povidone-iodine 7.5%	**Adults & Peds:** Apply to affected area. Wash vigorously for 15 seconds and rinse and dry.
Betadine Solution	Povidone-iodine 10%	**Adults & Peds:** Apply to affected area qd-tid.
MISCELLANEOUS		
Aquaphor Healing Ointment	Petrolatum, mineral oil, ceresin, lanolin	**Adults & Peds:** Apply to affected area prn.
Wound Wash Sterile Saline Spray	Sterile sodium chloride solution 0.9%	**Adults & Peds:** Apply to affected area prn.

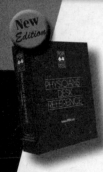
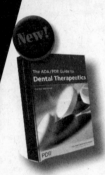
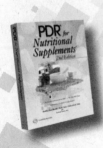
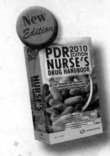
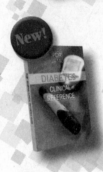
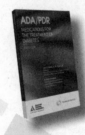
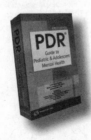
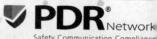

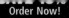

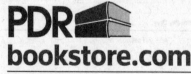
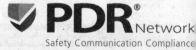

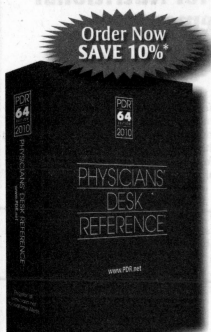
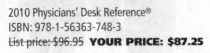
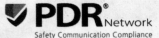